Cancer Diagnosis
What to Do Next

by W. JOHN DIAMOND, M.D.,
and W. LEE COWDEN, M.D., *with* BURTON GOLDBERG

ALTERNATIVEMEDICINE.COM BOOKS
TIBURON, CALIFORNIA

AlternativeMedicine.com, Inc.
1640 Tiburon Blvd., Suite 2
Tiburon, CA 94920
www.alternativemedicine.com

Editor: John W. Anderson
Associate Editor: Shila Alcantara
Art Director: Janine White
Production Manager: Gail Gongoll
Production Assistance: Victoria Swart

Manufactured in the United States of America.

10 9 8 7 6 5 4 3 2

Library of Congress Cataloging-in-Publication Data
Diamond, W. John, 1948-
    Cancer diagnosis: what to do next / by W. John Diamond and W. Lee
Cowden,with Burton Goldberg.
      p. cm.
    Includes bibliographical references and index.
      ISBN 1-887299-40-8 (pbk.)
          1. Cancer--Alternative treatment--Popular works. 2. Cancer—
Popular works. I. Cowden, W. Lee, 1952- II. Goldberg, Burton, 1926- III. Title.

RC263.D52 2000
616.99'406--dc21   00-027508
            CIP

Portions of this book were previously published, in a different form,
in *Alternative Medicine Definitive Guide to Cancer*.

for
John Harris

About the Authors

W. John Diamond, M.D.

Dr. Diamond earned his M.D. in 1973 from the University of the Witwatersrand in Johannesburg, Republic of South Africa. A board-certified pathologist, Dr. Diamond has extensive training in alternative medicine, including in medical acupuncture, classical homeopathy, and neural therapy. He is currently the medical director of the Triad Medical Center in Reno, Nevada, associate and alternative medicine consultant to the Bakersfield Family Medicine Center and Heritage Physician Network in Bakersfield, California, medical director of Botanical Laboratories, and director of the Associated Complementary Medicine Research Group, both in Ferndale, Washington.

W. John Diamond, M.D., Triad Medical Center, 4600 Kietzke Lane, M-242, Reno, NV 89502; tel: 702-829-2277; fax: 702-829-2365.
W. Lee Cowden, M.D., Conservative Medicine Institute, P.O. Box 832087, Richardson, TX 75083-2087; fax: 214-238-0327.

W. Lee Cowden, M.D.

Dr. Cowden received his M.D. from the University of Texas Medical School in Houston in 1978, followed by an internship and residency at St. Louis University in Missouri, and critical care and cardiology fellowships at the same hospital. Dr. Cowden is board certified in internal medicine, cardiovascular disease, and clinical nutrition.

Administering "crisis intervention medicine" convinced Dr. Cowden that to help people he needed to direct his efforts to preventive medicine. Dr. Cowden is accomplished in applied kinesiology, electrodermal screening, homeopathy, reflexology, acupuncture, acupressure, biofeedback, and color, sound, neural, magnetic, electromagnetic, and detoxification therapies. Dr. Cowden now conducts clinical research and teaches alternative medicine at the Conservative Medicine Institute in Richardson, Texas.

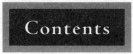

Contents

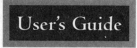

User's Guide

One of the features of this book is that it is interactive, thanks to the following icons:

 This means you can turn to the listed pages elsewhere in this book for more information.

 Many times the text mentions a medical term that requires explanation. We don't want to interrupt the text, so instead we put the explanation in the margins under this icon.

 This tells you where to contact a physician, group, or publication mentioned in the text. This is an editorial service to our readers. All items are based on recommendations from the clinical practice of physicians in this book. The publisher has no financial interest in any clinic, physician, or product discussed in this book.

 This sign tells you there may be some risks, uncertainties, side effects, or special contraindications regarding a procedure or substance.

 This icon highlights a particularly noteworthy point and bids you to remember it.

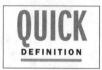 This icon asks you to give a particular point special attention in your thinking.

 More research on this topic would be valuable and should be encouraged to further substantiate a promising possibility of benefit to many.

Here we refer you to our best-selling book, *Alternative Medicine: The Definitive Guide*, for more information on a particular topic.

This icon will alert you to an article published in our bimonthly magazine, *Alternative Medicine*, that is relevant to the topic under discussion.

Here we refer you to our book *Alternative Medicine Definitive Guide to Cancer* for more information on a particular topic.

Here we refer you to our book *The Enzyme Cure* for more information on enzymes and how they can be used to relieve health problems.

Here we refer you to our book *The Supplement Shopper* for more information on nutritional supplements for various health conditions.

Important Information

Burton Goldberg and the editors of *Alternative Medicine* are proud of the public and professional praise accorded AlternativeMedicine.com's (formerly Future Medicine Publishing) series of books. This latest book in the series continues the groundbreaking tradition of its predecessors.

Your health and that of your loved ones is important. Treat this book as an educational tool which will enable you to better understand, assess, and choose the best course of treatment when a health problem arises, and how to prevent health problems such as cancer from developing in the first place. It could save your life.

Remember that this book on cancer is different. This book is about alternative approaches to health—approaches generally not understood and, at this time, not endorsed by the medical establishment. We urge you to discuss the treatments described in this book with your doctor. If your doctor is open-minded, you may actually educate him or her. We have been gratified to learn that many of our readers have found their physicians open to the new ideas presented to them.

Use this book wisely. As many of the treatments described in this book are, by definition, alternative, they have not been investigated, approved, or endorsed by any government or regulatory agency. National, state, and local laws may vary regarding the use and application of many of the treatments discussed. Accordingly, this book should not be substituted for the advice and care of a physician or other licensed health-care professional. Pregnant women, in particular, are urged to consult a physician before commencing any therapy. Ultimately, you must take responsibility for your health and how you use the information in this book.

AlternativeMedicine.com and the authors have no financial interest in any of the products or services discussed in this book, other than the citations to AlternativeMedicine.com's other publications. All of the factual information in this book has been drawn from the scientific literature. To protect privacy, all patient names have been changed. Branded products and services discussed in the book are evaluated on the independent and direct experience of the health-care practitioners quoted. Reference to them does not imply an endorsement nor a superiority over other branded products and services which may provide similar or superior results.

If It Were Any Good, My Doctor Would Know About It

OUR MESSAGE is simple, direct, and lifesaving: cancer can be successfully reversed using alternative medicine. The book you are now holding in your hands shows you how. A century ago, one in 33 people had cancer; today, it is more than one in three, and growing. When I was a child, cancer was the tenth leading cause of death among children—now it is second. No other health topic today has the urgency of cancer because no other health condition is escalating as fast. Although many of the alternative methods for treating cancer have been with us for perhaps 50 years, it is only recently that these approaches have achieved major clinical breakthroughs and moved into wider public awareness. I wish I had known more about them myself when my sister and my mother were dying of cancer. Seeing them ravaged not only by cancer but by the toxic treatments of conventional medicine made me think there must be a way to treat cancer without poisoning the body and destroying the immune system, and I vowed to find it.

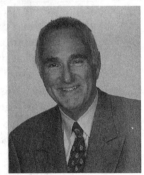

By meeting with hundreds of alternative doctors, I learned how they treat hundreds of health conditions using alternative methods. Their recommendations and views became Alternative Medicine: The Definitive Guide, a national best-seller that changed the lives of many readers by showing them, as I tell everyone I meet, you don't have to be sick. You can get better using safe, effective, inexpensive, and nontoxic methods from the world of alternative medicine. Let me give you an example. In chapter 1, you will read the story of Cheryl Wilkins, who used alternative medicine to reverse malignant melnoma. Instead of chemotherapy, which she had been told would probably not be effective for her cancer, she underwent a detoxification and nutritional therapy program. Today she is healthy and nearly cancer free.

A great deal of what you will read in this book will probably be new to you and you may well say, "If alternative medicine for cancer were any good, my doctor would know about it and would have told me." I offer you two reasons for why this is not the case. First, your doctor may not know about it. Very few physicians are taught in medical school even the rudiments of nutrition or the immune system. Until the mid-1990s, no conventional medical school ever discussed alternative approaches to treating illness. Too often, physicians blindly follow the conventions of their field and never look beyond to see what might work better. Sadly, while a great deal of new information about alternative approaches to cancer actually appears in mainstream medical journals, too few doctors seem to pay any attention.

Second, your doctor may not want you to know about it. Many powerful economic forces—pharmaceutical drug companies, physicians' trade groups, insurance companies, the Food and Drug Administration (FDA) and the National Institutes of Health (NIH), the latter two being taxpayer-funded organizations within the U.S. government—want health care to stay exactly the way it is because they're thriving under it. The reason alternative cancer treatments are not yet mainstream has little to do with alleged therapeutic ineffectiveness and far more to do with political control over the therapy marketplace. Successful alternative approaches to cancer are a direct financial threat to this system. The politics of cancer have an overriding influence on the science of cancer and, ultimately, on what the public thinks about cancer treatment options.

Alternative approaches are also a serious intellectual threat to the belief systems of conventional medicine. If nutrition and the immune system are so crucial to health and healing and they have never addressed either, this means conventional doctors will have to "go back to school" to catch up. For all their crowing about science, most conventional doctors are highly unscientific in their practices. They ignore results (in this case, the failure of such accepted treatments as chemotherapy) and refuse to change their methods based on results. The true meaning of being scientific is: observing patients and studying what works, then adjusting the therapy accordingly.

There is no single magic bullet cure for cancer. Many factors contribute to the development of cancer and many modalities and substances must be used to reverse it. To be successful, cancer doctors must become generalists and address the whole person along with the many interdependent factors that contributed to this cancer. Nutrition, diet, the vitality of the immune system, and the emotional life and beliefs of the person with cancer must all be examined. Safer, more effective ways of treating cancer must be utilized, from fields such as naturopathy, acupuncture, and homeopathy, which have long been recognized for their nontoxic holistic approach to treating illness.

In this book, you will learn about 33 contributing causes to cancer. You will see how each of these factors can weaken your immune system, start breaking down your health, and make you more susceptible to developing cancer following additional exposure to one or more of the causes. On the other hand, a healthy, strong, and vital immune system can withstand a great deal of such exposure and prevent cancer from ever starting.

Why is there so much cancer today? In simple fact, we are being slowly poisoned to death. The list of poisons includes pollution, pesticides, carcinogens in our food, air, and water, electromagnetic radiation, tobacco smoke, antibiotics, conventional drugs, hormone therapies, irradiated foods, nuclear radiation, mercury toxicity from dental fillings, diet and nutritional deficiencies, parasites, toxic emotions, X rays, and more. Most conventional doctors do not take these factors into consideration when treating cancer.

Here is a remarkable example. A man was diag-

You will quickly see why so few conventional cancer doctors today can honor the Hippocratic Oath—first, do no harm. Chemotherapy and radiation are toxic and often do as much damage to the body as the cancer itself.

nosed with prostate cancer. His tumor biopsy was examined by two different types of doctor: one a pathologist, the other a toxicologist. The pathologist saw only clear signs of cancer in the tissue sample, but the toxicologist found something more because she knew what to look for. She found abnormally high levels of a variety of carcinogenic chemicals including arsenic, chlordane, and DDT. In other words, there was evidence of pesticides and other environmental toxins in the tumorous tissue sample itself. If you know the toxin, you can remove it. But first you have to be looking for toxins and, here, conventional medicine is inexcusably lax. Most conventional oncologists disregard toxicity as a factor in cancer. The patient was overloaded with toxins and his liver could no longer detoxify his body. The pathologist missed the point entirely: he did not understand that in the tumor itself were the likely causes of the cancer. With this gap in understanding, the treatment he designed for the patient couldn't possibly be effective, because it would fail to address the root cause.

Cancer care will advance patient by patient. As each cancer patient recovers their health, thanks to alternative medicine, and tells a friend and the family doctor, this will transform Western medicine.

Not only do we show you the multiple causes that lead to cancer, we offer steps that lead to the removal of these causes. We do not offer a simplistic "cookbook" solution to cancer treatment. Rather, we emphasize the unique individuality of each case, with certain consistent elements in our approach: detoxify the body of its many cumulative poisons; fortify the body with nutrients; do everything possible to strengthen the immune system; stress the importance of early detection and preventive strategies; and honor the Hippocratic Oath—first, do no harm.

You will quickly see why so few conventional cancer doctors today can uphold this vow. Chemotherapy and radiation are toxic and often do as much damage to the body as the cancer itself. Even though conventional medicine presents and often forces these treatments (along with surgery) as the only options in existence for cancer, we wrote this book to prove to you that this is a lie. There are many successful alternatives to conventional care that can remove the root causes of cancer and restore you to health without further poisoning or damaging your body. There are also ways to minimize the side effects of chemotherapy, radiation, and surgery. Again, while mainstream medicine ignores this, we tell you how it is done. The information in this book is here to work for you, to empower and inspire you, and to show you ways you might experience a successful outcome in reversing cancer.

I urge you to give your doctors a copy of this book and insist they read it. Alternative medicine is good and your doctor should know about it. There is a famous saying I love to quote: Science and medicine advance funeral by funeral. This means old beliefs and practices die out and give way to new approaches only when the older generation of scientists holding them literally die off and leave the field. We no longer have time to wait for those who swear by conventional medicine to leave the field. The escalation of the rate of cancer demands this urgency. Doctors of all ages must open their minds to new possibilities, to alternative approaches that have been clinically proven to work. Otherwise, the toll of cancer deaths will continue to mount as thousands of cancer patients fail to hear about alternatives that could save their lives.

Let me adapt that previous famous quote to say: Cancer care will advance patient by patient. As each cancer patient recovers their health, thanks to alternative medicine, and tells a friend and the family doctor, this will transform Western medicine. Conventional physicians will have to start adopting new approaches because these approaches are the only ones consistently getting results and saving lives. If they don't, both their patients and more progressive colleagues will leave them behind in the archives of failed medicine. With your help, we can make this change happen quickly and decisively. God bless.

—Burton Goldberg

Visit our website at
www.alternativemedicine.com

CHAPTER

1

The Road to Recovery

"YOU'VE GOT CANCER"—they're the words you never want to hear. If you have just been diagnosed with cancer, your world may be turned upside-down and negotiating the roller coaster of emotions may leave you feeling overwhelmed. The initial shock may be followed by disbelief, denial, anger, and confusion. In this frame of mind, you may not be capable of making sound decisions about your health and treatment options.

First of all, don't panic. Now is the time when you need to be clear-headed, so that you can make the right choices. Acknowledge and experience the emotions you're going through—it's vital that you do this—then share your feelings and get support. While there is a strong focus on the physical aspects of cancer and how soon and what should be done, many alternative medicine physicians provide treatment that also addresses the compelling emotional, psycho-spiritual aspects of the illness as well.

Establish hope—there is reason for hope. Everyone responds differently to learning about their cancer, but an optimistic attitude is vital right from the beginning. A strong positive outlook cannot be underestimated in its power to contribute significantly to a successful outcome. Always keep in mind that others have been down this road before, received this diagnosis, have recovered, and are surviving today. No matter how frightened or upset or overwhelmed you may feel, know that you will get the care you need.

Unless the cancer requires immediate treatment, don't rush into making any decisions. Even though you may feel the need to immediately decide what kind of treatments you should have, very rarely is urgency warranted. There is almost always a chance to gather information. Don't be frightened into making decisions about your treatment until you know your options. As you will learn in this book, alternative medicine has established the causes of cancer—from radiation and dietary factors and pesticide residues to stress and dental factors and free radicals—and has safe, nontoxic, and effective therapies that can address each one.

Taking Positive Steps

When you were diagnosed with cancer, the first thing you may have said was 'Why me?' While you may feel like you've just been struck by lightning, you need to realize that this illness has happened because of various factors in your life. You'll need to look at your lifestyle and critically evaluate the way you live. To heal, it is necessary to understand how the illness was given an opening in your life and how you can eliminate it.

Cancer is an accumulation of imbalances—brought on by a combination of physical, environmental, and lifestyle stressors—and can be healed in the same way, through a process of identifying what went awry and stimulating the body to heal itself. Conventional medicine doesn't understand this way of looking at and treating cancer. Alternative medicine physicians, on the other hand, can assist you on this road to recovery. By identifying the underlying causes of cancer, using natural therapies to correct them, and addressing the psychological and emotional imbalances in you life, you will conquer your illness. There are a number of positive steps you can take right now to guide your own way on the journey through cancer.

Select a Physician and Get a Second Opinion
If your primary care doctor was the clinician who diagnosed your cancer, you may be comfortable continuing under their care. Be sure that your doctor is someone you trust and can communicate with. Think about the following when evaluating your choice of physician:
- Is the doctor well-qualified to treat you?
- Are they concerned with your personal needs in treatment?

- Does your doctor know alternative medicine in cancer treatment?
- Does your physician realize that your attitude and outlook are just as important as their treatment methods?
- Will your doctor be completely frank with you about the consequences and risks of every therapy (conventional and alternative), so that you can make the proper decision about your treatment options?

Even if you have complete confidence in your doctor, a cancer diagnosis may warrant one or even several second opinions. Generally, we encourage people to get tested again or find a second opinion to confirm the diagnosis. A second opinion can provide you with additional information that may help you feel more confident about the original diagnosis. Plus, a second physician may provide you with more treatment options to consider. The best choice for a second opinion would be someone with knowledge of both allopathic and alternative modalities.

Know What Causes Your Cancer

It is a good idea to gather as much information as you can about your type of cancer, its causes, and treatment options. Having this information will not only reduce your anxiety, but will help you select the best treatments for your recovery. This book is a good place to start—in Chapter 2: Cancer and Its Causes, we describe the cancer process and identify 33 underlying causes, many of them unrecognized by conventional medicine. There is no magic bullet for cancer. Rather, the alternative medicine approach systematically looks at contributing factors, such as toxins, dental factors, stress, and many others, then seeks to cleanse and support the body in the healing process. In later chapters, we describe, in detail, the alternative medicine treatment options available to you.

Ask your physician if they have any information for you to read or can suggest other good sources, such as websites, books, or magazine articles, that can provide you with a basic working knowledge of the type of cancer you are dealing with. Have your doctor explain any unfamiliar medical terms or anatomical processes. Don't be left in the dark by medical jargon. Illness has its own vocabulary and becoming familiar with technical terms allows you to gain a sense of strength in coping with the challenges of a long-term recovery process.

Ultimately, it is your decision as to what treatment program (conventional and/or alternative) you want to pursue and it is best for you to base that decision on sound advice and as much knowledge as you can acquire.

Choosing the *Right* Therapy

One of the primary messages of this book is that there are safe and effective alternatives to conventional, toxic treatments (chemotherapy and radiation) for cancer. Unfortunately, you probably won't hear about them from your conventional doctor. But a closed mind should not come between you and healing your cancer. In this book, you'll find out about using nutritional substances (vitamins, minerals, and essential oils) to fight cancer. You'll also discover the anticancer properties of herbs such as amygdalin, maitake mushroom, and algae, and about the benefits of innovative substances such as shark cartilage, hydrazine sulfate, and antineoplastons. Find out how detoxification, boosting the immune system, and physical and energy therapies fit into the holistic approach to cancer. Alternative medicine physicians can guide you on the wide range of natural therapies available as well as the judicious use of conventional treatments. The goal is to help you achieve a working balance between physical healing and emotional, mental, even spiritual aspects of your life.

For example, Robert C. Atkins, M.D., of New York City, says that the key to success in alternative medicine approaches to cancer is to gather as much data as possible on each patient, then to apply the "Hippocratic pecking order." This means using the more benign, nontoxic therapies first and saving the riskier, more invasive therapies for last, if ever. He studies the patient's immune system and the status of its key white blood cells in detail. Dr. Atkins also uses tumor markers (blood tests that detect the presence and extent of tumors) and sonographic or X-ray studies when needed. "The priority is to see whether we are getting a response to our initial treatments," says Dr. Atkins.

Dr. Atkins has observed that, in general, people diagnosed with advanced-stage cancers benefit more from nutrition and other biologic treatments (e.g., enzymes, botanicals, and glandular extracts) than from chemotherapy. For this reason, in most cases he suggests "holding off" on chemotherapy and conventional treatments unless it becomes clear that the safer treatments alone are not getting the job done. By employing nontoxic strategies first, Dr. Atkins is able to support his patients' immune capacity to reverse cancer before the system is ravaged by toxic treatments. Those patients who take this approach, says Dr. Atkins, tend to benefit the most from alternative cancer therapies. As one patient told him, "I've gotten to know about two dozen of your patients and the ones who went through chemotherapy before they saw you aren't here or alive anymore."

"Chemotherapy and radiation are completely unwarranted in this situation, and surgery alone, when combined with an integrated immune-enhancement and detoxification program, is almost always sufficient for curing breast cancer," says Robert C. Atkins, M.D.

But the either-or question many patients ask—"should I go with orthodox treatment or alternative treatment?"—is off the mark. This question is like asking which half of the card deck a person wants to play with, says Dr. Atkins. "As long as both halves are there, let's play with the whole deck," he says. "Patients with cancer who seek either orthodox or alternative approaches are entrusting their lives to doctors who are playing with half a deck."[1] In most cases of cancer, Dr. Atkins says that a complementary approach is needed, one which emphasizes alternative therapies along with limited and judicious use of conventional methods.

Although Dr. Atkins contends it is a fallacy to think all cancer resides within the boundaries of a tumor, he does find a role for surgery on a case-by-case basis. He finds it rarely necessary in prostate cancer, but in breast cancer, for example, surgery can be appropriate, where possible. "Surgical removal of breast tumors can lead to a complete remission of breast cancer," says Dr. Atkins. "Chemotherapy and radiation are completely unwarranted in this situation, and surgery alone, when combined with an integrated immune-enhancement and detoxification program, is almost always sufficient for curing breast cancer."

Dr. Atkins regards chemotherapy as otherwise dangerous and best avoided in treating the majority of cancers. "Only in situations in which chemotherapy is proven to be effective and curative would I recommend it," he says. "In general, this might be testicular cancer, many children's tumors, and extreme cases of Hodgkin's lymphoma. On the other hand, Ukrain can do everything chemotherapy does but without any side effects, so it renders chemotherapy largely unnecessary."

Radiation treatments are typically futile, too, says Dr. Atkins. "In some cases, however, we need to shrink tumors if they're encroaching or impinging on more vital parts of the body. In that case, a combination of radiation and hyperthermia [heat treatment delivered by ultrasound or microwave] can be effective." Dr. Atkins was among the first doctors in the U.S. to successfully combine radiation with hyperthermia to help treat prostate cancer.

For more on **Ukrain**, see Chapter 6: The New Cancer Pharmacology, pp. 188-212.

Will Your Chemotherapy Work? A Test Can Tell You

In the event you decide to include chemotherapy in your cancer treatment program, a new lab test can help you determine the most effective chemotherapy drug for your particular cancerous tissues. In addition, the test, called the Ex Vivo Apoptotic Assay, can identify the smallest dosage that will be sufficient to kill your specific cancer. Lower dosages can reduce the severity of chemotherapy's notoriously awful side effects. Without this test, chemotherapy prescription is a process of trial and error as doctors try to determine what kind and dosage of chemotherapy will work best.

The test, developed by Robert A. Nagourney, M.D., involves placing a biopsied piece of your own cancer tissue in a test tube with a concentration of one of more than 70 drugs available in chemotherapy regimens. The mixture sits for 72 to 96 hours to allow the cancer to "grow," after which time the physician can determine which drugs caused the most cell death. The test tube simulation provides a reasonable picture of the likely effect of the drug on the body of that individual. Generally, the assay's ability to predict outcomes was scored at 19 out of 21 in a test published in the *Journal of Hematology Blood Transfusion* in 1990.

The process, because it is tailored for each individual, is said to improve the outcome of chemotherapy by about two to three times. Also, the patient doesn't have to endure a battery of different drugs—and their side effects—in the hopes that one will work. Let's say your physician tells you that the use of Adriamycin (a chemotherapy drug) induces remissions in 38% of women with breast cancer. How can you tell in advance if you're part of the 38% for whom it works or the 62% for whom it has no effect? "We can now painlessly determine things in a test tube for a patient that they would only be able to find out if they went through the treatments," Dr. Nagourney says. "This is crucial since I've never seen a correctly administered chemotherapy for an 'average' patient."

Based on their cumulative results, Dr. Nagourney's team has compiled a bell-shaped data curve that shows the range of sensitivity and resistance to different drugs among individuals with the same kinds of cancer. From this he now knows that out of 100 women with breast cancer, perhaps 35 will have cancer cell death taking 0.15 mcg/ml of doxorubicin, while 25 will require only 0.05 mcg/ml, and still others will need 1.0 mcg/ml.

His test can determine the likely effect on human cancer tissue from any of about 70 chemotherapy drugs, given singly or in combination. It can also test botanical substances such as betulinic acid (from white birch bark), Alvium (a 12-herb formula), antineoplastons, interferons, or theoretically any substance capable of killing cancer cells. All that is required is a living tissue sample of cancer cells obtained from the patient by biopsy or a blood sample in the case of leukemias.

Robert Nagourney, M.D., a board-certified oncologist, hematologist and pharmacology professor, is founder and medical director of Rational Therapeutics of Long Beach, California, which provides the test. For more information about the **Ex Vivo Apoptotic Assay**, contact: Rational Therapeutics Cancer Evaluation Center, 750 East 29th Street, Long Beach, CA 90806; tel: 562-989-6455; fax: 562-989-8160; website: www.Rational-T.com.

Consultation is Key in Complementary Cancer Care

To the cancer patient, Martin Milner, N.D., of Portland, Oregon, makes the following recommendations:

■ Contact your conventional physician and inform him about your decision to augment your conventional treatment with natural therapies.

■ No patient should self-prescribe and no patient should use all of the therapies listed.

■ Certain therapies are contraindicated and cannot be used in combination with other therapies; further, some absolutely require supervision and close monitoring by the physician.

■ No one should assume that these therapies offer definitive treatment or a cure for cancer. The increased incidence of cancer requires both physicians and the public to carefully scrutinize natural cancer treatment options. Practitioners and patients alike have the opportunity to share information and resources in the challenge to find mixtures of natural therapies that reverse disease when possible and optimize each patient's quality of life.

Martin Milner, N.D.: Center for Natural Medicine, Inc., 1330 SE 39th Avenue, Portland OR 97214; tel: 503-232-1100; fax: 503-232-7751.

With so many alternative cancer therapy options, it is literally impossible to do "everything," says Michael B. Schachter, M.D., of Suffern, New York. This is where the art of medicine comes in and why it is critical to have a physician well-versed in alternative medicine. To understand patients and their total situation, as well as the current available information on alternative therapies, which literally changes every day, the physician must integrate all of the information and, together with the patient and patient's family, choose the elements of the program that will most likely work for that particular person. Then a reasonable trial should be given with careful observation. A willingness to shift gears and either remove or add elements of the program should be maintained in order to increase the chance of a successful result. Many of Dr. Schachter's patients are exposed to conventional therapies before receiving his treatment. He believes that patients receiving conventional cancer therapy while also on an alternative medicine supportive regimen do better than those who undergo conventional therapy without receiving such support.

Coping with the Emotional Roller Coaster

The emotional stages that you will typically undergo after a cancer diagnosis are well-documented, but are not any less jarring or painful once you experience them. Rest assured that this is a perfectly normal experience. Knowing what to expect may alleviate some of the anxiety that comes with the news of a healing crisis. While everyone will cope in their own way, there are several stages or emotions that commonly arise:

- Shock and disbelief
- Confusion
- Fear and anxiety
- Denial and anger
- Frustration and a sense of hopelessness
- Feelings of a loss of control
- Loneliness and depression
- Grief and mourning
- Acceptance

Be aware that you may experience some or all of these stages at different times throughout the treatment and recovery process. Your reaction may be strong or mild. Remember that there's no "right" way to feel and that it's important to let your emotions happen. Experiencing and expressing these emotions (in a support group, with a confidant, or by keeping a journal) are critical to healing your cancer.

While fear, depression, and other stressful emotional stages often follow the diagnosis of cancer, the continued presence of anger, grief, guilt, or perceived lack of self-worth (which may be present only at the subconscious level) stimulates the production of potentially destructive neurotransmitters or hormones (such as cortisone), which, in turn, can cause the cancer to spread. "People who carry around a lot of unexpressed fear and anger are the ones who generally don't do as well after a cancer diagnosis," says Lawrence Taylor, M.D., of Chula Vista, California. "The research I've seen on the psychosomatic basis for cancer survival suggests that these types of people may be six times more vulnerable to cancer and cancer mortality."[2]

To succeed in reversing cancer, you must get rid of the negative thinking. Continued negative emotions stimulate the adrenal gland to produce the hormones cortisone and adrenaline. This so-

Coping Style and Cancer Survival

Research suggests that coping style can help prevent the recurrence of cancer. A study of women with recurrent breast cancer found that joy, levity, and happiness are associated with longer periods of being free of symptoms;[3] a study of over 2,000 men, followed for 17 years, revealed that those who score highest on depression tests have twice the incidence of cancer-related deaths.[4] The high cancer rate among the more depressed men in this study cannot be explained on the basis of their drinking and smoking habits.

"People who carry around a lot of unexpressed fear and anger are the ones who generally don't do as well after a cancer diagnosis," says Lawrence Taylor, M.D.

called fight-or-flight reaction is desirable when you face a physical threat, but is to no purpose in this situation, in which case these hormones suppress the body's immune system and anticancer defenses. To win the battle against cancer, Dr. Taylor asserts that a total change in attitude is needed. The ideal anticancer attitude, he says, has two primary components: (1) it is hopeful, optimistic, and life-affirming; and (2) it is assertive regarding one's own needs.

"People need to realize that they can alter the course of their cancer by the way they think about themselves and the world around them," says Dr. Taylor. "When you have feelings of joy and happiness, you produce more endorphins, which make you feel good." Endorphins, the body's own natural painkillers, also contribute to the synthesis of the hormone DHEA by the adrenal glands, which stimulates the thymus gland to carry out its immune functions more effectively. In other words, the immune system is bolstered by faith, hope, and happiness.

Conduct a "Personal Inventory"

Look at your cancer diagnosis as an alarm, a wake-up call, to examine your life. One of the first steps towards reestablishing health is to take stock and identify what factors in your life have contributed to creating this illness. This "inventory" should include an examination of one's personality, lifestyle, and environmental factors that have created an opportunity for this serious illness to take hold. If you don't attend to the causative factors and those factors remain in your life, you will keep recreating the environment for cancer to thrive.

Take a close look at your life, including the quality and dynamics of you job, major relationships, living situation, and sexual habits. The more thorough the self-examination, the more likely you will recover and not suffer future relapses. As a starting point, ask yourself the following questions:

- What has my attitude been about myself?
- Do I really love and honor myself?
- What is my purpose in life?
- What are the primary goals I would like to accomplish?
- What makes me unique?
- Do I exist in an environment which is not conducive to health?

Am I exposed to toxins in my home or workplace?

- Do I have emotional factors in my personal life and relationships that thwart or suppress my immune system?
- Is my diet sufficient? Has my diet been appropriate to the task of creating immune competence?

For more about **causes of cancer**, see Chapter 2: Cancer and Its Causes, pp. 48-93.

Think about these areas of your life in a deliberate and organized way. Any one of these factors, or the cumulative effect of two or three, can potentially cause a cancerous condition. This illness may be your opportunity to rediscover what is truly important in your life and to make changes accordingly.

"The best approach to cancer is one that combines interventions for the mind, body, soul, and current emotional state," says Victor Marcial-Vega, M.D., of Coconut Grove, Florida. "The only way to fully recover from cancer is to identify and connect with those parts within oneself that are wounded, repressed, or in need of healing attention." A willingness to pay attention to inner signals is the first step toward greater self-awareness and a clearer, more expansive sense of self. True healing is largely a process of getting to know oneself, says Dr. Marcial-Vega.

Cancer is a sign that your life is out of balance. Many people are living in *dis*ease—eating in an unhealthy way, overloaded with toxins, overworked and overstressed, or in unhealthy relationships. When the human body is free from chronic distress, it is far more resistant to toxic insults from the environment that can trigger the onset of cancer. Evaluating the stressors in your life and determining which lifestyle factors as well as personality traits, such as being able to express emotions rather than contain them, will not only allow you to gain a greater understanding of yourself, but actually facilitate the healing process.

Create a New Personal Paradigm

Despite the difficulties of coping with a serious illness like cancer, survivors often say that it was not only a "wake-up call" but forced them to create a new way to relate to themselves and their lives. Cancer survivors have even been heard to say about the life-changing experience of having cancer: "The best thing that ever happened to me was my cancer, because it made me wake up" and "That's the point where I began to realize what was really important about life." This self-examination is in alignment with the principles of alternative medicine: in order to heal, it is necessary to marshal all of one's resources, whether they spring from the body, mind, or soul.

It is vital for you to feel that you are important enough to recover, that you have a purpose for living, for being here. We live in a society

Is There a Cancer Personality?

How do you react to conflicts or stressful situations in your life? Do you respond with hope or despair? With helplessness or commitment to resolve the situation? With pent-up anger or tranquility? How you respond, to some degree, reflects your personality type.

Behavioral patterns are commonly broken down into two basic types, Type As and Type Bs. Type A personalities are described as aggressive and competitive, easily angered, always in a hurry, and hostile. Type Bs do not exhibit these characteristics, but are more deliberate, thinking through a situation and formulating a plan of action. Beginning in the 1960s, studies began to show that personality type can have a profound influence on your health. One study followed 3,000 middle-aged men over an eight-and-a-half year period and found that Type As were twice as likely to develop heart disease as Type Bs.[5] A recent study of air traffic controllers found that Type As had three-and-a-half times more job-related injuries and 38% more illnesses overall than Type Bs.[6]

There may be a third type—the Type C or immunosuppressive personality—with certain personality characteristics that correlate with cancer susceptibility, says Douglas Brodie, M.D., of Reno, Nevada. "Cancer patients are typically conscientious, caring, intelligent, and hard-working. They tend to take on other people's burdens and accept extra obligations to such an extent that they have little time for themselves or for relaxation and pleasurable pursuits." Another feature of the cancer-prone psyche is that these individuals usually prefer to suffer in silence, bearing their burdens without complaint or even acknowledgment.

People who tend to develop cancer often are those who are plagued by depression, indecision, hopelessness, low self-esteem, chronic fatigue, and physical weakness.[7] Anxiety, grief, loneliness, or isolation can also depress immune function, possibly increasing one's susceptibility to cancer, contends Dr. Donovan. Fear is "the primary toxin" from which stem all other "toxic" emotions, such as anxiety, hostility, resentment, bigotry, and selfishness.

Burdens of their own as well as of others weigh heavily, sometimes subconsciously, upon these individuals, because they tend to internalize their cares, concerns, and problems, Dr. Brodie explains. "The carefree extrovert seems to be invulnerable or at least far less likely to develop cancer than the caring introvert. Also, stress causes a suppression of the immune system, but it does so more overwhelmingly in the cancer-susceptible individual. Excessive levels of stress combine with the underlying personality to promote the immune deficiency which allows cancer to thrive."

where many people will do just about anything to win the applause of other people, to get approval from others, but we never give it to ourselves. Patrick Donovan, N.D., strongly encourages all his cancer patients to do some soul-searching to facilitate their healing and avoid, reduce, or remove obstacles to growth and self-expression. Such obstacles can include genetic/metabolic disorders, functional/structural disabilities, and dysfunctional relationships. When these factors are not effectively minimized, they can exacerbate the cancer process. This is your opportunity to discover who you are and how you want to live the rest of your life.

Eliminating these factors can facilitate healing, reestablishing hope or vision of a positive future, faith in oneself or in a higher power, a sense of personal meaning, and the feeling of having choices and control in one's life. Taking a more assertive view toward your personal needs may also have its advantages in curbing the development of cancer. Research suggests a connection between the progression of certain cancers—breast cancer and malignant melanoma—and passivity in coping with stressful situations.[10] In addition, feeling a sense of control seems vital to health and resistance to all diseases. The greater the perceived impact of a stressful event—a hurricane versus a thunderstorm—the lower one's sense of control tends to be. When people feel that some major life upheaval is overwhelming, they are more inclined to feel hopeless, and such hopelessness increases their risk of cancer.[11] Research with breast cancer patients indicated that when a stressful life event was felt to be beyond the woman's control, the likelihood of relapse was greater.[12]

It is crucial to understand here that the cause of your cancer is not the presence of a carcinogen alone, but a combination with the body's weakened capacity to destroy cancer

The Spiritual Connection to Healing

Spirituality and a feeling of connection to a divine presence can cultivate a hopeful attitude and a sense of meaning in one's life, which can help promote healing and recovery even with an illness as serious as cancer. The particular way this is expressed, through a specific religious practice or time spent in nature, for instance, is not the important issue. Prayer (of any kind or denomination) has been proven to be a health-giving practice in over 250 studies and can be used as an effective means of aiding with physical wellness and healing.[8]

A recent study at the University of Michigan, in Ann Arbor, found that people who regularly attended religious services (at least once per month) lived significantly longer than those who didn't. The national survey followed 3,617 Americans over a seven-year period. The non-churchgoers were about one-third more likely to die over the study period. Churchgoers tended to be more physically active, at a healthy weight, and nonsmokers. Even eliminating these healthier lifestyle factors, the non-churchgoers still had a 25% greater likelihood of dying. Researchers speculated that the community involvement and religious rituals might promote feelings of hope, serenity, and optimism, all helpful in prolonging life. Attending religious services "extends the life span about as much as moderate exercise or not smoking," the researchers concluded.[9]

Disease does not arise solely from external effects on the body; it is the interaction between these effects and the body's immune system that counts.

Patrick Donovan, R.N., N.D.: University Health Clinic, 5312 Roosevelt Way NE, Seattle, WA 98105; tel: 206-525-8015; fax: 206-525-8014.

cells as they arise from the influence of carcinogens. Disease does not arise solely from external effects on the body; it is the interaction between these effects and the body's immune system that counts. By all indications, we should consider the mind to be an integral part of the immune system. That's why your attitude and taking positive actions to change your life can make all the difference.

Establish a Network of Support

Get support—this is critical to your recovery from cancer. A sense of isolation, of being alone in the cancer process, is the quickest way to deplete your immune system. "There is overwhelming evidence that people who have few social contacts are more likely to get sick and less likely to recover from an illness," says Erik Peper, Ph.D., Associate Director of the Institute of Holistic Healing Studies at San Francisco State University. People with the fewest social ties are two to three times more likely to die of all causes than those with the most social connectedness.[13]

These lifestyle factors seem to be especially important when the diagnosis is cancer. David Spiegel, M.D., a psychiatrist at Stanford University, demonstrated that women with breast cancer who participated in a weekly support group lived twice as long as those who did not.[14] These women were given the opportunity to express their feelings about their condition, their doctors, and anything else they were experiencing. It seems that this freedom to give vent to emotions gave support to the immune system. In a 30-year study, medical students characterized as "loners," who suppressed their emotions beneath a bland exterior, were 16 times more likely to develop cancer than those who expressed their emotions and, at times, took active measures to relieve anger or frustration.[15]

To help cope with the effects of long-term stress, establish an effective support network for yourself and your family. Alternative medicine physicians believe in the therapeutic value of support networks, whether they take the form of family and friends, support groups, or other social and religious affiliations. It has even been shown that a support groups can lessen your need for pain medications and other drugs for anxiety or depression. Support programs can improve your sense of being in control of the disease process and help you stick with your therapeutic regimen.[16]

It is also necessary for you to avoid those people who have a negative impact on you. Stay away from people who see you as a goner, as though you're not here anymore—the 'pity party'. Surround yourself with positive, open people to facilitate your healing. Support groups provide a safe place where you can acknowledge what you're going through in the presence of people who truly understand your experience. Support groups are also an excellent source of information on treatment options and other practical know-how for getting through the cancer process.

Proper attention to the mind/body realm is often overlooked in conventional cancer treatment programs, says Keith I. Block, M.D., of Evanston, Illinois. He tries to guide his cancer patients toward recovering a sense of meaning and fulfillment—a reason to go on living. Cultivating and sustaining this attitude is key to recovery.

A fundamental premise of Dr. Block's approach is that giving patients a sense of personal power and responsibility regarding their care is as important as prescribing the right medications. When they begin to enhance their own emotional and physical vitality, this sense of empowerment begins to grow quickly.

Dr. Block's insight in this area derives from his personal experience as a patient. His introduction to alternative medicine began at the other end of the stethoscope when a personal health crisis led him to explore dietary and botanical therapies. In the course of working through his own experience, Dr. Block became acutely sensitized to the emotional needs of patients. "I try to help people discover the chords in their being that connect them to a desire to live more fully," Dr. Block says. "If I can help them identify with that zest for life and tap into their own inner resources, then deeper healing of their inner being can occur."

Fostering Hope

There are a number of ways you can help yourself keep a hopeful attitude during treatment and recovery from cancer:

- Use life-enhancing language when speaking about your experience. For instance, refer to yourself as a cancer survivor, not as a cancer victim.

- Find other cancer survivors—their success stories will serve as encouragement.

- Avoid pessimistic people.

- Support your body with proper nutrition and exercise and pay attention to your psychological and spiritual needs.

- Make plans for the future.[17]

Daring to Heal My Cancer
with Alternative Medicine—
Cheryl Wilkens' Story

Cancer survivor Cheryl Wilkins writes:[18] What prompts a person with cancer to say no to chemotherapy and radiation? As suspicions build today that scientists are misfiring in their battle with cancer, more people like myself are investigating other ways of treatment. Two-thirds of Americans are now choosing alternative care, and not just those needing cancer treatment. But if you want to know about cancer, I have a firsthand understanding on why this is so.

My own medical experiences opened my mind to alternative medicine. It all began in July 1991, when a tumor on my knee and three moles on my back were surgically removed. The surgeon told me the tumor was merely fatty and the moles were benign. The following month the lump returned to the same place on my knee, but all he said was "it's scar tissue, don't worry about it."

In December, I was back in his office again because the lump had grown dramatically and it felt hot. No longer thinking it was scar tissue, he operated at once. He told me it was a high-grade malignancy, a kind of cancer called histiocytoma. He said he was sure he got it all with his scalpel. But the next day the lab said he had to cut out an even bigger chunk of my knee, which he did, leaving me with a 15-inch scar, somewhat disabled, and in constant discomfort.

Two weeks later, I sat in the oncologist's office. He glanced through my medical file then recommended the maximum treatment of chemotherapy and radiation over the next six months to kill any remaining cancer cells. He said he wanted to check with other institutions over the weekend for a second opinion. But when I saw him again the next week and asked him what he had learned, he said he had gone skiing instead. When I told him I'd be seeking a second opinion at the Mayo Clinic in Rochester, Minnesota, and with New York City physician Dr. Nicholas Gonzalez, he abruptly stood up and walked out.

One of the first shocks I got at the Mayo Clinic was that while my surgeon had said there was no evidence of a malignant melanoma, when the Mayo Clinic doctors examined the pathology slides for my moles they called it "a superficial spreading level three melanoma (skin cancer that has begun to spread or metastasize to the lymph nodes)." They also told me, for the first time, what the likely side effects of chemotherapy might be, such as damage to my kidneys, heart, and gallbladder.

Back home again, my surgeon asked me to visit his office. He "warned" me that I had been the topic of conversation for 15 top cancer specialists and that none of them had heard of Dr. Gonzalez' metabolic-nutritional therapy. They all said I shouldn't waste my time on a New York City "quack." The way the surgeon looked at me would have crushed the hopes of many patients, I'm sure, but when he saw I wasn't convinced, he looked uncomfortable, dropped his surly posture, and changed the subject.

He pulled out a report from the National Cancer Institute that said there basically weren't grounds for believing chemotherapy would be effective for my histiocytoma. Yet here he was telling me I should go through with it because alternative treatments were useless. Meanwhile, my knee wasn't working right because the surgeon had removed my patella tendon. Of course nobody told me about this until much later, when I discovered it by reading through my records. Now my knee wasn't strong enough for me to even walk up stairs.

I thought about things. I'm 43. There is cancer in my family. My father, grandfather, and great grandfather all died of cancer. With that kind of history, I thought: maybe it's time to take a different approach to treatment. When you are diagnosed with cancer, you are introduced to yourself. You find out what you are made of. And when you choose an alternative therapy, you find yourself living in a glass house. People watch what you do—they watch everything—and often with a skeptical eye.

In February the next year, or seven months after my first office visit for my knee problem, I walked into the Park Avenue offices of Nicholas J. Gonzalez, M.D., in New York City for my first two-hour appointment. I was reassured to learn that he tapes his office visits for future reference. I suppose I wasn't quite as desperate as many of his patients who come to him bearing prognoses of 2-3 months more to live, after having survived unsuccessful courses of surgery, radiation, and chemotherapy. Still, the results from his analysis of my blood and hair weren't good news. I had a great deal of cancer in my body, most of it in my lymphatic system.

I saw Dr. Gonzalez again the next day for two hours when he laid out the details of his comprehensive program of metabolic therapy. This is based on the 25 years of research by a dentist named Dr. William Donald Kelley, who developed a program featuring nutrition, detoxification, and supplements as a way of treating many degenerative diseases, including cancer. Dr. Kelley described ten categories of metabolic types. As he saw it, there are ten different body styles of needing and assimilating foods. Nutritional therapy should be based on this, he said. Dr. Gonzalez spent five years studying cancer patients in Dr. Kelley's program to be sure it worked.

As I drove back home, I thought that maybe more doctors should ask patients about their bowel movements. All my life I have been constipated. If I went once a week, I considered that normal. Now I see how abnormal and toxic that was, how it contributed to my illness. And I thought: if a body is smart enough to create a disease, then it makes sense that it must be smart enough to cure it, too.

I began to figure out how best I could make Dr. Gonzalez' program work for me. It called for a daily regimen of, literally, 150 vitamins, minerals, and enzymes, starting at 3:30 a.m. I had to do four coffee enemas a day, starting at 2 a.m., to help rid my system of the toxins being released as the tumor dissolved. This would especially help my liver and gallbladder, which would respond quickly to the caffeine and contract vigorously, releasing stored wastes.

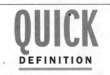

QUICK
DEFINITION

Kelley's Metabolic Therapy is a cancer treatment that consists of individualized nutrition, detoxification, and supplementation with pancreatic enzymes. Dr. Kelley, originally a dentist who made his discoveries in the late 1960s while seeking a cure for his own pancreatic cancer, recognized that individuals have different food requirements and ways of digesting and assimilating nutrients. On this basis, he classified ten different metabolic types for which dietary and nutritional programs must be specifically adjusted. Examples include slow-oxidizing vegetarians and fast-oxidizing carnivores. Specific foods that contain the raw materials needed to improve the blood levels identified in the testing are recommended, and the overall dietary pattern is designed to match the metabolic type.

About once a month I did a special bowel clean-out (Dr. Gonzalez calls it the "clean sweep") using psyllium seed husks and a bentonite liquid. This really scrubbed out my colon. Along with this I did a liver flush (using olive oil, apple juice, ortho-phosphoric acid, and other ingredients) to help purify my liver. Both of these procedures took about a week.

There were other practices I didn't have to do but that Dr. Gonzalez often prescribes to cancer patients. There is a detoxification program Dr. Gonzalez calls the "purge." You drink a mixture of citrus fruit juices and Epsom salts. This is to aid in the rapid removal of metabolic wastes from the body. Dr. Gonzalez also has patients do skin rubs, salt and soda baths, mustard foot soaks, and castor oil compresses—and again, all of this is to draw the toxins out of the body.

For more information on **Kelley's Metabolic Therapy**, see Chapter 4: Nutrition as Cancer Medicine, pp. 130-159.

I had to start eating organically grown foods and whole grains, only meats produced without hormones or antibiotics, raw vegetables and fresh fruits, fresh juices, especially eight ounces of carrot juice every day, and no canned, processed, or deep-fried foods. I figure that by the end of my first year on the Gonzalez program I drank the juice from over 2,000 pounds of carrots and an untold amount of apples. I avoided refined sugar out of consideration for my pancreas; I avoided aluminum cooking utensils, as well as aluminum-containing deodorants and lotions. White flour, soybean products, and peanuts also had no place in my diet as part of this program.

Sometimes I had doubts about it all. I would say to myself: "Who do you think you are that you can drink some carrot juice, pop vitamins, do coffee enemas, and get well when there are sophisticated technologies for cancer?" Except they aren't winning the cancer war with these supposed marvels.

My doubts usually came when I wasn't feeling well or was overtired. My husband was a strong support. "It's a done deal," he'd say whenever he saw me in these funks. He meant that, as far as he was concerned, this was the best and only way to whip cancer. That made me able to trudge on. How do you eat an elephant? One bite at a time. The same applies to completing a comprehensive regimen like this one. Just hit away at it one day at a time until it becomes second-nature to you—which took me about three years, by the way. Anyway, the alternative to the alternative—conventional medicine—doesn't really work.

Basic Tenets of Alternative Medicine

Although alternative medicine includes a wide range of treatment options of varying approaches, all the therapies are based on a common philosophy that includes the following elements:

- focuses on empowering you to accept responsibility for at least part of the task of recovery and health maintenance in the future

- emphasizes the importance of nutrition as an essential requirement for good health

- considers a balanced lifestyle (proper exercise, sleep, relaxation, and emotional tranquility) a prerequisite for optimum health

- attempts to ensure the efficiency of your body's organs and organ systems (through detoxification, nutritional supplements, and related whole-body approaches)

- recognizes that your musculoskeletal system provides a vital link between nerve transmission and energy pathways and is in direct relationship with internal and emotional states

- treats you rather than your symptoms

Looking back at the last 40 years of cancer research, it seems like digging in your pocket for a coin that's not there. Somewhere in my healing journey I took on the attitude of this Chinese proverb: "Man who says it will not work shouldn't disturb man who's making it work." And I thought: Until God opens another door, this alternative treatment is the best for me.

Perhaps my greatest discouragement comes from the fact that a program like this—that works—is not covered by insurance, even

Interest in Alternative Approaches to Cancer is Growing

Studies and polls in the U.S. indicate a steadily rising acceptance of alternative medicine as a treatment option for disease. The first major indication of this shift appeared in 1993 in a study published in the prestigious *New England Journal of Medicine*. This article reported that, based on interviews with 1,539 Americans, 34% had used at least one "unconventional" practitioner in 1990, and that one third of these had seen an exclusively alternative physician an average of 19 times in that year. The study also revealed that 72% of those consulting alternative physicians did not tell their conventional doctor of this choice. On the basis of this poll, the researchers estimated that Americans made 425 million office visits to alternative practitioners, spending about $13.7 billion, of which $10.3 billion was out of their own pockets.[19]

In 1992, U.S. government data showed that the number of alternative medicine offices grew by 163% over the previous five years compared to that of conventional doctors, which grew by only 56%. Between 1987 and 1992, the second fastest growing field in U.S. health care was alternative medicine, second only to home health care.[20] In 1994, *Self Magazine* reported that 84% of its readers had consulted an alternative medicine physician and 36% said they had more faith in alternative medicine than in conventional.[21] In 1995, 41% of people living in the San Francisco Bay Area tried alternative medicine at least once, 54% said they were "very satisfied" with the results, and 80% said they would do it again.[22]

Confidence in the efficacy of alternative medicine as a treatment option for cancer is similarly growing. The American Cancer Society estimates that 9% of U.S. cancer patients use complementary therapies,[23] although other researchers place the figures higher at 10% to 60%.[24] A study undertaken at New York Hospital revealed that about 30% of breast cancer patients polled said they had consulted an alternative practitioner while 25% were currently receiving some form of "unconventional" therapy such as shark cartilage, medicinal mushrooms, Chinese herbs, or vitamin injections.[25]

Yet another study estimated that from 10% to 50% of cancer patients try some form of alternative or complementary care; the same study reported that 5% of cancer patients abandon conventional treatment in favor of alternative approaches.[26] Estimates by the U.S. government place annual expenditures on alternative cancer treatments at $2 billion.[27] Based on the most conservative estimate that 10% of U.S. cancer patients consult alternative practitioners every year, this means that at least 100,000 cancer patients are under alternative care or using alternative substances as part of a cancer treatment program.[28]

though it costs less than chemotherapy. I paid for this out of my own pocket. The supplements ran me about $400 a month and my two sessions with Dr. Gonzalez cost $1,800. It was a huge financial burden, yet it was a price I was willing to pay to get well. Of course it meant I had to keep my full-time job during this period even though Dr. Gonzalez generally recommends you concentrate your time on healing.

Today, I am nearly cancer free. According to a standardized blood test used by conventional cancer doctors, I do not have any cancer. But according to the more refined test that Dr. Gonzalez uses, I still have some cancer activity. So I will always have to keep up a nutritional maintenance program.

Am I lucky? Yes, I am lucky—lucky to have taken control of my own health care. Lucky to have been introduced to this form of treatment. Lucky not to have burned up my body with chemotherapy and radiation. Let me tell you something a little grim. In the three years I've been on this program, I have known many people with cancer who chose chemotherapy and radiation. They are now either dead or on yet another chemotherapy series for a relapse. Yes, I am lucky!

Conventional Medicine is Losing the War on Cancer

The number of new cancers reported annually has increased steadily since the 1960s, as have cancer-related mortality rates for a variety of cancers. In 1900, a mere 3% of deaths were attributed to cancer, yet today, that number has jumped by eight times—to 24%. To put this in perspective, this is an 800% increase in less than a century.

The National Cancer Institute reports a 28% rise in the incidence of childhood cancers from 1950 to 1988. Against some of the more common cancers in the United States—lung, liver, pancreas, brain, and bone, as well as advanced cancers of the colon, breast, and prostate—little or no progress has been made in conventional medicine's expensive "War on Cancer" since it was declared in 1971 by then-president Richard Nixon.

Cancer is the number one health concern of every American, and for good reason. Each year, about 1.3 million people in the U.S. will be diagnosed with cancer and more than half this number will probably die from the disease or its treatment. That's about one American life lost to cancer every 45 seconds. "Despite some gains, cancer death rates remain unacceptably high, and the disease will kill 554,740 people in the U.S. this year," wrote J. Madeleine Nash in a special edition of *Time* magazine that summarized conventional cancer treatments.[29]

Cancer now kills more children between the ages of three and 14 than any other illness.[30] Of greater concern is the fact that the numbers of both new cancer cases and deaths continue to rise. From 1950 to 1980, there was an 8% increase in cancer deaths,[31] but from 1975 to 1989, the number of new cancer cases reported each year increased 13% and the mortality rate rose 7%.[32] Although mortality rates for a few less-common cancers declined, overall rates have continued to rise.[33]

A look at individual cancers paints a more ominous picture. From 1973 to 1987, melanoma (a form of skin cancer) increased by 83%, non-Hodgkin's lymphoma by 51%, and lung cancer by 32%.[34] Of these, lung cancer has become the leading cancer killer among men and women alike, surpassing breast cancer, which was the leading cause of death among women until 1986. Specifically, for the incidence of lung cancer in women, between 1973-1990, there was a 100% increase. In addition, rates of brain, kidney, breast, and prostate cancers have also risen.

Regarding prostate cancer, one estimate cites a 600% increase since 1985 in new cases—"the fastest rise in cancer detection ever recorded." One out of every five males born in the 1990s are likely to develop prostate cancer, compared to only one out of eight females who will probably develop breast cancer.[35] The 30-year trend (1960-62 to 1990-92) for deaths from lung cancer is up 85% for men and up 438% for women; up 29% for prostate; up 4% for breast cancer; up 12% for female pancreatic cancer. The rate of death from some cancers has dropped over this same period: colorectal, -9%; male pancreas, -5%; male leukemia, -9%; female colorectal, -31%; and ovary, -8%.[36]

Breast cancer is perhaps the best example of the changing global picture of cancer. For many years, the incidence and mortality rates for breast cancer have been highest in the U.S. and Northern Europe and lowest in Asia and Africa. In recent years, steep increases have been reported in Asian and Central European populations; thus the differences in rates between such countries as Japan and the U.S. is much less than previously. The annual incidence of breast cancer worldwide is predicted to be more than one million cases.

Scientists expect to see a further increase in cancer mortality rates. They also predict an estimated 10 million cancer patients and survivors alive in the U.S.[37] The hardest hit will be the elderly, who in the coming decades are expected to experience increases in incidence rates for all cancers, but particularly for those of the colon, rectum, pancreas, stomach, lung, bladder, and prostate; half of these people will probably die within five years. Although these are dismal forecasts, they should not be taken as guaranteed outcomes, given that they do

THE ROAD TO RECOVERY

not include successful alternative medicine therapies as part of the equation. They do indicate, however, that conventional medicine has failed to stem the tide of this disease.

According to John C. Bailar III, Ph.D., Professor of Epidemiology and Biostatistics at McGill University in Toronto, Canada, conventional medicine is decidedly losing the war on cancer. In 1993, he declared: "In the end, any claim of major success against cancer must be reconciled with this figure," referring to the steady increase in cancer deaths between 1950 and 1990. "I do not think such reconciliation is possible and conclude that our decades of war against cancer have been a qualified failure. Whatever we have been doing, it has not dealt with the broadly rising trend in mortality."[38]

Dr. Bailar's data, confirmed by the National Cancer Institute, holds that overall U.S. cancer death rates (adjusted for changes in the size and composition of the population with respect to age) went up by 7% between 1975 and 1990. From 1950 to 1990, the increase was from about 158 deaths to about 172 deaths per 100,000 people. In a review article discussing trends in cancer epidemiology, even as stalwart a defender of the medical status quo as *Scientific American* admitted of cancer that it is "a war not won." The casualty report "from the war on cancer shows that the effort has not slowed deaths from the disease in the U.S."

Cancer is crippling America's health-care system. Despite spending over $35 billion on cancer research in the last 25 years, conventional medicine has made little progress in understanding the underlying causes for the rapid rise of cancer rates or in finding safe and effective treatments. The cost to patients and taxpayers for years of waging "war" against cancer has been one trillion dollars.[39] In pursuit of the elusive goal of a cancer cure, Americans made an estimated 50 million cancer-related visits to doctors and were exposed to countless diagnostic procedures to find out whether they had the disease.

In recent years, about 10% of annual health-care expenditures in the U.S.—an unbelievable sum of $96 billion annually—has been spent on cancer treatment alone.[40] In appreciating these numbers, one must also factor in that the direct cost of hospital care for cancer is considerably higher than the cost of hospital care for other diseases. Most (83%) of the direct expenditures for cancer care are attributable to breast, colorectal, lung, and prostate cancer, in that order.

How does this translate for the person in need of cancer care? The average conventional treatment charge to Medicare (for all types) is $14,205 for the initial three months; after this, the cost is just over

$800 monthly. For the final six months of "terminal treatment" (for cancer patients who don't survive), the average Medicare charge is approximately $23,000.[41] These staggering costs have little to show for them in terms of having successfully stemmed the tide of human death and suffering from cancer.

Spokespersons for conventional cancer care frequently tout five-year survival rates as indicative of progress and money wisely spent. However, a critical analysis of these numbers reveals such claims to be illusory. The public relations experts of the American Cancer Society claim that more cancer patients are living at least five years after their diagnosis than ever before. The facts are that between 1974 and 1976 and 1981 and 1987, the five-year survival rates rose only 2%, from 49% to 51%, and for cancers of the liver, lung, pancreas, bone, and breast, rates are about the same as they were in 1965.[42]

The five-year mark is used as a yardstick for "cure" by conventional oncologists. It doesn't matter if you die one day after the five-year mark, you are still counted among the cases cured. Since many people die not long after five years, this can be a highly misleading statistic. For example, the five-year survival rate for breast cancer is about 75%, but the extended survival rate is less than 50%. Similarly, while the five-year survival for prostate cancer is about 70%, the ten-year survival rate is only about 35%.[43]

Even the small overall increase in five-year survival for all cancers may be an exaggeration, since many diagnostic tests in use today enable earlier diagnosis, which makes the survival time only appear longer than in the past. For instance, consider the woman whose breast cancer is diagnosed an average of three years earlier because of mammography; today she might live for seven years. In 1985, using the older diagnostic and treatment tools, this same woman would have appeared to live only four years. Nothing has changed in terms of the effectiveness of conventional therapy, and yet the breast cancer patient appears to live longer, owing to the improved screening measures. The "success" exists only on paper.

These statistics, flawed and misleading as they are already, do not factor in the far longer survival times commonly produced by physicians using alternative modalities of cancer care. Nor do they account in any way for the radical degree to which alternative medicine applied to cancer care could profoundly shift the outcomes from dismal to successful. A rational person will ask why this isn't already so. Powerful economic and political forces are arrayed against alternative medicine—generally, and for cancer specifically—precisely because of its promise of remarkable success at less cost.

Don't Settle for Conventional "Strategies of Containment"

About the best that spokespersons for the conventional cancer establishment can say in summarizing more than 25 years of cancer research is: "we're making headway." As *Scientific American* editors John Rennie and Ricki Rusting state, "There is no way to skirt the fact that the combined death rate for all cancers has yet to come down." Short of finding a "single cure" that would "kill the tumor"—which, *Scientific American* admits, seems unlikely—the article concludes that the current option is to settle for "strategies of containment."[44]

The message of this book is altogether different: you don't have to settle for strategies of containment while you wait for scientists to discover that single magical cure for cancer. Alternative medicine looks at multiple treatments and substances working together—synergistically—to effect major changes in the cancer process, from containment to remission to a life that is cancer free. "Synergy" in alternative medicine treatments means many substances work cooperatively in such a way as to enhance the overall effect, making it stronger than single substances could ever produce alone. More important, even though there are dismaying cancer statistics—see the table on pages 50-53—you do not have to become a statistic.

Cancer reversal is quite possible, but it requires some effort, commitment, and trust on the part of the person involved, and a comprehensive knowledge by the physician of the modalities available and their effectiveness as proven in clinical practice. Skilled alternative practitioners take the time needed to find the root causes of cancer and the patient also becomes actively involved in their treament. Mortality from certain cancers may seem statistically likely, but that is an illusion compounded by fear and ignorance. It's not only patients who fear cancer outcomes; probably most oncologists are equally in fear of this disease and shield themselves against the disturbing scenarios, statistics, and probabilities they know too well. This book offers patients the statistics of optimism. Men and women can and do survive cancer, and go on to live long, productive, healthy lives—cancer free.

For more on the **politics of cancer**, see *Alternative Medicine Definitive Guide to Cancer* (Future Medicine Publishing, 1997; ISBN 1-887299-01-7); to order, call 800-333-HEAL.

What Alternative Medicine Offers—Cancer Healing

With cancer claiming so many lives each year and bringing sickness and disability to so many more, the search for a cure has become a global industry. Yet, as enticing as the idea of a "magic bullet" for cancer may seem, because of the multiple factors related to the cause of the disease, conventional medicine will never find it. As this book explains, the concept of a single magic bullet is a conceptual, physiological, and medical mistake. A far more useful clinical model is that presented by alternative medicine: multiple interacting and interdependent factors contribute to the emergence of cancer and multiple modalities, substances, and practitioners contribute to its reversal.

Alternative therapies offer the advantage of bolstering the patient's own self-healing capacities while avoiding the toxic side effects that accompany conventional medical treatment for cancer. For most alternative medical doctors, the practical starting point is a change in a patient's diet, exercise, and attitudes. By helping to rejuvenate the whole person, these strategies also offer an improved quality of life and a sense of control in the healing process.

Unlike conventional therapies, which actually weaken the body, alternative therapies work to support the body's anticancer defenses and detoxification capacities as much as possible. This may explain why the phenomenon of "spontaneous remission"—the sudden, unexplained recovery from cancer, without any recognized (i.e., conventional) treatment—is so rare in the typical hospital setting. One study found that 88% of the spontaneous remission cancer cases involved a significant dietary change, mainly toward vegetarianism.[45] Many cases also entailed some form of alternative therapy, such as nutritional supplementation and botanical medicine.

A paradoxical situation exists in the language used to describe cancer outcomes. Conventional medicine speaks freely of "cures" when they discuss the fabled magic bullet, but they prohibit (and often punish) alternative practitioners from using the word; yet conventional oncology rarely cures cancer. There is a crucial distinction here, one that has special relevance to the problem of cancer.

Curing typically refers to a medical treatment that relieves the patient of the disease. Healing, by contrast, refers to an internal process of "becoming whole," a feeling of harmonious relationship with one's social and familial sphere—indeed, with one's entire environment. Thus healing pertains to all levels of a person's being, and the most powerful alternative cancer therapies are those aimed at strengthening all these levels at the same time—at reducing the body's toxic burden while also enhancing its multifaceted self-healing capacities and bringing the true character of the individual into focus and healthy expression.

How This Book Can Help You

Part of the process of healing from cancer is to learn as much as you can about your condition. While the demands of coping with cancer can be overwhelming, it is in your best interest to become as informed as possible about the nature of your cancer and the options available for treatment. Seeking the tools and knowledge may also provide a greater sense of control in the midst of this medical crisis. Having a basic understanding of the nature of cancer and how it develops or goes into remission is crucial to combat unrealistic fears you may have about your condition and also provide a sense of order in an otherwise chaotic time. And while your oncologist may or may not be open to the use of alternative therapies, use this book to educate yourself about the wide range of safe, nontoxic, and effective alternative treatments for cancer.

Cancer and Its Causes

In its simplest terms, cancer represents an accelerating process of inappropriate, uncontrolled cell growth—a chaotic process within the order of biology. Healthy cells stop functioning and mutations occur that encourage cancer growth. In Chapter 2: Cancer and Its Causes, we learn that doctors now know that the development and growth of cancer begins with specific, undesirable changes in the cell, in its DNA, or genetic components. Normally such changes are thwarted by a healthy immune system, but when these changes go unchecked, then the cancer process can continue to its next stage of uncontrolled rapid growth. The concept that cancer is the result of multiple factors impinging on an individual's mind and body is actually not a new one, but it is one that has been consistently ignored by conventional cancer specialists. To date, up to 33 factors have been linked to the creation of cancer, among them are sunlight, chronic exposure to pesticides, industrial toxins, dietary and dental factors, chronic stress, hormone therapies, free radicals, and radiation.

Early Detection and Prevention

The hallmark of alternative medicine is the notion that it is possible to reverse serious illness in its early stages through early detection and, by maintaining good health habits, prevent illness in the first place. In Chapter 3: Early Detection and Prevention, we examine the testing protocols used by alternative medicine physicians and how they are often superior to those used by conventional oncologists. These tests include the AMAS (anti-malignin antibody screen) test, darkfield microscopy, thermography, biological terrain assessment, and other innovative evaluations. In every instance, the intention is to test for the appropriate cancer markers in the blood, cells, or tissue and to map a treatment plan. Preventive strategies, including dietary recommendations, supplementation, exercise, and detoxification, are provided for prostate and breast cancers, along with stress reduction therapies.

Nutrition as Cancer Medicine

In Chapter 4: Nutrition as Cancer Medicine, we will describe in detail the many ways nutritional therapy is used successfully in treating cancer. The leading nutritional problem in the United States today is "overconsumptive undernutrition," or eating too many empty-calorie foods, says Jeffrey Bland, Ph.D., a biochemist and nutrition expert. Consuming a whole foods, largely vegetarian diet has been proved to be a good anticancer strategy. Because the diet is not always adequate as a nutrient source, supplementation is critical for those with cancer. This chapter will show how changes in your diet and supplementation—including vitamins, minerals, amino acids, probiotics, and essential fatty acids, among others—can bolster your immune system to prevent cancer or assist your body in fighting off the cancer that has invaded it.

Herbs for Cancer

Indigenous cultures around the world have relied on the healing power of herbs for thousands of years. Modern medicine is finally catching up by tapping into the powerful resources that can be found in herbs and botanicals such as aloe vera, echinacea, ginseng, and maitake mushrooms. Chapter 5: Herbs for Cancer, we explain how herbs treat cancer in a number of different ways: they can stimulate DNA repair mechanisms, fight cancer by producing antioxidant effects, promote the production of protective enzymes, or induce oxygenating effects, which help discourage cancer growth. This chapter will explore in detail a number of herbs and botanical compounds— algae, amygdalin, Essiac tea, grape seed extract, iscador, and others— shown to be highly effective in cancer treatment.

The New Cancer Pharmacology

Chemotherapy and radiation remain the primary treatments prescribed by the mainstream medical establishment despite its dismal success rate: 7% to 15% for only a few cancers. Alternative medicine physicians reject the mainstream prevailing concept that these toxic treatments are a viable way to treat cancer. In Chapter 6: The New Cancer Pharmacology, a new protocol is explored that includes innovative, nontoxic therapies, such as Carnivora, DMSO, shark cartilage, hydrazine sulfate, antineoplastons, and Ukrain, that have been found to be successful in treating cancer.

Stimulating the Immune System

Immunotherapy—therapies designed to support optimal immune function—can help enlist the body's own defense mechanisms to subdue cancer without the adverse side effects associated with conventional therapies. In Chapter 7: Boosting the Immune System, we review a number of methods used by alternative physicians to strengthen the immune system to overcome cancer. These include Coley's Toxins (in which bacteria are used to stimulate the body's anticancer defenses), anti-myoplasma auto-vaccines (a special vaccine cultured from the patient's blood), and Immuno-Augmentative Therapy or IAT (balances certain isolated blood proteins to subdue cancer), among others.

Revitalizing Metabolism to Fight Cancer

Metabolism is the sum total of all biochemical processes inside the body. When these chemical processes are balanced, normal cells thrive and cancer cells become depleted or die or revert back to normal. In Chapter 8: Enhancing Metabolism, you will learn about a number of therapies—oxygen, enzymes, hormones, and glandular/organ extracts—that can help normalize these life-sustaining metabolic functions, thereby helping to stop and reverse cancer, or prevent a recurrence.

Using Physical Support Therapies

Flushing toxins out of the body is a prime goal of alternative cancer therapy and, to achieve this, holistic physicians draw upon a variety of techniques, according to the needs of the individual patient. In Chapter 9: Physical Support Therapies, we look at a number of these techniques, including detoxification strategies, biological dentistry, water and heat therapy, bodywork, and *qigong*, as supportive therapies that help balance and strengthen the body to enhance its ability to ward off the cancer.

Energy Support Therapies

At the forefront of new alternative clinical approaches to cancer is the recognition of the role of energy, both as a means of diagnosis and treatment. Acting at a deeper cellular level than biochemical agents such as drugs, energy can make or break health. In Chapter 10: Energy Support Therapies, we explore the role of energy as it applies to cancer. In particular, we look at the diagnostic power of electrodermal screening (EDS), a device that can detect the abnormal energy signals (through the acupuncture meridian system) that accompany ill health. We also look at the use of magnets and magnetic fields as well as light therapy in cancer treatment.

Having a basic understanding of the

nature of cancer and how it develops or goes

into remission is crucial to combat

unrealistic fears you may have about your condition

and also provide a sense of order in an

otherwise chaotic time. And while your oncologist

may or may not be open to

the use of alternative therapies, use this book

to educate yourself about the wide range

of safe, nontoxic, and effective

alternative treatments for cancer.

CHAPTER

2 Cancer and Its Causes

ROM A BIOLOGICAL VIEWPOINT, cancer is fundamentally a rational process. Once its physiological and biochemical mechanisms are understood, however, therapeutic approaches can be successfully deployed against it, in many instances producing stabilizations, remissions, and, practically speaking, life after cancer. Without this understanding, however, appropriate treatments are unlikely, as is the case when rational treatment is approached solely by conventional medical thinking and practices.

A Chaotic Process in the Rational Order of Biology

Cancer is a disease process in which healthy cells stop functioning and maturing properly. A mishap occurs inside these cells. Perhaps it begins with a change (mutation) in the genetic blueprint, its DNA. The altered DNA makes copies of itself and passes its information and gene sequencing on to other cells, which then become cancer prone. As the normal cycle of cell creation and death is interrupted, the newly mutated cancer cells begin multiplying uncontrollably, no longer operating as an integrated and harmonious part of the body.

In its simplest terms, cancer represents an accelerating process of inappropriate, uncontrolled cell growth—a chaotic process within the order of biol-

In This Chapter

- A Chaotic Process in the Rational Order of Biology
- Cancer Classification, Types, and Stages
- How Cancer Can Become Life-Threatening
- What Causes Cancer?
- 33 Factors That Contribute to Cancer

ogy. Cancer cells, when examined under a microscope, are abnormally shaped, inconsistently formed, and disorganized and contain misshapen internal structures—the essence of biological disorder. Cancer, despite its horror for the individual, is a natural phenomenon: it represents the body's response to a continuous attack on its balancing and regulatory mechanisms by numerous factors.

Cancer may seem to us a modern epidemic, but traces of cancer have been detected in the bones and skulls of mummies from Egypt and Peru embalmed 5,000 years ago. Hippocrates (circa 400 B.C.), the renowned Greek physician, first coined the term *carcinoma* to indicate skin cancer; to him, this Greek word (*karkinoma* means "crab") is appropriate because of the way a spreading cancer extends clawlike extensions across the cell, tissue, or skin. What is different today is the incidence of cancer: it is steadily affecting more people each year, specifically one out of every three. It is no longer one serious disease among many, but the disease of our time.

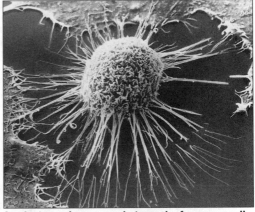

An electron microscope photograph of a cancer cell.

The development and growth of a cancer is called carcinogenesis. Physicians now understand that it involves many steps, beginning with specific, undesirable changes in the nucleus of the cell, specifically in its genetic components, the DNA. What distinguishes a cancer process from life-as-usual in the cell is that normally—in a state of health—DNA mutations are repaired or rendered harmless by the immune system, an intricate, multifaceted biochemical defense system. When undesirable genetic alterations remain uncorrected, then a cancer process can potentially escalate to its next stage of uncontrolled rapid growth.

It does this by making copies of itself. This replication, again, is a normal function of DNA, but the trouble here is that it is altered, mutated, and undesirable DNA that is copying itself. As more cancer cells are generated, the process continues to expand and form a tumor. The normal mechanisms of cell growth, replication, differentiation, and maturation then become unregulated, leading to chaos in the body.

Cancer Symptoms and Statistics

TYPE OF CANCER	POSSIBLE SYMPTOMS (If these occur, see your physician for a physical exam and/or lab tests.)
Bladder cancer	Blood in urine, making it look bright red or rust-colored; pain or burning upon urination; frequent urination; feeling the need to urinate but nothing comes out; urine may appear cloudy because it contains pus
Breast cancer	A lump or thickening of breast; discharge from the nipple; retraction of the nipple; change in skin of breast, such as dimpling or puckering; redness, swelling, feeling of heat; enlarged lymph nodes under arm
Colorectal cancer	Rectal bleeding (red blood in stools or black stools); abdominal cramps; constipation alternating with diarrhea; weight loss; loss of appetite; weakness; pallid complexion
Kidney cancer	Blood in urine; dull ache or pain in back or side; lump in kidney area; sometimes accompanied by high blood pressure or abnormality in red blood cell count
Leukemia	Weakness, paleness; fever and flu-like symptoms; bruising and prolonged bleeding; enlarged lymph nodes, spleen, liver; pain in bones and joints; frequent infections; weight loss; night sweats
Lung cancer	Wheezing "smoker's cough," persisting for months or years; increased, sometimes blood-streaked, sputum; persistent ache in chest; congestion in lungs; enlarged lymph nodes in the neck
Melanoma	Change in a mole or other bump on the skin including bleeding, or change in size, shape, color, or texture
Non-Hodgkin's lymphoma	Painless swelling in the lymph nodes of the neck, underarm, or groin; persistent fever; feeling of fatigue; unexplained weight loss of more than 10% in a 6-month period; itchy skin and rashes; small lumps in skin; bone pain; swelling in some part of abdomen; liver and spleen enlargement
Oral cancer (oral cavity, lip, pharynx)	May often feel a lump in the mouth with the tongue; sometimes a sore spot can be felt while eating or drinking; ulceration of the lips, tongue or other area inside the mouth that does not heal within two weeks; dentures may no longer fit well; or in advanced cases, oral pain, bleeding, foul breath, loose teeth, and changes in speech
Ovarian cancer	Frequently, few symptoms; abdominal swelling; in rare cases, abnormal vaginal bleeding; women over 40 may experience generalized digestive discomfort
Pancreatic cancer	Upper abdominal pain and unexplained weight loss; pain near the center of the back; loss of appetite; intolerance of fatty foods; yellowing of the skin (jaundice); abdominal masses; enlargement of liver and spleen

POSSIBLE RISKS	5-YEAR SURVIVAL RATES (all stages) PER CONVENTIONAL TREATMENT	ESTIMATED # OF NEW U.S. CASES PER YEAR
Twice as high in whites as in blacks; 2-3 times higher in men as in women; 2-3 times higher in cigarette smokers as in nonsmokers; machinists, truck drivers, and workers exposed to chemicals	80.7%	52,900
Increasing age; early menstruation; late menopause; not having a child or having first child after 30; family or personal history; inherited breast cancer gene	83.2%	185,700
Polyps, ulcerative colitis, or Crohn's disease; family history; residence in urban or industrial area; specific genetic mutations	61%	133,500
Being overweight; twice as high in men as in women; twice as high in cigarette smokers as in nonsmokers; coke-oven and asbestos workers	57.9%	30,600
Specific genetic abnormalities (e.g., Down and Bloom syndromes); excessive exposure to ionizing radiation and chemicals such as benzene; HTLV-1 virus exposure	68.6%	27,600
Cigarette smoking; secondary smoke; asbestos, radiation, radon, or other toxic exposure	13.4%	177,000
Sun exposure, particularly during childhood; sunburning or freckling easily; 40 times higher in whites as in blacks	86.6%	38,300
Lowered immune system function as with HIV and HTLV-1 viruses; recipients of organ transplants; possibly exposure to herbicides	51%	52,700
More prominent in males, with predisposing factors including tobacco and pipe smoking and chewing tobacco; radiation and other toxic exposures	not available	28,150
Increasing age; never pregnant; residence in industrial country (Japan excluded); family history of breast or ovarian cancer; inherited breast cancer gene	44.1%	26,700
Increasing age; cigarette smoking; higher in countries with high-fat diets; higher in blacks than whites	3.6%	26,300

TYPE OF CANCER	POSSIBLE SYMPTOMS (If these occur, see your physician for a physical exam and/or lab tests.)
Prostate cancer	Urination difficulties due to blockage of the urethra; bladder retains urine, creating frequent feelings of urgency to urinate, especially at night; may have difficulty stopping urination; urine stream may be narrow; bladder doesn't empty completely; burning, painful urination; sometimes bloody urine; tenderness over the bladder and dull ache in the pelvis and back
Uterine cancer	Abnormal vaginal bleeding of fresh blood, or a watery bloody discharge in a postmenopausal woman (70%-75% of all cases are postmenopausal); a collection of fluid may also occur in the uterus; painful urination; pain during intercourse; pain in pelvic area

*Cancer statistics obtained from *CA—A Cancer Journal for Clinicians* 45:1 (1995), 8-28: Report by the Surveillance Branch of the Department of Epidemiology and Surveillance, American Cancer Society, Atlanta, GA; and "Twelve Major Cancers," *Scientific American* (September 1996), 126-132.

Modern oncology (the study of tumors) needs to radically rethink its cancer model, which is based on the Halstead theory of cancer (developed by W. S. Halstead, 1852-1922). G. Zajicek, M.D., of the H.H. Humphrey Center for Experimental Medicine and Cancer Research at Hebrew University-Hadassah Medical School in Jerusalem, Israel, argues that the Halstead theory, whose central premise is that the primary fact about cancer is the tumor, not the patient as a living organism, must be dropped in favor of a more systemic model.[1]

The fact that the age-adjusted mortality rate for cancer has remained virtually unchanged for 60 years means that the standard treatments devised to kill tumors have failed because they are "based on false premises," says Dr. Zajicek. "This hypothesis implies that tumor removal should cure the patient, yet 60 years of intensive effort to remove the tumor did not change the biological outcome of the disease. Obviously, the hypothesis is wrong and should be modified." Focusing medical efforts at removing the tumor is fundamentally a mistake, argues Dr. Zajicek, and will not cure cancer because cancer is "a metabolically systemic deficiency" and "a chronic system disease."[2] Halstead's cancer theory is flawed, says Dr. Zajicek, because it emphasizes the tumor and ignores the patient.

POSSIBLE RISKS	5-YEAR SURVIVAL RATES (all stages) PER CONVENTIONAL TREATMENT	ESTIMATED # OF NEW U.S. CASES PER YEAR
Increasing age; 37% higher in blacks as in whites, with twice the mortality rate	85.8%	317,100
Cervical: cigarette smoking; sex before 18; many sexual partners; low socioeconomic status; mortality rate twice as high for blacks as whites Endometrial: Early menstruation; late menopause; never pregnant; estrogen exposure, estrogen replacement therapy without progestin; tamoxifen; diabetes, gallbladder disease, hypertension, and obesity	68.3%	49,700

Cancer Classifications, Types, and Stages

Among the 150 different types of cancer, five major groups are conventionally recognized. Carcinomas form in the epithelial cells that cover the surface of the skin, mouth, nose, throat, lung airways, and genitourinary and gastrointestinal tract, or that line glands such as the breast or thyroid. Lung, breast, prostate, skin, stomach, and colon cancers are called carcinomas and are solid tumors.

Sarcomas are those that form in the bones and soft connective and supportive tissues surrounding organs and tissues, such as cartilage, muscles, tendons, fat, and the outer linings of the lungs, abdomen, heart, central nervous system, and blood vessels. Sarcomas are also solid tumors, but sarcomas are both the most rare of malignant tumors and the most deadly.

Leukemias form in the blood and bone marrow and the abnormal white blood cells produced there travel through the bloodstream creating problems in the spleen and other tissues. Leukemias are not solid tumors; they are characterized by an overproduction of abnormal white blood cells.

Lymphomas are cancers of the lymph glands. Lymph glands act as a filter for the body's impurities and are concentrated mostly in the

Staging in Cancer

In terms of tumor size and severity, oncologists (physicians who specifically treat cancer) distinguish four different phases, which they call stages. Staging refers to an index used by cancer specialists to determine how much cancer exists in the body, its size, location, and containment or metastasis. Stage I, the earliest, most curable stage, shows only local tumor involvement. Stage II has some spreading of cancer to the surrounding tissues and perhaps to nearby lymph nodes; Stage III involves metastasis to distant lymph nodes; Stage IV, the most advanced and least easily cured, refers to cancer that has spread to distant organs.

neck, groin, armpits, spleen, the center of the chest, and around the intestines. Lymphomas are usually made up of abnormal lymphocytes (white blood cells) that congregate in lymph glands to produce solid masses. Hodgkin's disease and non-Hodgkin's lymphomas are the two most prevalent types of lymphoma in the United States, while Burkitt's lymphoma, rare in the U.S., is common in Central Africa.

Myelomas are rare tumors that arise in the antibody-producing plasma cells or hemopoietic (blood cell–producing) cells in various tissues in the bone marrow.

A key characteristic of cancer cells is their greatly prolonged life spans compared to that of normal cells. It's ironic, given that cancer can potentially prove fatal to its host and thus to itself as an unwelcome "parasite," that cancer cells are essentially immortal. Not only do cancer cells not die when they are supposed to, they also fail to develop the specialized functions of their normal counterparts. Masses of cancer cells may become like parasites, developing their own network of blood vessels to siphon nourishment away from the body's main blood supply. It is this process that, unchecked, will eventually lead to the formation of a tumor—a swelling caused by the abnormal growth of cells. If the tumor invades adjacent normal tissue or spreads through lymph vessels or the blood vessels to other normal tissues, this tumor is considered malignant.

Technically, many people carry harmless tumors within their bodies, even until their death from other causes. Such benign tumors are encapsulated by fiber, functionally insulating the body from their otherwise toxic effects. At a certain point, these tumors simply stop enlarging; since they do not "seed" other tumors, they are considered benign. A malignant tumor, which is not encapsulated by fiber, is capable of invading nearby cells and spreading to distant sites within the body. If the cancer cells do not spread beyond the tissue or organ where they originated, the cancer is considered to be localized; if the cancer spreads to other parts of the body, it is then said to have metastasized.

The pathological character of such tumors stems from their cells' ability to invade other tissues and travel through the blood and lymphatic vessels to other areas of the body. Most cancer victims die not from the initial multiplication of these abnormal cells, but as a result of this secondary process, metastasis—the spread of cancer to other organs and tissues of the body. This process represents the cancer cells' tendency to break off from the original tumor, float in the bloodstream, and colonize other tissues.

Cancers that metastasize quickly—that is, even when the total number of cancer cells is still small—are generally considered aggressive, which means more malignant. Aggressive tumors contain cells that are generally less "mature" from a cellular point of view; that is, they are less physically defined and lack some of a cell's standard constituents. It is often said of these cells that they are less well-developed or well-differentiated.

Looking more specifically at the subject of aggressiveness in cancers, oncologists usually allocate the following categories: an aggressive cancer has a doubling time of 60 days or less (meaning how long it takes for the cancer mass to double its size); a moderate cancer doubles in 61-150 days; an indolent cancer doubles in 151-300 days; and a very indolent cancer takes up to 300 days. For a sense of perspective, the average size of a breast cancer when first detected by mammography is about 600 million cells, or about ¼ inch across; the average size detectable by manual palpation has about 45 billion cells and may be 1¼ inches in diameter.

Another characteristic of cells that metastasize is that they exhibit little or no "cell-to-cell adhesion." Most normal cells, by contrast, tend to adhere to one another to form well-defined tissues. The notable exceptions

Differentiation in Cancer

Differentiation is a process by which unspecialized cells mature and become specialized to carry out specific tasks. At birth, a human infant has an estimated five trillion cells differentiated into about 100 different cell types. Differentiated cells—red blood cells, for example—have a preset life expectancy and are programmed to live, die, and be replaced on a precise schedule. In cancer, there is an abnormal control over the way in which a cell becomes specialized. Generally, a poorly differentiated cancer, in which the tumor cells bear almost no resemblance to normal cells of that particular tissue, is the most virulent and dangerous. Tumors that are moderately differentiated generally pose a more favorable outcome, with survival likelihood, even under conventional medicine, extending into years or decades. A well-differentiated cancer, though less common than a moderately differentiated one, can be indolent and sometimes nonmalignant.

to this are circulating blood cells, which move freely about the body. To a lesser extent, the degree of malignancy depends on the rate at which the cells reproduce and cause tumors to expand. Tumors can either be slow-growing or fast-growing; either way, the tendency is fairly fixed.

In other words, those that grow rapidly and are likely to metastasize will tend to remain aggressive, while those that are less aggressive do not commonly change their behavior; they usually remain slow-growing.[3] Larger tumors—those weighing a few pounds—usually require years to develop, since the body imposes various restraints on cell reproduction. However, prostate cancer is usually slow, but often after treatment, especially conventional treatment, it can become very aggressive.

Once metastasis has occurred, cancer is more likely to be fatal, unless checked or reversed by successful multimodal alternative therapies. Metastasis can lead to the formation of more tumors, which further sap the body's energy supply, weakening (and eventually poisoning) the patient with toxins that make one feel fatigued, achey,

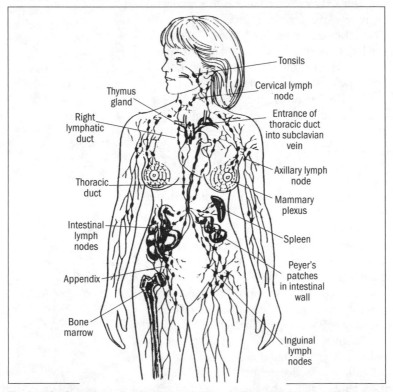

The lymphatic system, showing the major lymphatic organs and vessels.

Understanding Clinical Terms: What is a Cancer "Marker"?

A cancer or tumor marker generally refers to any of a variety of standard laboratory blood tests used to measure the level of a protein material or other chemical produced by cancer cells. These numbers become elevated in the presence of a cancer or tumor. Technically, X rays and scans (such as CT, or computerized tomography) are cancer markers because they can determine with specificity the presence and location of cancer in the body, but the term *cancer marker* usually indicates a blood test.

Here are a few of the cancer markers for different kinds of cancer:

- CEA (carcinoembryonic antigen) test for colon cancer
- AFP (alpha-fetoprotein) test for liver cancer (primary hepatocellular carcinoma)
- PSA (prostate specific antigen) for prostate cancer
- CA (carcinoma) 27.29 for breast cancer
- CA 125 for ovarian cancer

Ideally, after treatment, the numbers go down, indicating that the cancer has been eliminated. If the person is retested some time later and the numbers are again elevated, the indication is that the cancer has either recurred in that area, spread to lymph glands nearby, or metastasized to another organ.

For example, a man's PSA for prostate cancer might test above 4.5 units, which is at the upper end of the acceptable range. After being treated with alternative or conventional methods, his PSA might drop to 0.4 (0 is the bottom of the scale). If, some months later, his PSA jumps to 40, the cancer may have metastasized to the lymph nodes or bone, which are the most common areas of metastasis in prostate cancer. He could then be tested with a bone scan and/or a blood test to determine if the tumor has spread to the bone.

A less specific cancer marker is the AMAS (anti-malignin antibody screen), which detects cancer in the body in general. It has the advantage of being able to detect cancer in its early stages and also screens for all types of cancer (with the exception of leukemia).

depressed, and apathetic. Eventually, the unchecked growth overwhelms other body functions. Whatever the immediate cause, the cancer-related death is usually preceded by metastasis and by the establishment of "secondary cancers" that grow as a result of metastasis from the primary tumor site.

How Cancer Can Become Life-Threatening

Many, if not most, cancer deaths come as a result of infection by bacteria, viruses, and fungi—microbes that normally would be destroyed by the immune system. In the case of cancer, the immune system becomes severely suppressed, partly because of the systemic weakening brought on by the cancer process and partly because of the negative, toxic effects of conventional cancer treatment—chemotherapy, surgery, and radiation.

A tumor can directly interfere with the functioning of a vital organ, such as the lungs, liver, pancreas, brain, or kidneys, in effect, strangulating it. When a cancerous mass becomes too large, it steals nourishment from the organ, secreting toxins into it or causing some physical obstruction that effectively shuts the organ down.

Severe malnutrition or emaciation, which is a condition of cellular starvation called cachexia (pronounced cah-CHECK-see-yah) may affect up to 90% of all advanced cancer patients and account for 50% of all cancer deaths.[4] The cancer process effectively starves cancer patients, using up their energy reserves. These effects primarily result from the body's shifting to an inefficient use of fuel sources, as well as the person's loss of appetite.

Protein-calorie malnutrition is not uncommon among hospitalized patients in general, and can lead to overall weakness, apathy, increases in mortality and surgical failure, a reduction in immunity, and poor responsiveness to treatment. Some cancer patients die from hemorrhage (uncontrolled blood loss from a failure of the blood to clot), which is a frequent cause of death in leukemia, but can also occur when a tumor grows into a large blood vessel. Cancer can impair the blood's ability to form clots and internal bleeding can occur readily and persistently. Cancer can also cause excessive clotting and the formation of thrombi (blood clots attached to the interior wall of a vein or artery), cutting off the blood supply to a vital organ.

What Causes Cancer?

As much as science strives to identify single precipitating factors—such as genes or infectious organisms—practitioners of alternative medicine know there is no single cause for cancer, just as there is no single magic bullet therapy or substance to end it. Many interdependent factors contribute to the development of cancer. In fact, this chapter will present detailed information on 33 distinct contributing factors that, in various combinations, can begin a cancer process in a given individual.

The concept that cancer is the result of multiple factors impinging on an individual's mind, body, and organic systems is actually not a new one, but it is one that has been consistently ignored by conventional cancer doctors. For example, in 1958, Max Gerson, M.D., an alternative cancer treatment pioneer, explained in general terms how cancer results. First, there is a slow buildup of toxicity throughout the body, especially the liver, which is responsible for most of the body's detoxification, leading to a functional alteration of most systems, including the chemical balance between sodium and potassium in the cells. Next comes a lowering of electrical potentials in the vital organs, a further accumulation of poisons, a reduction in the activity and supplies of oxygen, and the preliminary mutation of some normal cells into cancer cells, according to Dr. Gerson. With this, "general poisoning increases, vital functions and energies decrease, and cancer increases," said Dr. Gerson. Next comes a further destruction of the metabolism (energy extraction from food) and liver functioning as the cancer rules and spreads.[5]

Today, we talk more in terms of immune system dysfunction and perhaps less in terms of sodium and potassium balances, but Dr. Gerson's basic insight of a progressive, systemic poisoning and weakening is still valid. In fact, it is even more valid today, as we are routinely subjected to far more toxins in our environment and have become increasingly aware of their harmful effects, particularly with respect to the cancer process.

As Robert O. Becker, M.D., noted authority on the health perils and medical promise of electromagnetic energy, explains, everyone is constantly exposed to substances and energies, from chemicals to X rays, that can potentially start a cancer process. "As a result, we are always developing small cancers that are recognized by our immune system and destroyed." The healthy body can normally handle individual carcinogenic influences, but when they become multiple and cumulative, the body begins to weaken, and this is the point at which harmful influences may gain the upper hand. "Any factor that increases the growth rate of these small cancers gives them an advantage over the immune system," says Dr. Becker, and cancer emerges.[6]

Dr. Becker's observation underscores a key concept involving cancer: cancer cells—an estimated 300, but more if the body has been exposed to carcinogens—are created every day in healthy human beings. What's a mere 300 out of an estimated 30 trillion cells that comprise the human body? Cancer cells, in moderation, are a legitimate part of nature. The difference between a person with cancer and a person with fleeting cancer cells is that, in the latter, the immune system is able to eliminate the aberrant cells before they are able to do any damage or start a growth process culminating in a tumor. As naturopathic physician and educator Joseph Pizzorno, N.D., explains,

"When the immune system is not working well, the result is frequent or chronic infections, chronic fatigue, and, eventually, cancer."[7]

On a microscopic level, cancer is Nature's way of removing defective genetic material, says cancer doctor Victor Marcial-Vega, M.D. Cancer reflects a change or mutation in the DNA, a cell's genetic makeup, but this process is defensive and occurs all the time. "The body is creating throughout life and every once in a while something goes amiss. At this point, the body says, 'Oh, this didn't come out that well, let's get rid of it.' The purpose of a cancer cell is to signal the body to get rid of matter in the body that did not replicate normally." The immune response is the body's way of cleaning up defective DNA.

Out of billions of DNA replications occurring in the body each day, several will become abnormal and may lead to cancer. In fact, in an average lifetime, the human body goes through an estimated 10^{16} (ten thousand trillion) cell divisions. Those who practice good diet, exercise, and other preventive lifestyle measures may reduce their cancer risk as low as 10%. Despite the astronomical number of cell divisions, the body's cellular defense system is able to hold cancer incidence down to one case in every 10^{17} cell divisions.[8] "This is the way Nature intended it. When cancer cells occur—and everyone has abnormal cells arising in their bodies throughout the day—they are readily detected and removed by a healthy immune system." The immune system helps maintain and revitalize the body by eliminating cancer or otherwise abnormal cells. Only when the immune system weakens can the cancer cells multiply and spread through the body, says Dr. Marcial-Vega.

What makes the immune system weaken is a multiplicity of stress factors, collectively known as carcinogens. Technically, carcinogens refer to chemicals or radiation with cancer-causing potential, but for the purposes of general understanding, we use the term *carcinogen* more broadly here. Carcinogens as we define them include chemicals, electromagnetic energy, faulty diet, free radicals, genetic predisposition, toxicity, radiation, parasites, strong emotions, and viruses, among others. There are dozens of potential influences, which we will review in this chapter. These are not so much "causes" of cancer, as facilitators: they edge the body into a condition of weakness, vulnerability, and immune dysfunction. In this condition, the ordinary production of a few cancer cells can gain the upper hand in the molecular life of the individual, and a cancer process is initiated.

Depending on a person's biochemical and psychological makeup, certain stressors will play a more primary role. The key concept is that the cumulative effect of many carcinogens and immune-suppressing agents acting together is a weakening of the immune system, thereby allowing cancer cells to proliferate. In this chapter, we'll chart the activity of carcinogens, from ones seemingly removed from the human being (sunlight and electromagnetic energy) to influences closer to the body (pesticides and polluted water), to those that change the nature of the body (food), to ones that work inside the body (free radicals), to ones that may have preceded one's birth (genetic influences).

Defining a Carcinogen—Initiators and Promoters

The term *carcinogen* is an umbrella term to denote a substance or energy that begins or promotes the cancer process. These can be put into two categories.

First, there are substances called initiators or triggers that damage genes which normally control the proliferation of cells. When a single cell accumulates various changes or genetic mutations over a period of months or years, it will eventually escape from the ordinary restraints on cell growth. Defects in the DNA become embedded in the genetic materials passed from one cell generation to the next, making it a permanent mutation. The cell grows and produces "offspring" or descendants that are increasingly free of the normal growth constraints. The result is a tumor.

Second, there are cancer promoters. These substances do not damage genes but support the growth of tumor cells or their precursors. After the initiation of the cancer process, the disease will often lie undetected for many years; during this phase, cancer promoters can selectively enhance the growth of tumor cells at the expense of healthy cells. In this way, they further the cellular damage, allowing cancer cells to continue spreading abnormally. Promoters can also hamper the removal of initiated cells by the immune system, make certain tissues a more favorable growth habitat for the tumor, and start the migration of cancer cells to other sites in the body, planting the cancer process like seeds (metastasis).

The probability is that if a person gets enough exposure to carcinogens, tumors can and will develop even if the immune system is fairly healthy. This is due to the concept of the total body tumor burden—that is, the sum of all factors suppressing the immune system including the cancer cells themselves. A tumor or leukemia develops when there is either an increased production of cancer cells because of excess facilitators (causes) or a decreased removal of cancer cells from the body because of clogged lymphatic drainage or weakened immunity.

The Immune System—First Line of Anticancer Defense

Most tumors never make it beyond the microscopic stage; they disappear before we have a chance to know they exist. In the language of orthodox oncology, these tumors "spontaneously regress." The obvious implication is that certain immune system components stop cancer in its tracks. Could it be that these immune factors largely determine the cancer patient's survival and help explain the anecdotal reports of "spontaneous remission"?

Given that each of us is constantly exposed to carcinogens in our food, air, and water, resulting in the production of cancer cells within the body, and that normally the immune system recognizes and destroys these cells before they have a chance to multiply, we can say this means that having abnormal cells develop is probably not the critical factor in determining the course of cancer. The primary threat of cancer may result instead from the body's inability to eliminate the abnormal cells even when they are few in number.

Many oncologists and medical immunologists now believe that cancer emerges as a result of a functional breakdown or imbalance in the immune system—indeed, as "a prime example of failure of the immune system."[9] The immune system may produce too much of a particular substance and not enough of another, resulting in a diminished ability to resist cancer and other immune-related illnesses.

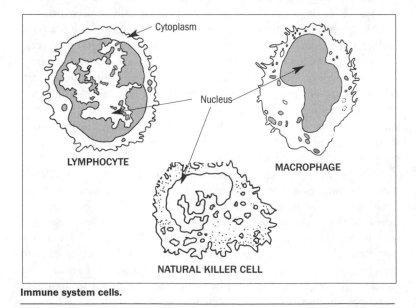

Immune system cells.

The immune system has a way to assess whether normal cells have been transformed into cancer cells. This is the job of the specialized white blood cells known as T lymphocytes, or T cells. Derived from the thymus gland, these cells travel throughout the body to detect unusual cells and tumor-associated antigens—foreign proteins released by tumor cells. Lymphocytes represent 25% to 33% of the total white blood cell count, which increases during certain infections.

Lymphocytes produced in the bone marrow actually come in two forms: the T cells that mature in the thymus gland and have many functions in the body's immune response; and B cells that produce antibodies to neutralize foreign matter in the blood and tissues. Each B lymphocyte produces a single and specific type of antibody. Certain types of T cells signal other white blood cells that cancer cells are present. Some lymphocytes can produce various anticancer chemicals known as cytokines, which include tumor necrosis factor, interleukin, and interferon. These are the body's own "chemotherapy," except they don't harm healthy cells as administered chemotherapy does.

Melanoma, a potentially deadly form of cancer, is one of the human tumors most extensively studied for its immunologic characteristics. Evidence for the immune system's involvement in melanoma includes the presence of specific T-cell and antibody responses upon exposure to melanoma cells; also, the more of these T cells present, the longer the melanoma patient's survival.[10] Again, the many anecdotal reports of "spontaneous remission" of cancer among "terminal" melanoma patients suggest that the body naturally has the means to rid itself of this cancer.[11]

One of the body's most immediate and powerful means of protection against cancer results from the action of natural killer (NK) cells (SEE QUICK DEFINITION). They are a specialized form of lymphocyte capable of migrating to the site of cancer and destroying the malignant cells before they can divide.[12] NK cells afford constant surveillance against cancer. Their "killer" reputation—it comes from the "attack" mentality of conventional medicine—is based on the fact that, without any prior exposure to the abnormal cells, they can cause cells to split or break apart.[13]

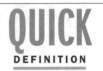

DEFINITION

Natural Killer cells are a type of nonspecific, free-ranging immune cell produced in the bone marrow and matured in the thymus gland. NK cells can recognize and quickly destroy virus and cancer cells on first contact. "Armed" with an estimated 100 different biochemical poisons for killing foreign proteins, they can kill target cells without having encountered them previously. As with antibodies, their role is surveillance, to rid the body of aberrant or foreign cells before they can grow and produce cancer or infection.

Macrophages are a form of white blood cell (originally produced in the bone marrow and called monocytes) that can "swallow" germs and foreign proteins, then release an enzyme that chemically either damages or kills the substance. The name means "big" (macro) "swallower" or "eater" (phage). Macrophages are the vacuum cleaners and filter feeders of the immune system, ingesting everything that is not normal, healthy tissue, even old body cells.

In the normal immune system, NK cells will descend directly on a minuscule tumor and begin devouring and disintegrating it. As a consequence, many tumors never make it beyond this asymptomatic stage; however, NK cells have little effect against large tumors. Their main value is in protecting against the spread of micrometastases, those tiny, blood- and lymph-borne accumulations of cancer cells that would otherwise seed new tumor growth.

Macrophages (SEE QUICK DEFINITION) support the body's detoxification channels by scavenging debris and storing wastes. These cells, a major part of the body's first line of defense, destroy cancer cells by splitting them apart and ingesting them; they also regulate cell reproduction as well as the activities of other immune cells. Macrophage function alone can ultimately determine whether tumor cells thrive or die.[14] The increased activity of macrophages has been associated with decreased tumor growth and decreased tumor incidence in animals.[15]

33 Factors That Contribute to Cancer

Sunlight
Solar radiation, or sunlight, particularly ultraviolet-B and ultraviolet-C radiation, is a common carcinogen, accounting for over 400,000 skin cancers of the overall estimated one million new cases of skin cancer ocurring annually in the United States. Today, even more ultraviolet radiation is present in sunlight because the ozone hole in the Earth's upper atmosphere has expanded, weakening the Earth's natural shield against it. Scientists believe that the ultraviolet component of sunlight can induce a permanent mutation at a specific point in the DNA (affecting a single gene called the p53 tumor suppressor gene)[16] of skin cells, especially in the skin of people with very fair (whitish) skin. Generally, the damaging effects of too much sunlight on fair skin, which produces a temporary but intense immunosuppression, can occur years before an actual tumor appears.

Chronic Electromagnetic Field Exposure
According to an Environmental Protection Agency study, there is growing evidence of a link between exposure to electromagnetic fields (EMFs)—which are generated by electrical currents—and cancer.[17] While EMFs are part of Nature and in fact are radiated by the human body and its individual organs, the quality and intensity of the energy can either support or destroy health. As a rule, EMFs generated by technological devices or installations tend to be much more harmful than naturally occurring EMFs.

33 Factors That Contribute to Cancer

■ Sunlight	■ Chronic Electromagnetic Field Exposure
■ Geopathic Stress	■ Sick Building Syndrome
■ Ionizing Radiation	■ Nuclear Radiation
■ Industrial Toxins	■ Pesticide/Herbicide Residues
■ Polluted Water	■ Chlorinated Water
■ Fluoridated Water	■ Tobacco and Smoking
■ Hormone Therapies	■ Immune-Suppressive Drugs
■ Irradiated Foods	■ Food Additives
■ Mercury Toxicity	■ Dental Factors
■ Nerve Interference Fields	■ Diet and Nutritional Deficiencies
■ Chronic Stress	■ Toxic Emotions
■ Depressed Thyroid Action	■ Intestinal Toxicity and Digestive Impairment
■ Parasites	■ Viruses
■ Free Radicals	■ Blocked Detoxification Pathways
■ Cellular Oxygen Deficiency	■ Cellular Terrain
■ Oncogenes	■ Genetic Predisposition
■ Miasm	

We are surrounded by stress-producing, electromagnetic fields generated by the electrical wiring in homes and offices, televisions, computers and video terminals, microwave ovens, overhead lights, and electrical poles. EMFs interact with living systems, affecting enzymes related to growth regulation, gene expression, pineal gland metabolism (regulation of the anticancer hormone melatonin), and cell division and multiplication—all of which can exert a major influence on tumor growth.[18]

"Only a few farsighted individuals have given much thought to the fact that the new electromagnetic environment created by 20th-century technology may be exerting subtle, yet very important effects upon biology," states John Zimmerman, Ph.D., president of the Bio-Electro Magnetics Institute in Utah. "This may include alterations in gene expression, immune function, viral pathogenesis, and future genetic tendencies."

Studies of human populations have consistently found associations between residential EMF exposure and cancer, particularly in the case of childhood leukemia.[19] Among adults, there is a stronger association between EMF exposure and brain cancer[20] and, to a lesser extent, breast cancer.[21] The National Council on Radiation Protection warned

Geopathic Stress and Feng Shui

Geopathic stress in home and work environments is a key factor in the onset of disease, as well as in the failure of some patients to respond to treatment, states Anthony Scott-Morley, H.M.D., Ph.D., of Dorset, England. Geopathic stress zones may be tiny, but shifting a bed a few feet in a geopathically troubled bedroom, can make, says Dr. Scott-Morley, the difference between cancer and no cancer for the susceptible individual. The growing popularity of feng shui (pronounced FUNG-shway), the Chinese science of landscape interpretation and household exterior and interior design, is bringing the concept of geopathic stress to a larger audience in the West.

that excessive exposure to EMFs may lead to cancer and that exposure to weak EMFs can disturb the brain's production of melatonin, which may lead to breast cancer.[22] The Council recommended that a maximum exposure limit of 0.2 microteslas (2 milligauss) be set for homes and offices. This level is substantially lower than the field strength of power lines and many common household appliances.

Geopathic Stress

Magnetic radiations from the Earth, presumably connected with geological fractures and subterranean water veins, have been associated with an increased risk of cancer in communities situated near these geopathic, pathogenic influences. According to some experts, the cause of geopathic stress is localized magnetic anomalies—unusual, sudden, local changes and quirks that can upset delicate human physiological balance and create problems.

In 1971, the theory of geopathic stress was supported by research showing that water flowing underground, especially subterranean streams that cross, produces measurable increases in magnetic anomalies; these conditions also increase electrical conductivity in the air and soil, and other physical changes. While the changes may be small, though measurable (in the vicinity of ten inches square), they are still capable of contributing to the development of serious illness, including cancer. One large-scale study by the U.S. government reported that geopathic stress may be a factor in between 40% and 50% of all human cancers and account for between 60% and 90% of all cancers attributed to environmental radiation.[23]

Sick Building Syndrome

In the early 1980s, physicians began using the term *sick building syndrome* (SBS) to refer to a host of symptoms produced by low-grade toxic environmental conditions found in living, work, or office spaces.

SBS symptoms are numerous: mucous membrane irritation of the eyes, nose, and throat, chest tightness, skin complaints (dryness, itching, abnormal redness), headaches, fatigue, lethargy, coughing, asthma, wheezing, chronic nasal stuffiness, temporary weight loss, infections, and emotional irritability. All of these depress the immune system, rendering the individual susceptible to long-term chronic illness and potentially to a cancer process.

"Indoor air pollution in residences, offices, schools, and other buildings is widely recognized as a serious environmental risk to human health," explains Michael Hodgson, M.D., M.P.H., of the School of Medicine, University of Connecticut Health Center, in Farmington. In most cases, problems with a building's engineering, construction, and ventilation system are the causes. Studies suggest that symptoms occur 50% more frequently in buildings with mechanical ventilation systems. Other sources of indoor toxic pollution include volatile organic compounds released from particleboard desks, furniture, carpets, glues, paints, office machine toners, and perfumes. All contribute to "a complex mixture of very low levels of individual pollutants," states Dr. Hodgson.

In addition, the carcinogenic effects of certain indoor air pollutants, such as asbestos, environmental tobacco smoke, radon, and formaldehyde, are well described in the clinical literature and are now considered cancer risk factors. The EPA estimates that indoor radon pollution may cause as many as 10,000 cancers a year in the United States.[24] Other data suggest that exposure to the radioactive decay products of radon in homes contributes to about 10% of annual lung cancers in the U.S. and that the average lifetime risk of lung cancer from environmental radon is one in 1,000.

Ionizing Radiation

Ionizing radiation consists of high-energy rays that are capable of ripping the electrons from matter, causing genetic mutations that can lead to cancer. This is the type of radiation used in X-ray technology, which may explain why radiologists (people who take many X rays each day) have historically had higher incidences of cancer, as have other workers exposed to low-dose radiation.[25]

Medical X rays may cause about 75% of breast cancer, according to estimates made by John W. Gofman, M.D., Ph.D., the director of the Committee for Nuclear Responsibility, Inc., and Professor Emeritus in the Department of Molecular and Cell Biology at the University of California at Berkeley. This shocker may be good news in disguise because it means potentially 75% of breast cancer could be prevented by avoiding or minimizing exposure to the ionizing radiation from mammography, X rays, and other non-nuclear medical sources such as radiation therapy. Given that over 180,000 new cases of female breast cancer occur each year, this means that a substantial number of breast cancers might result annually from unnecessary exposure to medical sources of radiation. X rays (or gamma rays) also emanate from fluorescent lights, computer monitors, and television screens, which add additional exposures in the lives of most people.

Nuclear Radiation

Working or living in the proximity of nuclear power plants presents a cancer risk. Among the hazards are the small amounts of radioactive gases released daily from nuclear reactors at levels deemed "permissible" by the U.S. Department of Energy. This low-level radioactive pollution returns to us in rainfall which then accumulates in the soils to contaminate the food chain. People who eat dairy products and other foods tainted by these radioactive releases may be unwittingly exposing themselves to dangerous carcinogens. Since dairy products tend to concentrate the radioactive fission products, avoiding such foods may lower your cancer risk.

According to one study, workers who were exposed daily to low-level radiation had a much higher risk of cancer, particularly leukemia.[26]

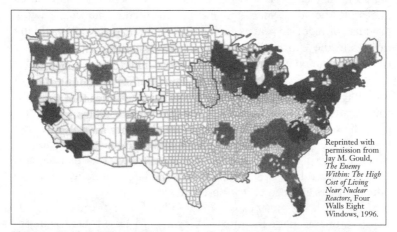

Reprinted with permission from Jay M. Gould, *The Enemy Within: The High Cost of Living Near Nuclear Reactors*, Four Walls Eight Windows, 1996.

Of the country's 3,053 counties, nearly half, or 1,321, are situated within 100 miles of nuclear reactor sites. The darker areas on the map indicate "nuclear counties" and represent the highest risk areas.

In the United Kingdom, a higher rate of leukemia has been reported in children living near nuclear facilities. The incidence of childhood thyroid cancer has increased 100 times in those areas of Ukraine, Belarus, and Russia most acutely exposed to the Chernobyl nuclear accident in April 1986, stated experts from the United Nations.

Ernest Sternglass, Ph.D., Professor of Radiation Physics at the University of Pittsburgh, found rising breast cancer rates among women in 268 counties located within 50 miles of nuclear plants. Age-adjusted cancer mortality rates for women living in these areas rose 10% from 1950 to 1989, compared with a 4% increase for the nation as a whole. The researchers propose that the cancer rates are linked to radioactive iodine and strontium, by-products of nuclear fission which tend to become concentrated in dairy products.[27]

Dr. Sternglass argues that nuclear radiation plays a major role in the recent rises in breast and other cancers not related to smoking, especially among older persons.[28] He further states that the conventional risk estimates for "acceptable" chronic, low-dose exposures may be underestimated by 100 to 1,000 times.

Dr. Sternglass' data proves that there is a direct, measurable, and causal dose/response relationship between extremely small doses and detectable health impacts; the prime carriers for fission products were municipal water and air, and to a lesser extent, fresh milk and dairy products. In fact, the radiation released by fission products appears to work synergistically (enhancing the negative effects of all factors) with other environmental carcinogens such as air pollutants, diesel fumes, dust, asbestos, cigarette smoke, and pesticides.

Chronic exposure to nuclear fission products through the diet and drinking water "may be the single largest factor in the increased incidence of most forms of malignancies" since 1945, says Dr. Sternglass. "In effect, the results presented here represent the outcome of an enormous, unplanned, double-blind epidemiological study in the United States involving some 200 million human beings exposed to fission products for nearly a whole generation," says Dr. Sternglass.

Since the first atomic bomb explosion in New Mexico in 1945 and the advent of nuclear power, nearly all of the continental United States has been irradiated by nuclear fallout. Today, 1,321 of the total 3,053 counties in the U.S. are nuclear counties, meaning the residents live within 100 miles of a reactor. In other words, more than 33% of those living in the continental U.S. are regularly exposed to nuclear radiation. These residents suffer higher than average rates of breast cancer, AIDS, and other immune deficiencies, and, among infants, premature births, low birth weights, reduced intelligence, and depressed thyroids.

Jay M. Gould, former employee of the Environmental Protection Agency, compiled data from the National Cancer Institute, state health departments, and the Centers for Disease Control. This data reveals that more than 1.5 million American women have died of breast cancer since the start of the "nuclear age," whereas prior to 1945, the rate of breast cancer incidence was actually declining. Gould marshals a huge body of health statistics to prove conclusively that those who live in proximity to active nuclear power stations or research facilities (which release radioactive gases, toxic liquid, and solid wastes) have far higher rates of disease than those who do not. The 1,321 nuclear counties account for more than 50% of all breast cancer deaths, says Gould.

Gould's research demonstrates convincingly that negative health effects such as breast cancer mortality are directly related to residential proximity to nuclear radiation. There has been an "overall decline in the health of all age-groups," says Gould, and this cannot be explained without "taking into consideration the great environmental changes" produced by the use of nuclear power.

Pesticide/Herbicide Residues

The scale of the pesticide residue problem is staggering. Since 1945, pesticide use has increased tenfold. Over 400 pesticides are currently licensed for use on America's foods and, in 1995, 1.2 billion pounds were dumped on crop lands, forests, lawns, and fields. Worldwide, in the past 50 years, some 15,000 chemical compounds and more than 35,000 different formulations have come into use as pesticides.[29] Many of those that are banned in the United States (including DDT) are sold to Third World countries, where they enter food products that are then imported into the U.S., such as coffee, fruits, and vegetables. "Although these chemicals for the most part have been banned or strictly regulated, they are durable and remain in the environment for a long time," says Samuel Epstein, M.D., Professor of Occupational and Environmental Medicine

at the University of Illinois School of Public Health. "Crops grown in soil contaminated with these chemicals will pass on their residue to the animals that are fed them, where they will accumulate in the fatty tissue."

For more information about **detoxifying the body of the effects of pollutants**, see Chapter 9: Physical Support Therapies, pp. 254-297.

About 50% of pesticide use is nonagricultural, used in building materials (wood preservatives), food containers, golf courses, parks, roadsides, utility rights-of-way, railroad track beds, school grounds and school buildings (as fumigants), restaurants, department stores, office buildings, airplanes, hospitals, mass transit areas, swimming pools, and hotels. Home and garden pesticides are another widespread source of contamination; research indicates that fumes from externally applied home and garden pesticides can seep into the home, contaminating residents.

The Environmental Protection Agency has identified at least 55 pesticides that could leave carcinogenic residues in foods. In a single meal, a person can conceivably consume residues of a dozen different neurotoxic or carcinogenic chemicals. "Many cancer-causing pesticides and industrial chemicals found in the environment and in our foods tend to accumulate in fatty tissues, whether in fish, cattle, fowl, or people," states Dr. Epstein.

The potential of pesticides, alone and in combination, to cause and promote cancer should be of grave concern to all physicians and public health officials. In 1989, the Natural Resources Defense Council (NRDC) announced that the residues of agricultural chemicals on fruits and vegetables eaten during a typical American childhood could be initiating between 5,500 and 6,200 cancers every year. The NRDC report estimated that the cancer risk could be as much as six times greater for children than for adults.[30] In light of these facts, a consortium of 75 EPA experts ranked pesticide residues among the top three environmentally derived cancer risks.

Israel Proves the Pesticide-Cancer Link

In 1978, following public outcry and threatened legal action, Israel banned many toxic chemicals such as DDT and PCBs which had been directly linked in a 1976 study with breast cancer. The study, conducted by the Department of Occupational Health at Hebrew University-Hadassah Medical School in Jerusalem found that when they compared cancerous breast tissue with noncancerous tissue from elsewhere in the same woman's body, the concentration of toxic chemicals, such as DDT and PCBs, was "much increased in the malignant tissue when compared to the normal breast and adjacent adipose tissue."[31]

Once Israel banned these chemicals, they began noting a significant decrease in the level of toxic chemicals found in human breast milk. Over the next ten years, the rate of breast cancer deaths declined sharply, with a 30% drop in mortality for women under 44 years old, and an 8% overall decline. Interestingly, at the same time, all other known cancer risks— alcohol consumption, fat intake, lack of fruits and vegetables in the diet— increased significantly. Furthermore, worldwide death rates from breast cancer rose by 4%.[32] The only answer scientists could find to explain this anomaly was the greatly reduced level of environmental toxics.

The National Academy of Sciences (NAS) estimates that the risk from a lifetime exposure to 28 pesticides in commonly eaten foods could amount to approximately six cancers per 1,000 people. The General Accounting Office found the FDA is testing less than 1% of all foods for pesticide residues. According to an NAS study, 64% of the ingredients in marketed pesticides had not been properly tested for toxicity, although the pesticide industry is legally required to do such tests.[33]

Home and garden pesticides—Americans spend an estimated $900 million a year on these products—represent another major source of toxicity. They have been linked to a variety of cancers, including childhood leukemia and brain cancer. Indoor pesticide use was found to result in a risk factor four times higher than normal for childhood leukemia.[34] Childhood brain cancer has been directly associated with adult use of chemical pesticides in the garden or orchard. Pesticides used to control pests in the home have also been implicated in this disease, including those found in no-pest strips, termite pesticides, home pesticide bombs, and flea collars for pets.[35]

Industrial Toxins

A great number of highly toxic chemicals, materials, and heavy metals are released by industrial processes and find their way into human tissue. Heavy metals, such as lead, arsenic, mercury, aluminum, nickel, cadmium, and many others that have no safe level in the human system may accumulate within the fat cells, central nervous system, bones, brain, glands, or hair, and may have negative health effects.

The claim that environmental chemicals can cause or promote cancer is supported by the fact that the distribution of toxic-waste dump sites closely correlates with the sites where the highest rates of breast cancer mortality have been registered, according to *Scientific American* (October 1995). A variety of chemicals found in the environment can mimic the activity of estrogen once inside the human body; they are now believed to contribute to many cases of breast cancer. By 1980, the Environmental Protection Agency had detected over 400 toxic chemicals in human tissue—48 in fat tissue, 40 in breast milk, 73 in the liver, and 250 in the blood.

Industrial workers are routinely exposed to potentially toxic chemicals and substances while on the job. Tanners, oil refinery workers, and insecticide/herbicide sprayers are exposed to arsenic and risk lung and skin cancer. Shipyard workers, demolition experts, and brake mechanics are exposed to asbestos, which places them at risk for lung cancer. Hospital and laboratory staff, as well as those involved in the manufacture of wood products, are routinely exposed to formaldehyde. Other carcinogens in the workplace, such as benzene, diesel exhaust, human-made fibers, hair dyes, mineral oils, painting materials, polychlorinated

The Toxic Kitchen Cabinet

Many common household items, including cookware, plastics, and cleansers, may be sources of carcinogens and are best avoided.

Aluminum Cookware: It is advisable to stay away from aluminum cookware, which can release traces of aluminum into the food. These traces can make their way into the bone matrix and create changes in mental functioning.[40] Food cooked in aluminum pans can pick up the element, but as to how much, the jury is still out,[41] especially with respect to anodized aluminum. "Anodized" cookware is constructed of aluminum that has been placed in an electrolytic solution and subjected to an electric current to seal the pores of the aluminum, a process which lessens—some say eliminates—the aluminum interaction with food. However, the safest cookware is probably glass.

Plastics: The safety of plastics used in storing and cooking various foods, particularly when cooking by microwave, is controversial, but it is known that many of the resins used in plastics are cancer-causing substances. Molecules from polyvinyl chloride (PVC), polyethylene (PE), polyvinylidene chloride (PVDC), and plasticizers in plastic wraps can, at the high temperatures achieved in microwave ovens, migrate into foods.

Kitchen Cleansers: Many dishwashing liquids, bleaches, chlorinated scouring powders, all-purpose cleaners, and drain cleaners contain petrochemicals. Nontoxic, environmentally-safe alternatives are available in every category of cleanser and detergent. In general, look for products that are water-based, free of phosphates, biodegradable, and free of propellants.

biphenyls, and soot, are linked with specific occupations, routine exposures, and various cancers.[36] It is estimated that 10% of all cancers are attributable to job-related exposure to carcinogens.[37]

Polluted Water

Tap water from municipal sources is increasingly becoming a health hazard in the U.S. It is not only pesticides and agricultural runoffs that contaminate public drinking water: according to the EPA, the tap water of 30 million Americans contains potentially hazardous levels of lead.[38] In addition, one out of every four public water systems has violated federal standards for tap water.[39] Municipal water can contain many different contaminants, including disease-causing bacteria, radioactive particles, heavy metals, gasoline solvents, industrial wastes, chemical residues, and synthetic organic chemicals.

A survey of 100 municipal water systems and suppliers found significant levels of cancer-causing arsenic, radon, and chlorine by-products, reported the Natural Resources Defense Council in October

1995. An estimated 19 million Americans drink water with radon levels higher than federal safety standards, and two-thirds of the 300 major water suppliers and agencies fail to give consumers information on their tap water. Polluted drinking water can further raise the risk of developing cancer.

Chlorinated Water

The most taken-for-granted chemical in our water supply is chlorine, which has been used for nearly one hundred years to "purify" drinking water. The disinfection of drinking water with chlorine is standard practice throughout the United States. While adding chlorine-type compounds to drinking water protects the public from several kinds of harmful bacteria such as *Shigella*, *Salmonella*, and *Vibrio cholera*, chlorine can form cancer-causing compounds in drinking water.

The EPA tries to downplay the cancer risk from chlorinated drinking water by asserting that the known risk of water-borne disease in humans, if water is not disinfected, is much greater than the theoretical risk of developing cancer. However, according to studies conducted jointly at Harvard University and the Medical College of Wisconsin, the consumption of chlorinated drinking water accounts for 15% of all rectal cancers and 9% of all bladder cancers in the U.S. Further, people drinking chlorinated water over long periods of time have a 38% increase in their chances of contracting rectal cancer and a 21% increase in the risk of contracting bladder cancer.[42]

Fluoridated Water

Fluoride, a poison second in toxicity only to arsenic, has routinely been added to public drinking water and toothpaste since the 1950s, despite mounting evidence of its health hazards. According to the scientific research, fluoride consumption creates multiple hazards with respect to cancer. Fluoride can produce cancer, transforming normal human cells into cancerous ones, even at concentrations of only 1 ppm (parts per million). Fluoride can increase the cancer-producing potential of other cancer-causing chemicals. A National Cancer Institute study compiling 14 years of data showed that the incidence of oral and pharyngeal cancer rises with increased exposure to fluoride by as much as 50%, accounting for 8,000 new cases per year.

For information about **water filtration systems**, see Chapter 4: Nutrition as Cancer Medicine, pp. 130-159.

Dean Burk, Ph.D., Chief Chemist Emeritus of the National Cancer Institute, compared the cancer death rates of the largest fluoridated and nonfluoridated cities. These death rates were similar prior to 1953 when the use of fluoride was introduced, then increased markedly among fluoridated cities. According to Burk's estimates, fluoride caused about 61,000 cases of cancer in 1995 and is likely to cause 90,000 cancer cases by 2015.[43]

The National Academy of Sciences has found that fluorine (a component of fluoride) slows down vitally important DNA repair activity as mediated by enzymes that normally correct for possible flaws or mutations in the genetic material. These biological effects can be induced by fluoride present even in concentrations as low as 1 ppm, the official "safe" dosage set by the U.S. Public Health Service for drinking water.

Tobacco and Smoking
About 30% of cancer deaths in the U.S. can be attributed to tobacco smoke, making tobacco smoke "the single most lethal carcinogen in the U.S.," according to researchers at the Harvard Center for Cancer Prevention at the School of Public Health, in Cambridge, Massachusetts. Passive smoking, or inhaling ambient tobacco smoke, also produces several thousand lung cancer deaths every year.[44]

It is estimated that 350,000-400,000 deaths occur each year in the U.S. as a result of tobacco use, and about 33% of these deaths occur from smoking-related lung cancer alone. Smoking has been linked to cancers of the head and neck, mouth, throat, vocal cords, bladder, kidney, stomach, cervix, and pancreas, as well as to leukemia; smokeless tobacco has been linked to cancers of the lip and tongue.[45]

Over 2,000 chemical compounds are generated by tobacco smoke, and many of them are poisons.[46] Carbon monoxide is released during smoking, reducing the amount of oxygen to organs like the brain, lungs, and heart. Tar, which is formed when organic compounds are burned, is the leading cancer-causing chemical found in tobacco smoke. Nicotine, an alkaloid found in tobacco, is not only addictive, but also acts as a cancer promoter, making it easier for cancer cells of all types to spread throughout the body.[47]

To make matters worse, smokers tend to have lower blood levels of vitamin C and several other antioxidants that would otherwise scavenge or neutralize free radicals. As a result, tobacco smoke offers the perfect formula for initiating and promoting cancer: carcinogens, toxins, free radicals, antioxidant deficiencies, and immune suppression.

Hormone Therapies
Drugs given to alter the natural hormonal cycle of women have been selectively implicated as capable of producing cancer. Regarding oral

contraceptives, a study showed that women who took birth control pills for more than four years were twice as likely as nonusers to develop breast cancer at age 50.[48] For women who start taking birth control pills before age 18 and continue for at least ten years, the risk of developing breast cancer before age 35 is three times higher, based on a study of 4,212 women, reports *Science News* (June 1995). Research reported as early as the late 1960s pointed to serious cancer risks associated with oral contraceptives. One study found that women on the pill had a 300% higher incidence of cervical dysplasia, usually benign changes in the shape of the cervix that, nonetheless, can be early indicators of possible later cancer.

The use of hormone replacement therapy and supplemental estrogens for menopausal women has been linked to endometrial and breast cancers. In 1989, Swedish researchers reported that women who had been on estrogen replacement therapy (ERT) for longer than nine years had a slightly increased risk of breast cancer, and those who took combined estrogen and progesterone replacement therapy had a higher risk than those women taking either alone. In 1995, researchers concluded that women aged 55-59 who took ERT for five years or more had a 40% higher risk of developing breast cancer; among women aged 60-64, the risk was 70% higher.[49]

Dairy milk may be another carrier of cancer-producing factors. Ever since recombinant Bovine Growth Hormone (rBGH) was approved by the FDA in 1993 for injecting dairy cows to increase milk yield, consumers have been alarmed about its possible negative health effects and the lack of solid scientific support for its safety. Many have also been outraged by the FDA's failure to require dairies to label milk and milk products as being derived from rBGH-treated cows. The problem with rBGH is that it contains a hormone common to cows and humans called IGF-1 (insulin-like growth factor), says Samuel S. Epstein, M.D., of the University of Illinois Medical Center in Chicago. IGF-1 causes cells to divide and grow, but when extra amounts enter the human body in the presence of milk protein, the body is unable to destroy it, and it is absorbed by the colon, which is known to have cell receptor sites for IGF-1. The hormone is also known to promote the growth of breast cancer cells. At least 17 scientific studies published since 1991 argue that rBGH milk may have cancer-producing effects.

For more information about **Dr. Epstein's rBGH research**, contact: Cancer Prevention Coalition, 2121 W. Taylor Street, Chicago, IL 60612; tel: 312-996-2297; fax: 312-996-1374.

Immune-Suppressive Drugs

The widespread, habitual, and chronic use of a great number of conventional drugs, antibiotics, and even vaccinations can have a seriously suppressive effect on the immune system, acting in concert with all the other factors to prepare the system for a cancer process. Drugs such as aspirin, acetaminophen, and ibuprofen taken for aches and colds, and glucocorticosteroids (such as cortisone) decrease antibody production and suppress immune vitality.

Antibiotics can directly hinder immune activity and increase the intestinal overgrowth of the yeast *Candida albicans*, which then can suppress the immune system. Vaccinations can suppress the immune system, sometimes for up to two weeks. Finally, cytotoxic agents or chemotherapy drugs used to stop cancerous growth have powerful immune-suppressive effects. They, in effect, render the individual even more susceptible to new, secondary cancers.

Irradiated Foods

The intent of food irradiation is to kill insects, bacteria, molds, and fungi, to prevent sprouting, and to thereby extend shelf life, but the results might be injurious to consumers as well. The process of irradiation leads to the formation of toxic substances, such as benzene and formaldehyde, and other toxic chemical by-products, that have been associated with cancer risk.

Food irradiation may increase the levels of aflatoxin, a deadly carcinogen;[50] it may allow the botulinum toxin (which causes botulism food poisoning) to remain undetected in irradiated foods;[51] over time it may induce some microorganisms to mutate, giving rise to new, dangerous species. Foods that have been irradiated lose much of their nutritional value; the vitamin C content of irradiated potatoes, for example, can be reduced by as much as 50%;[52] in cooked pork, a dose of irradiation equal to one-third the level permitted by the FDA reduced thiamin levels by 17%.[53]

The FDA estimates that 10% of the chemicals in irradiated food are not found in normal (nonirradiated) foods and often unknown to science.[54] As might be expected, the FDA, instead of acting to protect public health, acted to protect the food industry. Even though consumers have a right to know that food has been irradiated, the FDA permits foods exposed to gamma or ionizing radiation to be sold to consumers without any labels.

Food Additives

Over 3,000 chemical additives are added to the American food supply every year. The vast majority of them have been tested only on animals, not humans. Among the most common are saccharin and cyclamates,

Food Additives to Avoid

Aspartame: chemical sweetener used in NutraSweet® and Equal®

Bromated Vegetable Oil: emulsifier in foods and clouding agent in soft drinks

Butylated Hydroxyanisole (BHA) and Butylated Hydroxytoluene (BHT): prevents fats, oils, and fat-containing foods from going rancid

Citrus Red Dye No. 2: used to color orange skins

Monosodium Glutamate (MSG): flavor enhancer used in fast, processed, or packaged foods

Nitrites: used as preservatives in cured meats to prevent spoilage

Saccharin: artificial sweetener, used in Sweet 'n Low®

Sulfur Dioxide, Sodium Bisulfite, Sulfites: preserves dried fruits, shrimp, and frozen potatoes

Tertiary Butylhydroquinone: used to spray the inside of cereal and cheese packages

Yellow Dye No. 6: used in candy and carbonated beverages as a coloring

both used as artificial sweeteners and linked to greater incidences of bladder cancer; butylated hydroxytoluene, used as a preservative and linked to liver cancer; and tannic acid, found in wines and fruits and linked to liver cancer. Aflatoxins, which are found in milk, cereals, peanuts, and corn, have also been linked to liver, stomach, and kidney cancer.[55]

Among the many food additives that may be linked to an increased risk of cancer are gentian violet, nitrofurans, aldicarb, and aspartame.[56] Other food additives that may be carcinogenic include Blue Dye No. 2, Propyl gallate, and Red Dye No. 3.[57] Consumption of dairy products and meats contaminated with steroids and antibiotics also increases cancer risk.

Mercury Toxicity

Mercury, a toxic heavy metal that often comprises up to 50% of "silver" dental fillings, is a noted carcinogen and has the ability to impair immune function and create blockages in the autonomic nervous system and other tissues.

Evidence now shows that mercury amalgams are the major source of mercury exposure for the general public, at rates six times higher than that found in seafood. Since mercury vapors are continuously released from amalgam fillings, as long as you have mercury dental fillings, you inhale mercury vapor 24 hours a day, 365 days a year. After elemental mercury from amalgam fillings is inhaled or ingested, it is converted in the body to methylmercury, the organic form of mercury. Methylmercury, because it easily crosses the blood-brain barrier, has been associated with neurodegenerative diseases such as Alzheimer's, multiple sclerosis, and amyotrophic lateral sclerosis. As toxic as elemental mercury is, methylmercury is 100 times more toxic.

Mercury is a heavy metal. Heavy metals act as free radicals—highly reactive, charged particles that can cause damage to body tissues.

Like other heavy metals, mercury has been shown to cause damage to the lining of arteries and nerve bundles (ganglia), particularly those near the prostate, thereby contributing to cancer. "This means that if amalgam fillings are present, your circulatory system is constantly being exposed to the damaging effects of this heavy metal and free radical," explains Daniel F. Royal, D.O., medical director of the Nevada Clinic and the Royal Center of Advanced Medicine, both in Las Vegas, Nevada.[58]

The problem of amalgam toxicity is so serious that a growing number of doctors routinely advise their cancer patients to have their mercury amalgams replaced. Mercury amalgams weaken the immune system and, because individual teeth (with their toxic fillings) sit on different acupuncture meridians, it can become imperative for this cancer-contributing cause to be eliminated from a patient's body. The cumulative weakening effect these toxic "insults" can have on a body makes it more vulnerable to cancer initiation.

Studies by the World Health Organization show that a single amalgam can release 3-17 mcg of mercury per day,[59] making dental amalgam a major source of mercury exposure.[60] A Danish study of a random sample of 100 men and 100 women showed that increased blood mercury levels were related to the presence of more than four amalgam fillings in the teeth.[61]

Dental Factors

Alternative health practitioners familiar with the principles of biological dentistry have long noted a link between dental problems and degenerative illness. When a tooth is inflamed or infected or otherwise compromised, it can block the energy flow along one or more of the body's acupuncture meridians, causing the deterioration of a corresponding organ or tissue and, in time, leading to cancer. According to Thomas Rau, M.D., medical director of the Paracelsus Clinic in Lustmühle, Switzerland, in about 90% of breast cancer patients he has treated there is a dental factor. This means a problem in a tooth can focus its energy imbalance elsewhere in the body, in this case, the breast; hence the term *dental focus*.

"Each tooth relates to an acupuncture meridian," Dr. Rau states, noting that over the years, he has compiled a dental chart mapping the precise relationship among teeth, meridians, and illnesses. The breast, for example, lies on the Stomach meridian. Accordingly, if you have a problematic tooth (such as a root canal or an infected jaw) situ-

For more on **biological dentistry**, see Chapter 9: Physical Support Therapies, pp. 254-297.

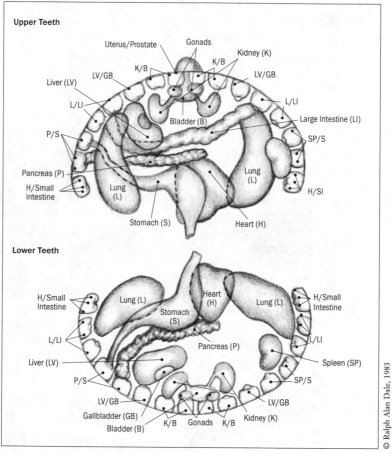

Upper Teeth

Uterus/Prostate   Gonads
Liver (LV)   LV/GB   K/B   K/B   Kidney (K)   LV/GB
L/LI   Bladder (B)   L/LI   Large Intestine (LI)
P/S   SP/S
Pancreas (P)   Lung (L)
H/Small   Lung   H/SI
Intestine   (L)
Stomach (S)   Heart (H)

Lower Teeth

H/Small   Lung (L)   Heart   Lung (L)   H/Small
Intestine   (H)   Intestine
Stomach
(S)
L/LI   Pancreas (P)   L/LI
Liver (LV)   Spleen (SP)
P/S   SP/S
LV/GB   LV/GB
Gallbladder (GB)   K/B   Gonads   K/B   Kidney (K)
Bladder (B)

© Ralph Alan Dale, 1983

Organ and teeth correspondences on acupuncture meridians in the mouth.

ated on this meridian, which passes through the jaw, it blocks the flow of energy and can cause degeneration and eventually cancer. To a lesser extent, a dental focus is also involved in the development of prostate and other cancers.

Nerve Interference Fields

Dysfunctions and imbalances in the autonomic nervous system (ANS) can contribute to a cancer process. Imbalances can be caused by skin scars from old accidents or surgeries; poisoned nerve bundles (called ganglia) in the nervous system made toxic from an accumulation of mercury, parasite toxins, solvents, and many other substances; restriction in blood flow (ischemia) to the ANS from strokes or carbon monoxide poisoning;

and general trauma to the ANS from events such as gunshot wounds, surgical injury, or skull fracture. Dysfunction in the autonomic nervous system often causes arterial spasm in the part of the body supplied by that ANS ganglia or nerve branch; this starves the tissues of oxygen and leads to tissue damage and poor flow of lymphatic fluid.

According to Dietrich Klinghardt, M.D., Ph.D., most cases of chronic illness involve changes in the ANS, especially in the electrical activity of the ganglia and fibers. A nerve ganglion is a group of nerve cell bodies located outside the central nervous system, except for those in the brain, Dr. Klinghardt explains. The majority of the body's ganglia are associated with the ANS. Each ganglion is composed of a mass of neurons and nerve cell bodies enabling it to act as a "little brain" within the body. "Just like thermostats, they can increase or decrease autonomic 'outflow' to the organs they innervate, depending on the needs of the organism."

Ganglia are adaptable, Dr. Klinghardt says, which means if an organ or tissue is inflamed, the toxins may be transported to the nearest nerve ganglia, which can then store them, transport them elsewhere, alter them, or create antitoxins to neutralize them. "Although this creates a toxic ganglion which is operating chronically at a higher and more dysfunctional neurological threshold, it saves the organ, and therefore the organism." As stated above, illness or a chronic condition can upset the electrical activity of ganglia.

Diet and Nutritional Deficiences

Food can make or break our health and, increasingly, factors related to food—its quality, its nutritional constituents, even how it is grown and processed—are considered a primary agent for contributing to the initiation and promotion of cancer. According to the National Academy of Sciences, 60% of all cancers in women and 40% of all cancers in men may be due to dietary and nutritional factors.[62]

One of the major factors accounting for the steady rise in cancer incidence and mortality rates is nutritional imbalances. The rise of degenerative disease has paralleled the adoption of an overly refined and adulterated, high-protein, high-fat diet over the past 100 years. After World War II, the U.S. population shifted away from regular consumption of whole grains and fresh vegetables, and instead increased its consumption of less wholesome, overly refined foods.

This so-called affluent diet is high in fat, which can more readily concentrate such chemicals as pesticides, preservatives, and industrial pollutants. The National Research Council's extensive report, titled

Diet, Nutrition, and Cancer, provided strong evidence that much of the rise in cancer incidence may be related to typical U.S. dietary practices, among other factors.

Excessive intake of animal protein—The high intake of animal protein is associated with an increased risk of breast, colon, pancreatic, kidney, prostate, and endometrial cancer. Excessive protein may produce large amounts of nitrogenous waste in the intestine, some of which can be converted to the highly carcinogenic compounds nitrosamines and ammonium salts. Heavy-protein diets may also cause the buildup of metabolic acids in the body and cause large amounts of calcium to leach from the bones, a serious detriment in the case of bone cancer, when bone-calcium reserves tend to be mobilized and depleted.

A causal relationship between red meat consumption and cancer is supported by several large studies conducted in the U.S. Specifically, women with the highest level of meat consumption had double the rate of breast cancer compared to those who consumed small amounts of meat.[63] Men who ate red meat over a five-year period were nearly three times more likely to contract advanced prostate cancer than men consuming mainly vegetarian fare.[64] High rates of colon cancer have recently been linked to regular intakes of beef, pork, or lamb.[65] In each of these studies, the meat-eating risks are associated with fat intake as well, since American meats are typically high in fat.

Worldwide, a clear association consistently appears between the highest rates of breast, colon, and prostate cancers and nations that have the fattiest diets.[66] But the link between cancer and meat eaters' exposure to toxic chemicals goes even deeper. All fried and broiled foods contain mutagens, chemicals that can damage cellular reproductive material, but fried and broiled meats have far more mutagens than similarly prepared plant foods.

Be wary of contaminated fish—Industrial and agricultural pollution has resulted in chemicals such as mercury, nickel, oil, hydrocyanic acid, and lactronitrile getting absorbed by ocean-borne plankton. From there, the toxins travel up the food chain, becoming concentrated in the tissues of large, fatty predatory fish, like tuna and swordfish. Industrial chemicals such as PCBs (polychlorinated biphenyls) and methylmercury tend to accumulate in significant amounts in some fish and most shellfish. According to toxicologists, it takes only ¹/₁₀ of a teaspoon of PCBs to make a person severely ill or possibly cause cancer.

Excessive fat intake—Fat intake, especially animal fat, is one of the key factors consistently implicated in higher cancer rates.[67] The cancers most closely associated with high fat intake include breast, colon, rectum, uterus, prostate, and kidney.[68] Partially hydrogenated vegetable oils, commonly found in processed foods, are considered a major contributor to the carcinogenic effect of fats.[69] Some evidence suggests that saturated fat consumption may be a factor.

In breast cancer studies conducted on laboratory mice, tumor growth was enhanced by a high-fat diet only after a chemical carcinogen had been introduced.[70] This suggests that fat is probably not an initiator but a promoter of cancer. Studies of fat's suppressive effects on the immune system, as well as fat's ability to generate free radicals, support this interpretation.

Eicosanoids—Eicosanoids are hormone-like substances produced from the metabolism of arachidonic acid and other fatty acids. Produced by nearly every cell in the body, eicosanoids are highly potent substances: as little as one billionth of a gram can have measurable biological effects.[71] The human body produces a variety of eicosanoids that direct a diverse range of functions, including immune-cell activity, platelet aggregation, inflammation, steroid hormone production, gastrointestinal secretions, blood pressure, and pain sensation.

Evidence suggests that one of the eicosanoids, PGE2, promotes the development of various cancers by paralyzing certain key parts of the immune system (specifically the natural killer cells), stimulating inflammatory processes, and promoting the proliferation of tumor cells. Omega-3 fatty acids appear to reduce PGE2-induced inflammation, inhibit tumor cell proliferation, and enhance immune system function, as demonstrated in a study in which omega-3 fatty acids slowed or delayed the development of metastases in breast cancer patients. Specifically, women who had high fatty tissue content of alpha-linolenic acid (the main omega-3 EFA) were five times less likely to develop metastases than women with a low content.[72]

Excessive intake of refined carbohydrates/sugar—Sugar and white-flour products are believed to have a direct effect on cancer growth, as well as acting to nullify the positive effects of protective foods such as fiber.[73] In addition, they can significantly add to the risk of breast cancer, says cancer researcher Wayne Martin, of Fairhope, Alabama. "When someone eats sugar, the body produces insulin, and insulin can promote breast cancer just as estrogen does," he explains.

Sugar is remarkably effective at lowering the immune system's ability to work properly. Eating only three ounces (100 g) at one sitting can reduce the ability of the immune system's white blood cells to destroy bacteria. The immune-suppressive effect starts within 30 minutes after sugar ingestion and can last for up to five hours. As the average American consumes about five ounces (150 g) of sucrose (granular sugar found in processed foods) daily, the immune system of many people is chronically suppressed from dietary factors alone.[74]

Excessive intake of iron–Iron overload refers to an excess of body iron. A Danish study found that iron overload significantly raises the risk of developing cancer.[75] Two other reports suggest that even moderately elevated iron accumulations in the body may increase cancer risk.[76] Much of the cancer in the U.S. population today may be related to overconsumption of red meat, a rich source of iron.

Neal Barnard, M.D., of the Physicians Committee for Responsible Medicine, states: "Although it is unclear whether the iron in the meat promotes tumor growth any more than the fat does, iron definitely contributes to free-radical production, which only increases one's risk of getting cancer."[77] Cooking in iron pots or skillets, fortified bread, rice, and pasta products, and multivitamins with iron are further sources of exposure. Iron fortification is largely unnecessary as iron deficiency is uncommon in the U.S., except occasionally in menstruating women.

Excessive intake of alcohol–Regular, heavy consumption of alcohol, including beer, is associated with an elevated cancer risk.[78] According to Charles B. Simone, M.D., of Princeton, New Jersey, an alcohol habit can greatly increase the risk for cancers of the breast, mouth, throat (pharynx, larynx and esophagus), pancreas, liver, and head and neck. Alcohol can accelerate the growth of an existing cancer by suppressing NK cells, immune cells that would otherwise help repel cancer.[79]

Excessive intake of caffeine–Found in coffee, tea, colas, and chocolate, caffeine is thought to be a factor in the development of cancer of the lower urinary tract, including the bladder. Studies have found the rates for these cancers to be significantly higher in people who drink more than three cups of coffee a day.[80] Caffeine can cause damage to genetic material and impair the normal DNA repair mechanisms, thereby adding to the potential risk for cancer.[81]

Chronic Stress
Stress can be defined as a reaction to any stimulus or interference

that upsets normal functioning and disturbs mental or physical health. It can be brought on by internal conditions, such as illness, pain, emotional conflict, or psychological problems, or by external circumstances, such as bereavement, financial problems, loss of job or spouse, relocation, or many of the cancer-contributing factors described in this chapter such as ionizing radiation, geopathic stress, and electromagnetic fields.

For more on **stress reduction techniques**, see Chapter 3: Early Detection and Prevention, pp. 94-128.

Under emotional distress, the brain may signal the adrenal glands to produce chemicals called corticosteroids, hormones which weaken the immune response. Cancer-related processes are accelerated in the presence of these chemicals[82] as well as other stress hormones like prolactin.[83] Certain cancers have also been associated with distressing life events. In one study, the risk of developing breast cancer was five times higher if the woman had experienced an important emotional loss in the six years prior to the discovery of the tumor.[84]

Toxic Emotions

Since the 1970s, research in the field of psychoneuroimmunology has documented direct links between emotions and biochemical events in the body, thereby establishing on a scientific basis what folk healers have always known: emotions can manifest themselves as physical symptoms. Noted women's health expert, Christiane Northrup, M.D., of Yarmouth, Maine, coined the term *toxic emotions* to indicate the powerful, strongly held, and often unconsciously active beliefs and emotions that help generate symptoms that keep illnesses in place. "A thought held long enough and repeated enough becomes a belief," says Dr. Northrup. "The belief then becomes biology." In the view of Dr. Northrup as well as other alternative practitioners working with cancer patients, beliefs and emotions can be legitimate toxins, contributing to an overall weakening of the immune system.[85]

Although scientists have long debated the role of repressed emotions in cancer, at least three studies offer compelling evidence validating that role. In each of these studies, people were followed over time to determine their rates of disease in relation to various behaviors or exposures. Taken together, the results indicate a link between cancer resistance and emotional expression or its suppression.

Emotional repression may also influence one's survival from cancer—that is, how well a cancer patient fares after being diagnosed. In eight separate studies of patients with various cancers, each reported a significant association between hopelessness or passive coping

The Role of Emotions in Cancer

During the 1960s, psychotherapist Ronald Grossarth-Maticek administered questionnaires to 1,353 inhabitants of Crvenka, Yugoslavia. After following the subjects for a decade, Grossarth-Maticek concluded that nine out of ten cases of cancer could be predicted on the basis of "an overly rational, anti-emotional attitude" and a tendency to ignore signs of poor health. People with low anti-emotional scores were 29 times less likely to develop cancer than those with high anti-emotional scores.[89]

Patrick Dattore and colleagues followed 200 disease-free individuals for ten years and compared the psychological tests of 75 veterans who eventually got cancer with the 125 who remained cancer free. Contrary to expectations, those who developed cancer appeared less depressed than the others; however, these same individuals were also more likely to suppress their more intense or upsetting feelings. Again, those who openly expressed their feelings were less likely to develop cancer.[90]

The longest study to date, initiated in 1946, focused on students from the Johns Hopkins School of Medicine. Researchers divided 972 of the students into five groups based on various psychological measures. Over the course of three decades, students characterized as "loners" who suppressed their emotions beneath a bland exterior were 16 times more likely to develop cancer than those who gave vent to their feelings. In an earlier report, based on 1,337 students, cancer death rates correlated significantly with a lack of closeness with parents.[91]

responses—not taking an assertive position toward one's illness and recovery process—and poor cancer survival rates.[86]

The connection between emotional stress and cancer survival can be explained by recent findings in psychoneuroimmunology (PNI).[87] Its research suggests that the persistence of cancer cells depends in part on internal body controls that retrain or stimulate tissue growth; psychological factors appear to regulate these controls through neurological, hormonal, and immunologic pathways.[88] These and other mind/body links could play a major role in determining a person's ability to survive cancer and mind/body therapies should be employed to alleviate these psychological factors.

Depressed Thyroid Action

An underactive or dysfunctional thyroid gland (a key endocrine gland located in the neck) may contribute to a cancer process. Broda O. Barnes, M.D., observed in his clinical practice a myriad of patients with typical hypothyroid (underactive thyroid) symptoms and found evidence that suggests a relationship between low thyroid activity and cancer. Research in 1954 by Dr. J.G.C. Spencer from Bristol, England, showed that there was a consistently higher incidence of cancer in areas of 15 countries and four continents where goiter (enlargement of the thyroid gland) was more prevalent among the population than in the non-goiter areas of the same localities. Dr. Barnes noted that Austria, a country with a high incidence of goiter, had the highest incidence of cancer of any country reporting malignancies at that time, further supporting the link between hypothyroidism and cancer.

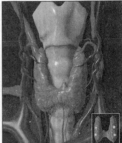

The thyroid gland is the body's metabolic thermostat, controlling body temperature, energy use, and, for children, the body's growth rate.

Intestinal Toxicity and Digestive Impairment

Many illnesses, such as a number of cancers, most allergies, infections, liver disease, acne, psoriasis, and asthma, start in the intestines. The intestines become clogged, toxic, and diseased by what and how we eat and by how poorly we eliminate waste material. Once the bowel is toxic, it creates toxicity for the entire body and an inability to absorb the nutrients necessary for health.

Around 1900, most people in the U.S. had a brief intestinal transit time. That means it took only about 15-20 hours from the time food entered the mouth until it was excreted as feces. Today, many have a seriously delayed transit time of 50-70 hours. This means there is more time for the stool to putrefy, for harmful microorganisms to flourish, for probiotics to die off, and for toxins to develop and poison the tissues.

When you eat mucus-producing foods, this further slows down the transit time. Mucus-producing foods are nearly all foods aside from most vegetables and fruits; however, the most mucus-producing foods are milk products. Other foods include meats, fish, fowl, eggs, soybeans, oily seeds and nuts, and cooked beans and grains (but not beans and grains that have sprouted). Fruits and vegetables tend to cause the mucous material in the intestines to break down and be eliminated.

As this sticky mucoid false lining builds up in the small intestine, it blocks absorption of essential nutrients into the bloodstream and it produces a hiding place for bacteria, fungi, yeast, and parasites that are harmful to human health. When these abnormal life forms start growing too freely in the intestines, they kill off *Lactobacillus acidophilus* and other "friendly" bacteria. They also create a situation called dysbiosis (an imbalance among intestinal microflora), in which the contents of the intestines putrefy and harmful chemicals are generated.

For information on **intestinal detoxification** and **parasite elimination**, see Chapter 9: Physical Support Therapies, pp. 254-297.

The result is a toxic bowel and a body-wide condition of toxicity as toxins leak out of the intestines into other tissues. If there are too many toxins, the lymphatic system becomes blocked and overloaded and can no longer drain and filter poisons efficiently. As toxins build up in all the tissues, the result can be swelling of the torso and legs and damage to the immune system, liver, and other organs.

An additional cause of intestinal toxicity results from the decreased production of hydrochloric acid and pepsin in the stomach as people age.[92] Undigested proteins that pass into the small and large intestines without being broken down into their constituent amino acids produce toxicity. This is because bacteria convert these proteins into nitrosamines and other cancer-causing agents, or because the undigested food proteins are absorbed intact through the intestinal wall into the bloodstream, creating "circulating immune complexes." These complexes put an unnecessary strain on the immune system so that it becomes less capable of identifying and attacking cancer cells. This makes it easier, and more likely, for a cancer process to gain a footing in the organism.

Parasites

The presence of parasites in the body, mostly in the intestines, is a little appreciated but major health problem. People assume they are vulnerable to parasites only if they travel in tropical areas, but this is a dangerous misconception. Anyone can get them (and many probably already have) from merely staying at home.

Parasite damage can be extensive. They can destroy cells faster than they can be regenerated; they can release toxins that damage tissues, resulting in pain and inflammation; and, over time, they can depress, even exhaust, the immune system. Of the dozens of specific parasites of concern to human health, the major groupings include microscopic Protozoa, roundworms, pinworms, and hookworms (Nematoda), tapeworms (Cestoda), and flukes (Trematoda).[93]

According to naturopathic physician Hulda Regehr Clark, Ph.D., N.D., who practices in Tijuana, Mexico, a single parasite—the fluke, a flatworm called *Fasciolopsis buskii*—may be responsible for cancer. Under completely healthy conditions, the body, thanks to the liver, is able to trap and destroy flukes before they have grown large or completed their growth cycle. However, the presence of the solvent propyl alcohol in the body makes the immune system unable to destroy the flukes. The pressure of the fluke population causes the release of a special cell growth factor called ortho-phosphotyrosine, which marks the beginning of the cancer process, Dr. Clark states. Two studies in the *Annual Review of Biochemistry* (1985, 1988) confirmed that this chemical is a reliable cancer marker for different kinds of malignancies.[94] Ortho-phosphotyrosine is a metabolic by-product of some parasites and a growth factor stimulator for parasites and cancer cells.

Viruses
According to some researchers, up to 15% of the world's cancer deaths are attributable to the activities of viruses, bacteria, or parasites. Among the cancer-producing viruses that work through a host's DNA-synthesizing and protein-building mechanisms are human papilloma viruses type 16 and 18 (which are sexually transmitted) associated with cervical cancer, among others, and the hepatitis B virus, associated with liver cancer. Worldwide, viral infections, especially hepatitis, may cause up to 80% of liver cancers. Epstein-Barr virus, which produces mononucleosis, is also carcinogenic, linked to about 50% of cancers of the upper pharynx, 30% of Hodgkin's, and 10% of non-Hodgkin's and certain gastric cancers.[95]

Blocked Detoxification Pathways
In a healthy individual, the body's normal detoxification systems, especially the liver, are generally able to eliminate toxins and thereby prevent illness. But these systems can be overwhelmed by a multiplicity of toxins—any combination of the factors described in this chapter—and become functionally incompetent to complete the necessary detoxification. A blocked detoxification system might involve a clogged lymphatic drainage system, in which thickened lymph accumulates in the lymph nodes without being emptied into the blood for removal from the body. It may also involve chronic intestinal constipation and liver enzyme dysfunction.

As Joseph Pizzorno, N.D., explains, to prevent cancer, the liver's detoxification system must be working optimally. When it is not functioning well, it is unable to process and eliminate the multiplicity of carcinogens entering the body, and we become more susceptible to cancer. "High levels of exposure to carcinogens coupled with sluggish detoxification enzymes significantly increase our susceptibility to cancer."

Free Radicals
A free radical is an unstable molecule that steals an electron from another molecule and produces harmful effects. Free radicals are formed when molecules within cells react with oxygen, as part of nor-

mal metabolic processes. If not controlled by antioxidants, free radicals can break down cells and damage enzymes, cell membranes, blood lipoproteins, unsaturated fatty acids in cell membranes, and DNA or chromosomes.

Free radicals are produced both by external harmful influences, such as radiation and environmental pollution, and by internal processes, such as metabolism and immune defense. Free radicals are generated by energy production and fat metabolism, from the immune response by white blood cells, and by the liver's own detoxification procedures. However, uncontrolled free-radical production plays a major role in the development of at least 100 degenerative conditions, including cancer. Sources of free radicals include carcinogens, pollution, smoking, alcohol, viruses, radiation, most infections, allergies, stress, low blood supply, burns, certain foods, and inflammation.

An antioxidant (meaning "against oxidation") is a natural biochemical substance that protects living cells against damage from free radicals. Antioxidant nutrients include vitamins A, C, and E, beta carotene, selenium, coenzyme Q10, pycnogenol (grape seed extract), L-glutathione, superoxide dismutase, and bioflavonoids. Plant antioxidants include *Ginkgo biloba* and garlic. What makes the difference between normal functioning of the immune system, which includes the deactivation of free radicals, and the initiation of a potential cancer process is the amount of antioxidants available in the system. "When free-radical production exceeds the ability of the neutralizing systems, progressive cellular damage occurs," states Dr. Pizzorno. When this damage becomes chronic, the next step is degenerative disease, including cancer.

Cellular Oxygen Deficiency

One of the most provocative theories of cancer causation was originally put forth by Nobel laureate Dr. Otto Warburg. He was a German biochemist who won the Nobel Prize in 1931 for the discovery that oxygen deficiency and cell fermentation are part of the cancer process. "From the standpoint of the physics and chemistry of life, the difference between normal and cancer cells is so great that one can scarcely picture a greater difference," Dr. Warburg wrote.

According to Dr. Warburg's theory, when cells are deprived of oxygen, they can revert to their "primitive" state and enter into glucose reactions, deriving energy not from oxygen, as normal plant and animal cells do, but from the fermentation of sugar. Oxygen is dethroned in cancer cells and replaced by an energy-yielding reaction of the

For information on **oxygen and cancer**, see Chapter 8: Enhancing Metabolism, pp. 232-253.

lowest living forms, namely, a fermentation of glucose.[96] It is a highly inefficient method, as the rapid reproduction of the cancer cells uses up large amounts of glucose, breaking it down into lactic acid. Lactic acid is a waste product that puts a strain on the body and causes an imbalance in the acid/base ratio, or pH level. As the acidity of the body rises, it becomes even more difficult for the cells to use oxygen normally. Cancerous tumors may contain as much as ten times more lactic acid than healthy human tissues.[97]

One possible reason for the dramatic increase in cancer rates over the past century, according to Dr. Warburg's theory, may be the decreasing levels of oxygen and the increasing levels of carbon monoxide in urban air. Carbon monoxide (CO) has a higher affinity for hemoglobin (which transports oxygen to the cells) than does oxygen; for this reason, when we breathe in CO, our hemoglobin binds more CO and less oxygen. By contrast, according to this same oxygen deficiency theory, cancer cells cannot exist in an oxygen-rich environment. Humans can become oxygen deficient through several routes, including long-term exposure to air pollution (tobacco smoke, auto exhaust, factory emissions), devitalized foods (overcooked, processed, preserved, all of which deplete oxygen), shallow breathing, and inadequate exercise.

Cellular Terrain

European practitioners of biological medicine first coined the term *cellular terrain* to refer to the general vitality, activity, and biochemical condition of the cells in the body. At the core of biological thinking is the concept of the body's internal environment, the condition of the cells, known as the terrain, explains Thomas Rau, M.D., medical director of Parcelsus Clinic in Lüstmuhle, Switzerland. When the cell becomes imbalanced, conditions are set for infection, illness, chronic disease, or cancer to begin; when they are rebalanced, conditions are set for healing and a return to health. "As we see it," says Dr. Rau, "sickness is not caused by bacteria, but the bacteria comes with the sickness. Bacteria, viruses, or fungi can only develop if they have the suitable cellular

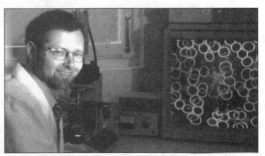

Dr. Rau examines a live sample of a patient's blood using darkfield microscopy.

conditions." Of course, infections may enter the body from outside, but if the body is healthy and its cellular terrain balanced, they will not thrive or even survive.

Outside influences, such as faulty diet, inadequate nutrition, exposure to carcinogens, chronic organ toxicity, stress, or trauma provide the impetus to throw the cells out of balance, says Dr. Rau. Once imbalanced, disease processes can take root, potentially leading to cancer.

Oncogenes

The predominant emphasis in conventional cancer research today is to find individual genes capable of causing, initiating, or triggering tumor growth. First identified in the 1970s, these causal genes are referred to as oncogenes (meaning the gene that starts the *onkos*, or tumor mass). An oncogene is a gene believed to transform normal cells into cancer cells, thus initiating the development of cancer. Some of these genes have reportedly been identified in cancer-causing viruses. Proto-oncogenes are genes in a neutral, inactive stage that activate cell division; under certain conditions, they mutate and become oncogenes, which then activate cell proliferation that soon becomes uncontrolled.

Researchers now believe that about 20% of all human cancers, including cancers of the lung, colon, and pancreas, are partly brought about by mutations in oncogenes. In healthy people, the activities of oncogenes are counterbalanced by tumor suppressor genes, also called anti-oncogenes. Under normal conditions, they act to prevent uncontrolled cell growth that could lead to tumors. However, oncogene mutations (when a proto-oncogene becomes a carcinogenic oncogene) inactivate the tumor suppressor genes so that, paradoxically, they actually contribute to tumor growth. Other factors that can inactivate tumor suppressor genes include DNA changes, chemical carcinogens, and electromagnetic energy.

Genetic Predisposition

The theory of gene causation for cancer inevitably leads researchers into speculations about inherited cancers—gene configurations or mutations that might predict if a given individual will develop cancer. The term *family cancer syndrome* is now used to describe the tendency of particular cancers (such as breast, colon, or ovarian) to show up in succeeding generations of the same family. For example, many scientists now believe that the following inherited cancers may be linked to mutations in certain related tumor suppressor genes: melanoma and pancreatic cancer (MTS1, p16); breast and ovarian cancer (BRCA1);

breast cancer (BRCA2); colon and uterine cancer (MSH2, MLH1, PMS1, PMS2); and brain sarcomas (p53). Inheritance of "flawed" genes probably accounts for about 5% of all cancers in the U.S.[98]

Miasm

More than 200 years ago, German physician Samuel Hahnemann, the founder of homeopathy, used the term *miasm* to indicate a deeper predisposition to chronic disease. Showing remarkable foresight, Hahnemann's concept of miasm accurately prefigures today's description of oncogenes: a miasm represents an energy residue of an illness from a previous generation, while an oncogene represents a molecular residue of an illness from a previous generation. Miasms are broad-focused, predisposing individuals to certain families of illness, whereas oncogenes are coded specifically not only for a single type of illness (cancer) but actual varieties of that illness (breast, ovarian, lung, pancreatic cancers).

According to Hahnemann, three miasms underlie all chronic illness, and these parallel broad stages in the history of the human experience with primary disease states. The *Psoric* miasm is the earliest and thus the most fundamental predisposing layer. In fact, according to this theory, the *Psoric* miasm is the foundation of sickness underlying all the diseases experienced by humans—cancer, diabetes, and arthritis as well as serious mental disorders such as epilepsy and schizophrenia. The *Syphilitic* miasm came next in the history of human diseases and derives from syphilis. The *Sycotic* miasm, the third layer, arose as a residue of gonorrhea. In recent years, homeopaths have added a *Cancer* miasm to Hahnemann's original three; the *Cancer* miasm is a combination of the effects (or taints) of the *Psoric*, *Sycotic*, and *Syphilitic* miasms.

CHAPTER

3 Early Detection & Prevention

ONE OF THE HALLMARKS of the alternative medicine approach to treating and reversing cancer is to detect signs of cancer at the earliest possible time and to take all practical steps to prevent its recurrence, or to keep it from developing in the first place.

Prevention is the most important and reliable cancer-fighting tool that exists today. The fact that cancer can be treated and reversed and that it can be detected early and prevented are the most important messages of this book. Foremost among the preventive measures is to maintain a strong and healthy immune system. This can be accomplished in a number of ways, such as maintaining a diet that ensures the optimal intake of immune system–enhancing nutrients and decreasing your intake of immune system–suppressing foods. Living a life free from constant emotional or mental distress is also important, as is avoiding carcinogenic toxins, geopathic zones, and harmful electromagnetic fields in your home and work environment.

The following case study illustrates how early detection and prevention work well together in keeping cancer at bay.

Success Story: Early Warning Signal for Cancer

Sue, 35, felt a stinging sensation in her shoulder blade as she reached to scratch it in the shower. When a spot of blood appeared on her washcloth, she realized she had chafed a mole slightly wider than the diameter of a pencil eraser. Upon closer inspection, she saw that one half of it was shaped differently than the other and had slightly jagged edges.

Several weeks later, when the mole still appeared to be irritated, Sue decided to consult a physician who was a proponent of alternative medicine. The physician examined the mole carefully, then advised Sue to have it removed and sent to the lab for analysis. Noting her pale complexion and low energy levels, he placed Sue on a low-fat, high-fiber diet, and nutrient supplement program.

A few days later, Sue's doctor informed her that she had malignant melanoma, a potentially deadly form of skin cancer. Upon removing the tissue around and under the mole, the surgeon had determined that this cancerous lesion had penetrated several layers of skin and the underlying layer of fat. According to biopsies at the time, the cancer had apparently not spread to the lymph nodes—good news for Sue. Sue underwent a complete series of nutrient and enzyme tests to provide optimal support for her body's anticancer defense systems. However, her physician recommended that she take the AMAS (anti-malignin antibody screen) test, which is designed to pick up cancers well in advance of other signs and symptoms.

Cancer Detection and Prevention Tests in This Chapter

- AMAS
- PSA
- Pap Smear
- PAPNET
- Mammography
- Thermography
- Hemoccult Test
- Darkfield Microscopy
- Biological Terrain Assessment
- CBC Blood Test Report
- Maverick Monitoring Test
- ToxMet Screen
- Individualized Optimal Nutrition (ION)
- Oxidative Protection Screen
- Pantox Antioxidant Profile
- FORCYTE Cancer Prognostic System
- T/Tn Antigen Test
- Lymphocyte Size Analysis

The result from the AMAS test, which was repeated twice, revealed that cancer still existed in Sue's body. Furthermore, the nutrient and enzyme tests indicated several deficiencies that could compromise her body's ability to fight the cancer. Since the cancer was still at an early stage, the doctor recommended that she try a vegetarian diet based on the Gerson therapy, which has shown considerable success in the treatment of malignant melanoma. He also expanded her supplement program, which had included vitamins C and E, coenzyme Q10, selenium, and zinc, to now include germanium and various enzymes, glandulars, and botanical medicines such as Essiac tea, echinacea, and maitake mushroom.

Eight Telltale Signs of Cancer

The message of prevention is that you can beat cancer before it becomes advanced. The key is to detect the presence of cancer early enough so you can treat it with the immune-enhancing, nontoxic treatments of alternative medicine. These methods work best when the body's tumor burden is relatively small—in the earliest phases of the cancer's development. Here are signs that may indicate the presence of cancer.

1. A Lump or Thickening in the Breast or Testicles. Self-examination of the breast and testicles offers women and men the best protection against breast and testicular cancer. A lump or thickening in the breast, or any noticeable change in the testicles, are early warning signs. Such signs are immediate grounds for a medical examination.

2. A Change in a Wart or Mole. Changes in warts or moles may be indicative of melanoma or squamous carcinoma. Skin cancers may appear as dry, scaly patches, as pimples that never go away, or as inflamed or ulcerated areas. Warts or moles that grow or bleed should be checked, as should sores in the mouth that persist.

3. A Skin Sore or a Persistent Sore Throat That Does Not Heal. Sores that do not heal may also be indicative of melanoma. A persistent sore throat, hoarseness, lump in the throat, or difficulty swallowing, may indicate cancer of the pharynx, larynx, or esophagus. These cancers are readily treated when caught early.

4. A Change in Bowel or Bladder Habits. Continuing urinary difficulties, constipation, chronic diarrhea, abdominal pains, rectal or urinary bleeding, or dark tar-like stools should not be ignored; they should be regarded as signals to seek professional help.

5. A Persistent Cough or Coughing Blood. Coughs that become chronic, especially in smokers, should be checked. If there is a cancer in the air passages into the lungs, they may be partially obstructed or irritated or even bleed. Coughing may be a sign of this obstruction or irritation.

6. Constant Indigestion or Trouble Swallowing. Difficulties in swallowing, continued indigestion, nausea, heartburn, bloating, loss of appetite, and bowel changes all may be symptoms of colon cancer or cancer of the stomach or esophagus. Unexplained weight loss is also an indicator.

7. Unusual Bleeding or Vaginal Discharge. The early stages of uterine endometrial cancer and later stages of cervical vaginal cancer exhibit signs of unusual bleeding or vaginal discharge. Prompt attention to these symptoms means a better chance of catching cancer at its most treatable stage. In the case of cervical cancer, Pap tests can detect problems before the later stages cause bleeding.

8. Chronic Fatigue. General feelings of chronic fatigue will often accompany any type of cancer that is rapidly progressing.

If you are experiencing any of these signs and symptoms, contact your physician immediately.

Ten months later, Sue's AMAS test indicated that she no longer had cancer. All her nutrient and enzyme levels had returned to the optimal range and her doctor declared her to be in excellent health. She continued with the nutrient treatment regimen for several months longer and decided to maintain a primarily vegetarian diet and regular exercise program thereafter. At the same time, she decided to spend less time in the bright sun, exposure to sun being a risk factor in developing melanoma.

Fortunately, Sue caught the cancer early. Malignant melanoma is now the most common cancer among women ages 25-29 and second only to breast cancer in ages 30-34. From 1975 to 1992, the overall number of melanoma cases reported annually in the United States has tripled, increasing more than any other cancer; the disease now claims at least 7,000 American lives each year and accounts for 75% of all skin cancer deaths. Finally, it is more likely than other skin cancers to spread to other parts of the body, making it more difficult to arrest and cure.

In light of these facts, Sue's emphasis on early detection and prevention serve as an excellent example for others to follow. Sue took two crucial steps that gave her an excellent chance for long-term survival. First, she took action early, embarking on a nutritional and botanical program to strengthen her immune system at a point when the melanoma had not yet grown to a dangerous degree. Second, after the cancer had apparently been eliminated from Sue's body, she adopted an active preventive strategy. In other words, she made a conscious decision to reevaluate aspects of her former lifestyle and environment that could have contributed to the weakening of her immune system. She opted to stay with her new diet program, exercise regularly, reduce her exposure to sunshine, and generally monitor her stress level. These important changes enabled Sue to keep the cancer at bay for good.

AMAS: Accurate Blood Test for Early Cancer Detection

Until recently, there was no single blood test that could reliably and accurately indicate whether cancer was present, either for an initial diagnosis or for monitoring a recurrence. The tests available were sometimes positive when cancer was not present (a false positive), and sometimes negative when it was known that the person had cancer (a false negative).

Many oncologists and cancer specialists use blood tests called cancer markers, which detect substances present in abnormal amounts in

Prevention is the most important and reliable cancer-fighting tool that exists today. The fact that cancer can be treated and reversed and that it can be detected early and prevented are the most important messages of this book.

The AMAS test is most suited to detecting cancers in their earliest developmental stage, before gross tumor masses are observable, and for determining whether all signs and activities of cancers have disappeared following treatment. It is not suitable for detecting advanced cancers with severe immune suppression.

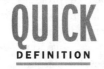

DEFINITION

An **antibody** is a protein molecule containing about 20,000 atoms, made from amino acids by B lymphocyte cells in the lymph tissue and set in motion by the immune system against a specific foreign protein, or antigen. An antibody is also referred to as an immunoglobulin and may be found in the blood, lymph, colostrum, saliva, and the gastrointestinal and urinary tracts, usually within 3 days after the first encounter with an antigen. The antibody binds tightly with the antigen as a preliminary for removing it from the system or destroying it.

the blood or urine of a person with cancer. But cancer markers can be unreliable for a variety of reasons. Some fail to indicate the presence of the new, previously undetected cancers and show only whether known cancers are shrinking or expanding. Others register levels of substances that could be produced by diseases other than cancer. Still others are not sensitive enough to pick up cancers in a certain percentage of patients.

For many years, researchers have been hoping for a cancer marker that could serve as a reliable indicator for a variety of cancers. Possibly the most accurate cancer marker was unveiled in the 1990s, thanks to the efforts of Harvard-trained biochemist and physician Sam Bogoch, M.D., Ph.D., who labored for 20 years before finally uncovering the secret to detecting all forms of cancer in its earliest stages. Known as AMAS (anti-malignin antibody screen), the test analyzes a sample of blood to reveal whether antibodies (SEE QUICK DEFINITION) to cancer are present.

Generally speaking, the test is called an immunoassay, which means it measures the amount present of a specific antibody, in this case, anti-malignin, an antibody that acts against the inner protein layer of a cancer cell, called malignin. Dr. Bogoch found that the anti-malignin antibody serves as a reliable marker for cancers of all kinds. "If there are any cancers that don't respond to the [AMAS] test, we haven't found them yet," says Dr. Bogoch.

Although it was approved by the FDA in 1977, it wasn't until late 1994 that the clinical trials with 4,278 patients were completed, validating the test's effectiveness. Now this patented, FDA-approved anti-malignin antibody screen is available to doctors worldwide through Dr. Bogoch's Oncolab. According to Dr. Bogoch, AMAS is 95% accurate on the first test, and 99% when repeated; the test can detect cancer up to 19 months before conventional medical tests can find it.

The AMAS test is reliable, except in advanced stages of cancer, in which, as Dr. Bogoch explains, "the anti-malignin antibody is wiped out," meaning there is nothing for the test to pick up. The person who is initially diagnosed with advanced-stage cancer typically appears ill or will show various outward physical signs of disease.

For more information about **AMAS**, contact: Oncolab, 36 The Fenway, Boston, MA 02215; tel: 800-922-8378; fax: 617-536-0657.

In these advanced cases, other types of medical testing are recommended—cancer markers (but not the AMAS), biopsies (surgical samples of cancerous tissue to determine the degree of malignancy), and various scans, depending on the type of cancer. With brain cancer, for example, CT (computerized tomography) scans and physical examination are typically used, and an MRI (magnetic resonance imaging) scan can give even more specific information. X rays and bone scans are useful for detecting metastases to the bone; ultrasound and liver scans can be used to detect metastases in the liver.

Ultrasound, in general, is one of the least invasive and most helpful ways to diagnose tumors of the kidney, uterus, ovaries, gallbladder, and pancreas; ultrasound is able to detect very small tumors. It is also useful in detecting cancer in younger women, whose breast tissue is dense.[1] Unlike X rays or mammograms, ultrasound delivers no harmful radiation that could either seed cancer or further its course.

Orthodox Screening Methods and Their Relevance to Prevention

In most cases, cancer takes years or even decades to develop into a visible tumor. But even if a tumor is not yet visible by conventional means, it is still active as cancer and a serious health threat waiting to announce itself. Knowing that early detection of the growing tumor allows for early treatment and better chances of survival, holistic-minded physicians have begun seeking ways, such as the AMAS test, to diagnose precancerous conditions—those that precede the actual appearance of the cancer.

Two common statistical measures of the usefulness of a screening test are sensitivity and specificity. Sensitivity refers to the probability that a test will show a positive result when cancer exists; specificity is the probability that a negative test result occurs when cancer is absent. A test that has high sensitivity and high specificity is far more useful than one with low readings for either or both of these measures. For example, PSA (prostate specific antigen, a specific marker for potential prostate cancer) has low sensitivity (68%) and specificity (60%).[2] In contrast, recall that the AMAS has high sensitivity (95%) and specificity (95%).[3]

A fundamental difference between the AMAS test and other diagnostic tests is that the AMAS detects all types of cancer whereas most tests target only one kind of cancer. For example, PSA detects only prostate cancer and the Pap smear picks up only cervical cancer, albeit at an early stage of the disease. By using a test that picks up all cancers early on, it is more likely to catch cancers that would otherwise be missed by the more specific tests. We'll briefly review the three most common screening methods for the early detection of cancer—PSA, Pap smear, and mammography—and show how they can be used, misused, and misinterpreted.

Prostate Specific Antigen: Early Detection and Prevention of Prostate Cancer

Prostate cancer is the second leading cause of cancer-related deaths among American men and the most frequently diagnosed malignancy (other than skin cancer) in this segment of the population. The number of new cases almost doubled from 1990 (106,000) to 1994 (200,000).[4] The important point here, however, is that this surge of new cases appears to be related to the increased popularity of prostate cancer screening via the use of a prostate cancer marker, the prostate specific antigen, or PSA. In recent years, doctors have looked to the PSA as a way to catch prostate cancer early. The disease can develop and spread with little or no warning signs, and many cases are discovered too late, that is, after they have spread beyond the prostate and are extremely difficult to reverse.

Although the PSA may help detect tumors too small to raise a bump on the prostate, the test is fraught with problems. To begin with, a high PSA reading (a positive or "high" result is greater than 4) is by no means proof that cancer is present, since factors other than cancer—an enlarged prostate (benign prostatic hyperplasia), mechanical pressure on the prostate, or inflammation of the prostate (prostatitis)—can cause the level to rise. Not surprisingly, then, the so-called false positive test results for PSA are extremely common, occurring in approximately 50% of all PSA test results. On the flip side, many men who actually have cancer may show a low or normal PSA reading at the time of testing.[5]

PSA may still have value when used in conjunction with other methods, namely digital rectal examination and ultrasound-guided biopsy of the prostate. When combined with these diagnostic techniques, PSA improves early detection, albeit by only 25%.[6] It is possible that the PSA now may be unnecessary as an initial screening device, thanks to the existence of the AMAS test.

Prostate cancer is generally classified as: (1) latent or benign; (2) moderately progressive; and (3) rapidly progressive and extremely malignant. Some experts now believe that the PSA screening is valuable only for the moderately progressive form, stating that "tumors of the first form need never be detected and tumors of the third form progress so rapidly that timely screen detection is nearly impossible, and, when accomplished, may be valueless."[7]

The latent, harmless form of prostate cancer is the most prevalent. Autopsies of thousands of men who died suddenly from automobile accidents, heart attacks, or other non-cancer-related causes have found that approximately 15% of men in their fifties have some cancerous cells in their prostates.[8] The number jumps to 40% for men in their seventies, and to 50% for men 80 and older.[9] This means that roughly 12 million American men are walking around today with microscopic signs of prostate cancer. For most of these men, the PSA may cause unnecessary worry and premature treatment, because it picks up prostate tumors that are likely to remain inactive for life.[10]

When prostate cancer is detected in its early stages, prevention should be emphasized before treatment. At this juncture, the wise physician will recommend "watchful waiting," which entails careful observation and monitoring to assure that small, slow-growing tumors remain so. Watchful waiting is considered appropriate for men in their upper sixties and older, who have a high PSA reading or positive result on the digital rectal exam, but are likely to die of another cause before their prostate tumor becomes a grave threat. Watchful waiting (compared to treatment) has lowered the death rate from prostate cancer among men with non-metastasized prostate tumors.[11] Unfortunately, since treatment in the form of surgery and radiation generates huge amounts of money for conventional physicians and hospitals, watchful waiting is not always encouraged. Fewer than 10% of all doctors

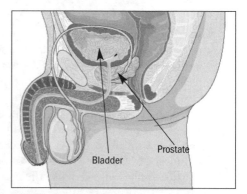

Bladder

Prostate

The prostate gland.

Recommendations for Prevention of Prostate Cancer

For preventing prostate cancer from developing, the following represent key findings to keep in mind:

- Vegetables rich in beta carotene—including broccoli and other green vegetables, carrots, and squash—may lower the risk of prostate cancer.[13]
- Tomatoes appear to reduce prostate cancer rates by 45% for those who have at least ten servings a week.[14]
- Fish oil supplementation (containing eicosapentaenoic acid, or EPA) may suppress the growth of prostate cancer cells[15] and inhibit the promotion of prostate cancer.[16]
- Selenium inhibits the growth of carcinoma cells in the prostate[17] and also blocks the stimulatory effects of the heavy metal cadmium on prostate cancer.[18]
- Soy foods, by virtue of their high genistein content, may help keep latent prostate cancer from developing into an invasive form.[19]
- Modified citrus pectin was found to reduce the number of metastases in laboratory animals.[20]
- Physically active men have a much lower risk of prostate cancer than their less active counterparts for the same age group.[21] The deep breathing of oxygen and increase in lymph flow caused by exercising may explain the benefit of exercise.
- Being overweight, smoking, and consuming alcohol may increase the risk of prostate cancer.
- A large body of evidence suggests that chemical toxins combined with poor nutrition may overwhelm the detoxifying mechanisms of the liver—in particular, the activity of an enzyme called glutathione S-transferase or GST—GST may play a key role in defending normal prostate cells against carcinogenesis.[22]
- Reducing one's exposure to toxins (mainly by eating a low-fat, vegetarian diet) and attending to other risk factors can improve the chance of surviving prostate cancer.

who recommend surgical removal of the prostate even discuss watchful waiting as a viable option with their patients.[12]

If you do have an elevated PSA (a reading greater than 4), then a repeat test and a digital rectal exam are needed. Since the digital rectal exam can raise the PSA, have the blood drawn before the rectal exam. It may be advisable to also undergo an ultrasound or sonogram of the prostate and a prostatic acid phosphatase blood test, which increases the accuracy of the PSA and digital examination in finding cancer. During a prostate sonogram, a blunt probe about the size of a thumb is inserted into the rectum and sound waves from the probe create images of the prostate on a screen so that tumors may be seen. Prostatic acid phosphatase is an enzyme made from protein in the prostate gland and becomes elevated usually when the prostate develops cancer, infections, inflammation from toxins, or benign prostatic hyperplasia.

If these tests also indicate prostate cancer, an ultrasound or guided needle biopsy will usually provide the definitive diagnosis. If the cancer is confirmed at this point, it is also advisable that you immediately adopt a low-fat, high-fiber diet, among other important lifestyle changes. Many studies have shown that people who eat diets high in fat, especially animal fat, are more likely to develop prostate cancer.[23] U.S. men have prostate cancer rates that are 30-40 times higher than men in China and about 6-10 times higher than men in Japan; Asian males consume less than half the saturated fat eaten by their U.S. counterparts, who get their fat mainly from red meats and dairy products.[24] Men consuming meat five times a week were two to three times more likely to develop invasive prostate cancer than those who eat meat once a week.[25] This increased risk of prostate cancer from eating meats and dairy may be related to the high pesticide content of these foods.

Many cancer experts contend that the diet that apparently helps prevent cancer—one low in fat and high in fiber and antioxidants—will tend to slow or even block cancer's development. This line of reasoning is summarized by noted cancer epidemiologist Lawrence Kushi, Sc.D., who states: "If we believe that dietary factors act as promoters of carcinogenesis, then the influence of diet on tumor growth and spread should not necessarily be much different before or after clinical expression of the tumor."

Regarding conventional treatment of prostate cancer, called androgen ablation, new research suggests that suppressing the male sex hormone may be counterproductive. Since the 1950s, oncologists have believed that prostate cancer cells require testosterone, the primary male sex hormone or androgen, to grow, so that blocking or removing testosterone should cause prostate cancers to shrink. However, physicians note that in about 80% of cases treated with anti-testosterone therapy (androgen ablation: either the testicles are removed surgically or a chemical is administered to block the male hormone action), while the cancers initially disappear, they almost always return in 1-3 years. More worrisome has been the discovery that the prostate cancer cells, after this 1-3 year period, can now grow independently of testosterone and no longer respond to ablation therapy. According to Shutsung Liao, Ph.D., a biochemist at the University of Chicago, the use of anti-testosterone drugs may be a dangerous mistake because it "may stimulate cancer growth by preventing testosterone from killing tumor cells that are androgen-independent but sensitive to the hormone's lethal effects in small amounts."

If the PSA is persistently elevated (a reading of 10 or higher) after two months of the "watchful waiting" strategy noted above, a prostate needle biopsy can indicate the status of tumor cells. The cell patterns are graded from 1 to 5, where a score of 1 indicates highly differentiated cells (meaning a relatively benign tumor) and 5 shows very poor differentiation (meaning a highly aggressive tumor). In this case, surgery combined with hormone therapy may be needed, together with the alternative strategies outlined in this book. Conventional strategies such as surgical removal of the prostate and/or radiation therapy should be considered a "last resort."

Pap Smear vs. PAPNET: Early Detection and Prevention of Cervical Cancer

Over 15,000 women develop cervical cancer each year, and nearly 5,000 die from it.[26] Even so, cervical cancer accounts for only about 3% of all new cancer cases in the U.S. and about 2% of all cancer-related deaths. The early form of the disease, called cervical dysplasia, is almost always reversible; however, once it becomes invasive or malignant, the cure rate drops by 50%.

The traditional Pap smear, introduced some 50 years ago (by George N. Papanicolaou, M.D., Ph.D.) for early detection of cervical cancer, generally means about 70% fewer deaths from cervical cancer. The Pap smear examines stained cells from the mucous membrane of the cervix for precancerous changes in cells. It is estimated that one-third of the women who die from cervical cancer do so because it was not accurately detected soon enough for successful treatment.

For more information about **PAPNET** and labs that use the system, contact: Neuromedical Systems, Inc., 2 Executive Blvd., Suffern, NY 10901; tel: 914-368-3600 or 800-PAPNET-4; fax: 914-368-3896.

Unfortunately, false negatives are common with this test, occurring in about 30% of all cases. The Pap smear registers between 50,000 and 300,000 cells in a single smear but those indicating potential cancer may be limited to a dozen or fewer cells. It is no wonder that identifying these few cells amidst many thousands is a formidable task that can result in false negatives.

A screening procedure developed in the late 1980s, called PAPNET Testing, successfully identifies abnormal cells in 97% of cases. Using an automated microscope, a full-color camera, and a high-speed image-processing computer, the PAPNET system meticulously screens slides for evidence of abnormalities. Once abnormal individual cells or cell clusters from a single Pap smear have been pinpointed, their images are stored in the computer. When the entire Pap smear has been rescreened, the 128 "cell scenes" judged most significant by PAP-NET are selected for evaluation by trained technicians. Researchers at the University of California at Los Angeles proved that PAP-NET is more accurate at reclassifying potential positive Pap smears than manual, visual evaluation. When lab technicians studied 62 Pap smears by standard manual methods, 31% of negatives needed further review; PAP-NET reclassified 83% of them and found about one half to be abnormal.

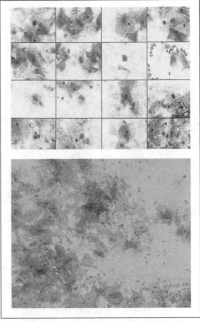

The PAPNET system presents 128 "cell scenes" from the original Pap smear, 16 of which are highlighted (top); also shown are details of a single scene (bottom).

If you are diagnosed as having evidence of cervical dysplasia, consider yourself fortunate. A balanced nutritional program alone often results in cancerous cervical cells reverting to normal. Again, nutritional changes generally call for a predominantly vegetarian, low-fat, high-fiber diet. Results from a study of 30 patients with this precancerous condition indicated that supplementing with beta carotene (30 mg per day for six months) suppressed cervical dysplasia; in addition, local application of a form of vitamin A (B-trans retinoic acid) was found to reverse moderate but not severe cervical dysplasia.[27] Research suggests that regular supplementation with vitamin C, vitamin E, and selenium, helps protect against cervical dysplasia and cervical cancer.[28]

Supplementation with folic acid has been shown to reverse cervical carcinoma *in situ*.[29] Folic acid seems to inhibit the human papilloma virus, a sexually transmitted co-carcinogen that increases a woman's chances of developing cervical cancer. Folic acid may act as a cancer promoter, so women should take it only in later stages of the disease under professional guidance. Women are also advised to

Smoking and Cervical Dysplasia

Women smokers with cervical dysplasia should stop smoking immediately. Heavy smokers may be four times more likely to develop cervical cancer: light smokers have about twice the risk.[30] A British study drew the following conclusions about the effect of smoking on cervical dysplasia and cervical cancer:

■ Precancerous lesions (cervical dysplasia) shrank by at least 20% in most women smokers who either quit smoking or greatly reduced the number of cigarettes they smoked.

■ The lesions disappeared in four out of 28 women who quit smoking or cut back on the habit.

■ About one out of every three women who kept smoking showed an increase in the growth of precancerous lesions.

■ Lesions did not disappear in any of the women who continued smoking.[31]

avoid oral contraceptives and douching with any liquid other than water.

Early Detection and Prevention of Breast Cancer: The Problems with Mammography

Breast cancer is the second leading cause of cancer-related death among women, and for women diagnosed between the ages of 15 and 54, it is the most common cause of cancer-related death. In 1992, the last year for which accurate statistics are available, 43,068 breast cancer deaths were reported. It is estimated that 184,300 new cases of breast cancer will be diagnosed in U.S. women annually and 44,300 will die from the disease.[32] In fact, in the U.S., every 15 minutes, five new cases of breast cancer are diagnosed and at least one woman dies of the disease.[33]

Remember, though: this is the cancer world according to conventional medicine. Given the right combination of therapy and prevention, far more people can survive cancer and live long, productive lives than conventional cancer experts would ever deem possible.

Breast Self-Examination

Given the rising incidence of breast cancer and the fact that early detection is one of the primary strategies for successful treatment, it is imperative that women conduct monthly breast self-examinations. One study found that self-examination was responsible for a greater percentage of cancer discoveries than mammograms. A 1996 survey of 281 women by Breast Cancer Action in San Francisco, California, revealed that of the 226 women (of whom 70% were aged 40-59) who had breast cancer, 44% discovered this through breast self-examination, 37% through mammograms, and 8% through a physician's exam.

A breast self-examination must be done each month at the same time in your menstrual cycle, in the same physical positions, and using the same sequence of steps. Some lumps are easier to find when lying down and others are more apparent when sitting or standing, so it is advisable to do an examination in several positions. Using the flat part of the fingertips, feel each area of the breast, systematically moving around it and noting any changes. Some women draw a sketch each time to record what they feel. Becoming familiar with the composition of your breasts is central to effective breast examination because it makes detection of abnormalities easier.

What's Wrong with Mammography?

Although mammography is the most widely employed screening method for breast cancer, there are a number of compelling arguments for adopting other methods in its place. Current research within conventional medicine itself provides five strong reasons why the use of mammogram screening for detection of breast cancer ought to be reconsidered.

■ Mammograms Add to Cancer Risk—Perhaps most damning, mammography exposes the breast to damaging radiation. As we noted previously, John W. Gofman, M.D., Ph.D., an authority on the health effects of ionizing radiation, spent 30 years studying the effects of low-dose radiation on humans. Dr. Gofman's findings are worth repeating: he estimates that 75% of breast cancer could be prevented by avoiding or minimizing exposure to the ionizing radiation from mammography, X rays, and other medical sources. Other research has shown that, since mammographic screening was introduced in 1983, the incidence of a form of breast cancer called ductal carcinoma *in situ* (DCIS), which represents 12% of all breast cancer cases, has increased by 328%, and 200% of this increase is due to the use of mammography.[34] In addition to exposing a woman to harmful radiation, the mammography procedure may help spread an existing mass of cancer cells. During a mammogram, considerable pressure must be placed on the woman's breast, as the breast is squeezed between two flat plastic surfaces. According to some health practitioners, this compression could cause existing cancer cells to move (metastasize) from the breast tissue. Even if cancer is not present in the breast, mammogram screening is uncomfortable and even painful.

■ High Rate of False Positives—Mammography's high rate of false-positive test results wastes money and creates unnecessary emotional trauma. A Swedish study of 60,000 women, aged 40-64, who were screened for breast cancer revealed that of the 726 actually referred to oncologists for

For more on the health hazards of **low-level ionizing radiation**, see Chapter 2: Cancer and Its Causes, pp. 48-93.

HOW TO PERFORM A BREAST SELF-EXAM. This exam should be conducted once a month (for pre-menopausal women, just after your period). Start by standing in front of a mirror and looking carefully at each breast and the chest muscle above it. (1) Look for anything out of the ordinary, such as puckering, dimpling, or scaling skin, nipple discharge or retraction, lumps, or asymmetry of breasts. (2) Raise your arms or clasp them behind your head and check for the same in this position. (3) Do the same check with your hands on your waist, pulling your shoulders and elbows slightly forward. (4) Feel for lumps in the lymph node area, from your breast into your armpit. (5) Squeeze each nipple to check for discharge. (6) Some women prefer to do this stage of the breast exam standing up, perhaps in the shower using soapy water so the fingers will glide more easily. In either case, with your right arm behind your head, examine your right breast with the fingers of your left hand. Using the pads of three or four fingers to press firmly into the breast, feel for lumps and cover the entire breast by following the patterns shown here. Some women prefer the radiating pattern (6a), thoroughly examining the breast by moving outward from the nipple in straight lines. Others prefer the circular pattern (6b), starting from the nipple and moving outward around the breast, or vice versa. Repeat on the left breast. If you notice anything abnormal or something you're not sure about at any point in the exam, consult your physician.

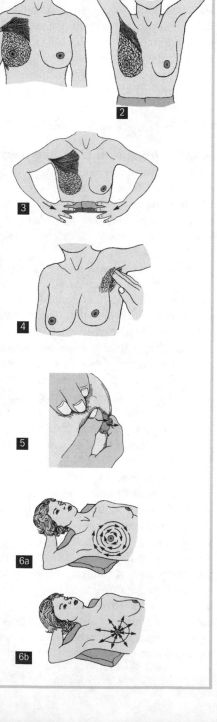

treatment, 70% were found to be cancer free. According to *The Lancet*, of the 5% of mammograms that suggest further testing, up to 93% are false positives. *The Lancet* report further noted that because the great majority of positive screenings are false positives, these inaccurate results lead to many unnecessary biopsies and other invasive surgical procedures.[35] In fact, 70% to 80% of all positive mammograms do not, on biopsy, show any presence of cancer.[36] According to some estimates, 90% of these "callbacks" result from unclear readings due to dense, overlying breast tissue.[37] Similarly, fibrocystic breast tissue can be mistaken for tumors and lead to unnecessary biopsies, and the biopsy itself is injurious to healthy breast tissue.

■ High Rate of False Negatives—Mammography also produces a high rate of false-negative test results. While false positives cause unnecessary distress and intervention, false negatives can be fatal. The breast tissue of women under 40 is generally denser than in older women, making it more difficult to detect tumors via mammography. In addition, tumors grow more quickly in women in this age group, so cancer may develop between screenings.[38] As for women aged 40 to 49, even the National Cancer Institute notes that there is a high rate of "missed tumors" in this age category; that is, 40% false-negative test results. Despite these findings, the American Cancer Society still recommends a mammogram every two years for women ages 40 to 49.[39]

■ Estrogen Distorts Breast X Rays—Estrogen therapy confuses mammogram results. According to a study of 8,800 postmenopausal women, aged 50 and older, the use of estrogen replacement therapy (ERT) leads to a 71% increased likelihood of receiving a false-positive result on mammogram screening, according to Mary B. Laya, M.D., M.P.H., study leader at the University of Washington at Seattle, who published the results in the *Journal of the National Cancer Institute* in 1996. Dr. Laya also found that women on ERT were more likely to get false-negative readings.

■ High Cost—In addition to the expenses accrued as a consequence of faulty mammogram results, mammograms themselves are costly (from $50-$120). Given their lack of accuracy, this level of expenditure is a doubtful investment.[40] In summary, mammograms are costly and can directly endanger a woman's health. Faulty test results further endanger her health, exact a heavy emotional toll, and can lead to expensive and unnecesssary tests. A study reported in *The Lancet* (July 1995) concludes that breast cancer screening via mammography for women under 50 years old is inappropriate due to the low accuracy level. The study further states that, in general, "the benefit is marginal, the harm caused is substantial, and the costs incurred are enormous, [so] we suggest that public funding for breast cancer screening [mammography] in any age group is not justifiable."[41]

Thermography: Safe and Accurate Imaging

A nontoxic, highly accurate, and inexpensive form of diagnostic imaging does exist and has been used by progressive physicians in the U.S. and Europe since 1962. Called thermography, it's based on infrared heat emissions from targeted regions of the body. As the body's cells go through their energy conversion processes, called metabolism, they emit heat. Thermography is able to register these heat emissions, display them on a computer monitor, and thereby provide a diagnostic window into the functional status of a given body area, such as the female breast. For breast cancer, thermography offers a very early warning system, often able to pinpoint a cancer process five years before it would be detectable by mammography. Most breast tumors have been growing slowly for up to 20 years before they are found by typical diagnostic techniques. Thermography can detect cancers when they are at a minute physical stage of development, when it is still relatively easy to halt and reverse the progression of the cancer.

Philip Hoekstra, Ph.D., of Thermoscan, in Huntingdon Woods, Michigan, is a pioneer in the use of thermography. Dr. Hoekstra's clinic has screened more than 50,000 women since 1971, at a typical cost of $55 for imaging and interpretation. The average mammogram, in contrast, can cost between $50 and $120. While a price differential of about $50 may seem insignificant, the risks associated with low-dose radiation exposure from mammograms in addition to their extra cost makes thermography the obvious choice for breast cancer screening.

The procedure is simple and noninvasive, says Dr. Hoekstra. The woman stands bare chested about ten feet from the device; the imaging takes only a matter of minutes, as results are displayed instantaneously on the monitor; and generally the data can be rapidly interpreted with image-analyzing software. No rays of any kind enter the patient's body; there is no pain or compressing of the breasts as in a mammogram.

Dr. Hoekstra points to the errors, false negatives, and radiation exposure dangers of mammograms, as discussed above. "Mammography is not an acceptable way of screening breasts; the only reason it's tolerated is that it is a major source of steady income for radiologists," Dr. Hoekstra says. "They have come to covet mammography and want no competition from other approaches." He believes that once women start making demands on their physicians for a different imaging approach, thermography can become the preferred initial screening method. Then mammography will be used only as needed to pinpoint the precise location of breast tumors.

While mammography tends to lose effectiveness with dense breast tissue, thermography is not dependent upon tissue densities. For this reason, Dr. Hoekstra says thermography is especially useful for screening younger women (who typically have denser breast tissue). Dr. Hoekstra adds that thermography is 86% to 96% accurate for indicating cancer in premenopausal women. When there is a mistake with thermography, it is almost never a false negative, but rather a false positive (suspecting a cancer process when in fact there was none).

Breasts That Glow in Infrared—From the viewpoint of thermography, the body is like a walking beacon—we glow in infrared. The glow is based on heat emissions from our tissues as they convert (metabolize) food into energy and as the energy is picked up by the blood circulation. Our circulatory system acts as a giant radiator to distribute and equalize body heat derived from metabolism. The thermographic image shows us areas of diminished energy flow.

During a typical thermography session, the subject stands in front of the heat-sensitive thermography camera while the operator takes a set of computerized pictures of the body's internal heat patterns. The subject then places both hands in cold water as a "challenge" to the nervous system. This sudden exposure to cold causes healthy blood vessels to constrict as an adaptive response intended to cool the skin. Blood vessels associated with cancerous growths, however, lack a smooth muscle layer and therefore cannot constrict. When a second set of pictures is taken, any cancerous area of the breast will scan as higher in temperature than the surrounding tissue, due to the relatively greater amount of blood flow (hypervascularity) in the area.

In addition to hypervascularity of blood vessels, cancerous growths tend to give off more infrared energy. That's because cancer itself is by definition an uncontrolled growth; it can't use its energy as efficiently as other cells in the body. This lack of energy efficiency in a cancerous growth, added to the inflammation of surrounding tissues—a result of the body's natural immune reaction against a cancerous mass—helps to emphasize the difference in infrared energy between cancer cells and healthy cells and thereby to accurately pinpoint the tumor process. The inflammation itself, produced by breast tissue injury from the tumor, gives off excess heat.

Philip Hoekstra, Ph.D.: Therma-Scan, Inc. 26711 Woodward Ave., Suite 230, Huntington Woods, MI 48070; tel: 248-544-7500; fax: 248-544-7276. For a **referral to a thermography technician**, contact: American Association of Thermology, 2740 Chain Bridge Road, Vienna, VA 22181; tel: 703-938-6140; fax: 703-938-1482.

The thermography diagnosis is then based on a comparison of the pictures taken before and after the cold water treatment. The thermography technician normally expects to see body temperature go down by about 0.25° C after the challenge to the system. If it stays essentially the same or actually goes up—this means there is no cold-water-induced constriction—then the technician starts suspecting cancer. Often with cancerous tissue, the blood flow increases as a result of the cold water challenge and the blood vessels in that area register thermographically as emitting more energy and a lighter image.

If the energy flow pattern (vascularity) in one breast is higher than in the other breast (usually by at least 1.5° C), this is a warning sign. Typically, five irregularities are screened for as indicators of a cancer process, but generally if even two of these are present, then there is about a 96% certainty of cancer, says Dr. Hoekstra.

Depending on the results of the thermography test, subjects are classified into the following categories: TH1, there are no abnormal features; TH2, some unusual metabolic activity is present, but probably due to causes such as hormonal imbalance; TH3, abnormalities are present in metabolic function, but the results are inconclusive; TH4, abnormalities are found which are possibly cancerous, but it's too soon to diagnose with certainty (approximately 38% of TH4 patients develop cancer within five years); and TH5, metabolic abnormalities suggest a very high probability (about 96%) of cancer. Usually thermography technicans request that TH3 patients return for a follow-up within 90 to 120 days.

According to Dr. Hoekstra's estimates, and those of independent clinical studies, thermography screening has an accuracy rate of between 86% and 96%, compared to the 40% to 60% accuracy rate of traditional mammography. At present, there are about 1,000 thermography devices in the U.S. for providing this detailed, clinically valuable information.

The AMAS Test Compared to Mammography

For more information on **breast cancer and screening tests**, contact: Breast Cancer Action, 55 New Montgomery Street, Suite 323, San Francisco, CA 94105; tel: 415-243-9301; fax: 415-243-3996.

The AMAS test has been extensively evaluated with respect to early detection of breast cancer.[42] Unlike mammography, which does not distinguish between benign and malignant breast tumors, the AMAS detects malignant growth only and has far greater sensitivity and specificity than mammography. If the AMAS is positive, a mammogram or ultrasound may be done to ascertain the location of the tumor for surgical purposes and a needle biopsy (perhaps with ultrasound) may be recommended.

If two consecutive AMAS test results are negative, then a mammogram is unwarranted. Mammography should be used only to confirm suspicions of the breast self-examination and AMAS results. Additional mammograms, performed to clarify the probability of malignancy, become unnecessary with the AMAS. Moreover, the AMAS can be used to follow breast cancer patients who are in remission, since the AMAS returns to normal within three months after the breast tumor are removed or eradicated.[43]

Thermographic Breast Images

1) TH2 Category. This patient demonstrates benign (non-cancerous) fibrocystic disease. The light grey bands represent blood vessels, while the darker areas suggest the presence of benign growths. Because cancer cells are energy inefficient, giving off more heat than healthy cells, the darker shading of these growths indicates that cancer is probably not the cause. It is common for women to develop growths and abnormalities in the breast, but most do not result in cancer.

2) TH3 Category. Warning signs: the light bands (blood vessels) form an irregular, complicated pattern throughout the breast, widening and narrowing erratically. This pattern may suggest metabolic processes that are "out of control," a key characteristic of cancer cells. After a few months, this patient will return for a follow-up evaluation of this possible cancerous situation.

3) TH5 Category. The cancer can be identified by the light area located in the top portion of the right breast. Warning signs: the "hot" spot is concentrated in one place, indicating a localized growth; the difference in shading occurs in only one breast, suggesting that this is not a routine abnormality.

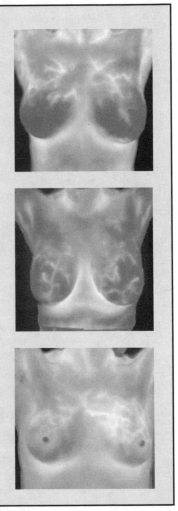

Breast Cancer Prevention

There are many ways to reduce one's risk of developing breast cancer. If you have an immediate family relative with breast cancer—especially more than one—you should take an active role now to modify these risk factors. Your risk is particularly high when breast cancer occurred in your mother, especially if your mother had cancer in both breasts or was premenopausal when the cancer was diagnosed.[44] Women who wish to keep their risk of breast cancer to a minimum should pay attention to the following established risk factors:

High-Fat Diet and High-Caloric Intake—Evidence shows that high-fat diets and high-calorie diets—fat is high in calories, so the two factors are typically inseparable—raise the risk of breast cancer.[45] Fat is a source of estrogens, free radicals, and (invariably) pesticides, all of which can promote breast cancer.

Estrogen Replacement Therapy (ERT)—This is often recommended for postmenopausal women as a way to reduce the risk of osteoporosis, but studies indicate that long-term use of ERT can significantly increase the risk of developing breast cancer.[46] The use of estriol, a relatively harmless form of estrogen, and natural progesterone may help resolve this problem.[47]

Pesticides and Other Compounds—Higher breast cancer rates have been found in the offspring of women who took DES (diethylstilbestrol) and among women with high breast-tissue concentrations of PCBs (polychlorinated biphenyls) and DDE (dichloro-diparacholophenyl-ethylene: a metabolite of the infamous DDT pesticide).[48] DDE levels tend to be higher among African-American breast cancer patients than African-American women without cancer.[49] Higher levels of PBBs (polybrominated biphenyls) and certain pesticides have been found in fatty tissue samples from women with breast cancer compared with women who had benign breast disease.[50]

The difficulty in calling these pesticides and other organohalogen compounds "risk factors" is that chronic low-level exposure is prevalent in the general population; about 90% of the organohalogen exposure that has been linked with breast cancer is traced to food, either as deposits or residues.[51] Pesticide use represents a "hidden killer" because these chemicals not only directly promote tumor growth, but can suppress the immune system, thereby increasing susceptibility to disease.[52]

Other Key Risk Factors—Among the strategies for reducing your risk of developing breast cancer are the following:

■ minimize exposure to low-level ionizing radiation

■ increase intake of dietary antioxidants (from fruits, vegetables, and vitamin supplements)

■ exercise regularly but in moderation

■ have a baby (pregnancy reduces a woman's lifetime estrogen exposure)

■ breastfeed your baby (lactation helps discharge pesticides and other toxins from the breast)

■ avoid magnetic fields from power lines, electrical appliances, computers, and geopathic lines, as electromagnetic fields may alter the brain's repairing, protein synthesis, and melatonin production; melatonin appears to help protect against breast cancer.[53]

The Hemoccult Test

Colorectal cancer (cancer of either the colon or rectum) is the second most common cancer in the United States and surely one of the deadliest. In fact, about one out of every five cancer deaths (20%) in the U.S. is attributed to colorectal cancer and almost half of all colorectal patients will probably die, according to conventional medical statistics. One reason for this heavy death toll may be that the majority of colorectal cancer cases are diagnosed at a late stage of the disease.

Detected early, progression of this disease is entirely preventable. Among the more reliable early signs of colorectal cancer is blood on the surface of or mixed in feces. If not visible to the eye, colorectal blood can be detected by chemical tests. In some cases, pain and tenderness are felt in the lower abdomen, but often no symptoms appear until the tumor grows so big that it causes obstruction or rupture of the intestine; at this point, surgery and aggressive forms of treatment become necessary.

For this reason, many doctors now recommend the hemoccult test, in which a sample of feces is applied to a card imprinted with a solution of guaiac, a plant gum. The presence of hemoglobin, hence the name hemoccult (i.e., blood in the feces), is indicated by a color change. The test will sometimes yield false positive results if the person has recently consumed fresh fruits or vegetables, red meat, iron tablets, aspirin, nonsteroidal anti-inflammatory drugs, or vitamin C supplements.

A positive finding with the hemoccult test warrants having a sigmoidoscopy, another tool used to detect polyps and tumors. This procedure involves the use of a flexible tube, about the diameter of a pencil, that is inserted into the colon. Using this lighted instrument, the physician explores the lower interior portion of the colon, called the sigmoid. Research indicates that two out of every three cases of colorectal cancer are accessible to detection by this means.[54]

To lower the risk of colorectal cancer, those over age 50 who have a poor diet and heavy meat-eating background should consider switching, if they haven't already, to a more vegetarian diet. Many oncologists recommend sigmoidoscopy at least every three to five years once people reach age 50. However, if you are physically active, have a normal 2-3 bowel movements daily, follow a low-fat, high-fiber diet, and have no symptoms, this practice should not be considered necessary.

If colorectal cancer is detected early, dietary treatment along with the other alternative therapies may constitute the best line of attack.

The number one risk factor for colorectal cancer is the consumption of red meat (but not fish or white meat) and refined sugar-containing foods or white flour products; a diet low in fruits and vegetables also increases the risk.[55] Dietary antioxidants (notably vitamin E), calcium, vitamin D, and folic acid may reduce the risk or aid in reversing this cancer in its early stages.

It is advisable to remove all dairy from the diet, except for low-fat yogurt on an occasional basis. A diet rich in cereal grains, fresh vegetables and fruits, legumes, and fish will be the healthiest strategy for anyone at risk for colorectal cancer or already diagnosed with the disease. Garlic, onions, chives, and cruciferous vegetables (broccoli, Brussels sprouts, cabbage, bok choy, etc.) are the most protective.[56]

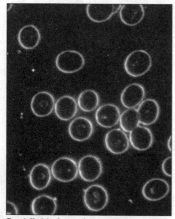
Darkfield view of normal blood.

Along with avoiding red meat, dairy, and processed meats, one should abstain from alcohol and smoking, which have been shown to amplify the risk of colorectal cancer or cause a recurrence.[57] Chlorinated water is associated with an increase in the incidence of colon and rectal cancers.[58]

Darkfield Microscopy

Until recently, scientists assumed that the only diseases generated by microbes were infectious disorders such as AIDS, influenza, or tuberculosis. It was assumed that blood contained no living organisms that could contribute to cancer since the use of standard microscopes had failed to detect any sign of such microbes. When the powerful electron microscope is used, live organisms are placed in a vacuum and subjected to deadening protoplasmic changes—meaning it is virtually impossible to observe living organisms.

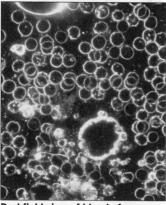
Darkfield view of blood of someone in early stages of cancer.

Based on the findings from more sophisticated light microscopes, there is now compelling evidence that such microbes do exist and may play a major role in cancer. This advance now enables forward-thinking physicians to see signs of cancer in living blood, even if it is only energetic traces or indications, before it manifests as a palpable tumor. French Canadian biologist Gaston Naessens invented an optic microscope called the Somatoscope, which enabled him to view tiny particles in the blood never before seen. He called these particles somatids, which means tiny bodies. What Naessens called somatids, the German bacteriologist Gunther Enderlein called "protits" and Virginia Livingston Wheeler, M.D., called *Progenitor cryptocides*. Whatever the name, the research cited here tends to confirm the pleomorphic or form-changing nature of microorganisms believed to underlie the cancer process.

The use of darkfield microscopy was a major change in the diagnostic routine of Maarten Klatte, M.D., a Dutch homeopathic physician and founding director of Vitality Research in The Hague, Netherlands. Like many physicians, he had assumed that all the essential components of blood could be detected by an electron microscope. "Instead of looking at blood, I looked at numbers," Dr. Klatte says. "These days, I look at the form and motion of the blood components, which include living organisms. I now realize that the old blood analyses, based on measurements, told us relatively little about the true condition of the blood."

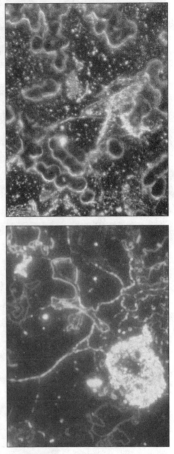

Darkfield view of blood of a person with advanced cancer (top) and another with very advanced cancer (bottom).

Using the darkfield microscope, what is normal quantitatively can be abnormal in a qualitative or "functional" sense, says Dr. Klatte. Even though the white cell count in a particular patient is normal, he maintains, the condition of the white blood cells may be revealed by the darkfield microscopy to be far from healthy. "If most of the cells look paralyzed and broken," says Dr. Klatte, "then the 'normal' cell

For more information on the **application of darkfield microscopy and pleomorphic theory**, see Chapter 7: Boosting the Immune System, pp. 214-231.

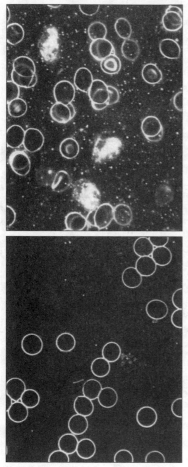

Darkfield microscopy photographs of two patients—a 49-year-old female suffering from osteoblastic metastasis (top) and a 66-year-old female suffering from primary lung carcinoma (bottom).

count means nothing. Motion tells me a lot more about the cells' function. Form tells me whether the cells are damaged or whether there are cell-wall deficiencies." A cell-wall deficiency means that the membrane surrounding the cell is porous or fragmented, allowing inappropriate or foreign substances to exert harmful effects. Poor cellular function is indicated by a lack of responsiveness to foreign microorganisms.

Dr. Klatte, like many physicians, used to think that in healthy people, the blood and urine are basically sterile. Through the darkfield microscope, he has become aware that the blood is full of living microorganisms. "Thanks to Gaston Naessens, Guenther Enderlein, and others, we now understand much more about the living particles in our blood," says Dr. Klatte, who has worked with Naessens and confirmed the form-changing cycle of Naessens' somatids.

In fact, this cycle reveals the physical states of health and disease, according to Dr. Klatte. The somatid cycle indicates early signs of cancer, usually 6-18 months before the onset of clinical symptoms such as a swollen lymph node or lump in the breast. "When the pleomorphic cycle appears, we can take action and reverse the cycle with therapy. If the cycle does not reverse, we know that the therapy is not working." In the physician's hands, the darkfield microscope is an early detection tool and a way to evaluate the effectiveness of a therapy.

Douglas Brodie, M.D., makes use of darkfield microscopic principles by way of a simple yet versatile procedure called live blood analysis (LBA). Dr. Brodie uses LBA for obtaining a quick and accurate assessment of his patient's blood composition and viability. With a single sample, taken by a pinprick of the fingertip, LBA is able to provide a composite of numerous factors from living blood. With our increasing awareness of the importance of a strong immune system, the LBA is a valuable tool, providing dynamic assessment of the degrees of cancer resistance a person possesses. Physicians can use it to determine blood imbalances that do not show up in the conventional procedure, known as the complete blood count (CBC). "In many cases, the live blood analysis provides information that enables us to predict which direction the cancer patient's body is heading," says Dr. Brodie. "We then make specific adjustments in nutrition and other modalities to optimize the healing process."

For more information on the **Live Blood Analysis** system used by Dr. Brodie, contact: NutriScreen, Inc., James R. Privitera, M.D., director, 105 North Grandview, Covina, CA 91723; tel: 626-966-1618; fax: 626-966-7226. Dr. Privitera provides detailed instruction manuals in darkfield microscopic interpretation and nutritional prescribing to licensed health-care professionals.

Assessment of Biological Terrain

French biologist Louis Claude Vincent, Ph.D., discovered that the key to healing was not the use of powerful drugs, but rather knowing the patient's biochemistry and the optimal conditions or "terrain" for body function. In 1958, Dr. Vincent was hired by the French government to determine why people living in certain regions of France had high cancer rates. This assignment led him to examine the relationship between the external environment—molded by a person's emotional and physical stress exposure, dietary choices, and other lifestyle habits—and the internal environment of the body.

Biological terrain is a phrase used to describe the conditions, general health, and activity level of cells. This includes the status of microorganisms at the cellular level: some are beneficial to life and health, others are not. Each type of bacteria, fungus or virus thrives in a precise biochemical medium. Viruses require a fairly alkaline environment, whereas fungi favor a more acidic environment; bacteria can thrive under various conditions, but their growth is stimulated in high-sugar conditions. An excess of toxins in one's diet and environment tends to increase the production of acid within cells, forcing the body to compensate by producing a strong alkaline reaction in the blood—this favors the growth of cancer cells.

Dr. Vincent concluded that the components of the blood, urine, and saliva afford insight into the way the body functions. By monitoring biochemical changes in these fluids and by making appropriate changes in diet, lifestyle, and medical treatment, health can be reestablished and disease processes retarded or possibly reversed.

Stress Prevention for the Cancer Patient

Stress can become harmful to the body when it is prolonged or chronic. It affects the body in very real, physical ways by influencing the immune and hormonal systems. A basic premise of mind/body medicine is that chronic stress contributes to illness and that relaxation techniques and learning positive ways of coping with stress will improve your health. This can be especially important to the person with cancer and a number of therapies are available to help deal with the stress and emotional trauma of this disease.

Research in psychoneuroimmunology, or PNI, has shown that the immune and nervous systems are linked by extensive networks of nerve endings in the spleen, bone marrow, lymph nodes, and thymus gland (a primary source of T cells). At the same time, receptors for a variety of chemical messengers—catecholamines, prostaglandins, thyroid hormone, growth hormone, serotonin, and endorphins—have been found on the surfaces of white blood cells. Such connections serve to integrate the activities of the immune, hormonal, and nervous systems, enabling the mind and emotional states to influence the body's resistance to disease.[59]

Meditation—Meditation is a safe and simple way to balance a person's physical, emotional, and mental states. It is easy to learn and can be useful both for treating stress and in pain management. Meditation is any activity that keeps the attention focused in the present. When the mind is calm and focused in the present, it is neither reacting to past events or preoccupied with future plans, two major sources of chronic stress. There are many forms of meditation, but they can be categorized into two main approaches, concentration meditation and mindfulness meditation.

Concentration meditation focuses the "lens of the mind" on one object, sound (mantra), the breath, an image, or thought, to still the mind and allow greater awareness or clarity to emerge. The breath is one of the most popular objects of focus in this type of meditation. As the person focuses on the ebb and flow of their breath, the mind is absorbed in the rhythm and becomes more placid, tranquil, and still.

Mindfulness-based meditation entails bringing the mind to a still point, tuning out the world and bringing the mind to a halt as much as possible. Mindfulness meditation helps us practice non-judgment. The meditator sits quietly and witnesses whatever goes through the mind, not reacting or becoming involved with thoughts, memories, worries, or images. This helps the person gain a more calm, clear state of mind.

Neuro-Linguistic Programming— Neuro-Linguistic Programming (NLP) helps people detect unconscious patterns of thought, behavior, and attitudes that contribute to their illness. These unconscious patterns are then reprogrammed in order to alter psychological responses and facilitate healing. NLP was developed in the early 1970s by a professor of linguistics and a student of psychology and mathematics, both at the University of California at Santa Cruz. They studied the thinking processes, language patterns, and behavioral patterns of accomplished individuals. They found that body cues—eye movement, posture, voice tone, and breathing patterns—coincided with unconscious patterns of a person's emotional state. Based on their findings, they developed the NLP technique to help people with emotional problems.

People who have difficulty recovering from physical illness have often adopted negative beliefs about their recovery. They perceive themselves as helpless, hopeless, or worthless, expressed in statements like "I can't get healthy" or "There's no hope." NLP tries to move the person from their present state of discomfort to a desired state of health by helping reprogram these beliefs about healing. NLP practitioners ask questions to discover how the person relates to issues of identity, beliefs, life goals, and health, then observe the person's language patterns, eye movements, postures, muscle tension, and gestures. These relay information about how the person relates to their condition in both conscious and unconscious ways, revealing what limiting beliefs may exist. These belief structures can then be altered using NLP. The practitioner will ask the person to see herself in a state of health. By doing so, an outcome is set that facilitates the healing process. The brain's natural response is to duplicate whatever images or beliefs are created about getting better.[60] The brain then triggers the necessary immunological responses to guide the body toward health. NLP has proved successful in treating people with AIDs, cancer, allergies, and arthritis.

For more information on **Neuro-Linguistic Programming**, contact: NLP University/Dynamic Learning Center, P.O. Box 1112, Ben Lomond, CA 95005; tel: 408-336-3457; fax: 408-336-5854; website: www.nlpu.com. For **guided imagery**, contact: Academy for Guided Imagery, P.O. Box 2070, Mill Valley, CA 94942; tel: 800-726-2070 or 415-389-9325; fax: 415-389-9342; website: www.healthy.net/agi. For **flower remedies**, contact: Flower Essence Society, P.O. Box 1769, Nevada City, CA 95959; tel: 800-548-0075 or 916-265-9163; fax: 916-265-6467.

Guided Imagery/Visualization

Using the power of the mind to evoke a positive physical response, guided imagery and visualization can modulate the immune system and reduce pain. By directly accessing emotions, imagery can help an individual understand the needs that may be represented by an illness and can help develop ways to meet those needs. Imagery is also one of the quickest and most direct ways to become aware of emotions and their effects on health, both positive and negative.

Imagery is simply a flow of thoughts that one can see, hear, feel, smell, taste, or experience. According to Martin L. Rossman, M.D., of the Academy for Guided Imagery, in Mill Valley, California, while the sensory phenomenon that is being experienced in the mind may or may not represent external reality, it always depicts internal reality. What Dr. Rossman means is that the sensations in the body that imagery creates are very real phenomena that can be measured via laboratory devices. Research using brain scans indicates that imagery activates parts of the cerebral cortex and centers of the brain. "If you are a good worrier," states Dr., Rossman, "and especially if you ever 'worry yourself sick', you may be a good candidate for learning how to positively

continued on next page

affect your health with imagery, as the internal process involved in worrying yourself sick and 'imagining yourself well' are quite similar."[61] Imagery is a proven method for pain relief, helps people tolerate medical procedures, reduces side effects of treatments, and stimulates the body to heal.

Flower Remedies

Flower remedies directly address a person's emotional state in order to facilitate both psychological and physiological well-being. By balancing negative feelings and stress, flower remedies can effectively remove the emotional barriers to health and recovery. Flower remedies comprise subtle liquid preparations made from the fresh blossoms of flowers, plants, bushes, even trees, to address emotional, psychological, and spiritual issues underlying physical problems. The approach was pioneered by British physician Edward Bach in the 1930s, when he introduced the 38 Bach Flower Remedies, based on English plants.

Today, an estimated 20 different brands of flower remedies, based on plants native to many landscapes, from Australia to India to Alaska, offer about 1,500 different blends for a diverse range of psychological conditions. The flower remedies each address a particular emotional issue: for example, Vine helps to increase feelings of self-worth, Impatiens is recommended for feelings of impatience with others and yourself, and Aspen is for feelings of fear. An individual formula can be made by combining four to six of the remedies and taking them orally or rubbing them into the skin. They can be taken for a short time to cope with a crisis or for a period of months.

Robert Greenberg, D.C., of the Whole Health Centre in Chesterfield, Missouri, developed an approach to assessing health known as biological terrain assessment, or BTA. This test enables him to determine the optimal conditions for a specific patient's internal environment. According to Dr. Greenberg, the healthy body must satisfy three criteria to function at the highest level: (1) optimal pH (acid-base balance); (2) optimal oxidation-reduction potential; and (3) resistivity. Through BTA, these factors are measured in blood, urine, and saliva, to yield a total of nine measures.

"The pH reading tells us whether enzymatic activity in the body is occurring properly and if digestion and absorption of nutrients is adequate," says Dr. Greenberg. "It can also alert us to the presence of environmental contaminants, substances that prove very damaging to the body's delicate chemistry."

Oxidation-reduction potential (abbreviated as redox) refers to the degree of "oxidative stress" on the body, or

For information about **BTA-S-1000**, contact: Biological Technologies International, P.O. Box 560, Payson, AZ 85547; tel: 520-474-4181; fax: 520-474-1501.

how much free-radical burden (oxidation of tissues) the body is exposed to. "Because of the effects of stress, poor air, poor food quality, and lack of exercise, these values are generally lower than they should be to sustain health," says Dr. Greenberg. "If the values remain low for extended periods of time, the person will be more susceptible to cancer."

The third factor, resistivity, is a measure of a tissue's resistance to the flow of electrical current, which indicates the ability to conduct electrical current through a cell, nerve, or muscle. With low resistivity (high conductivity), there is typically a buildup of mineral salts. High resistivity (low conductivity) means a lack of minerals, which indicates the need to evaluate the individual for specific deficiencies.

The BTA analysis is carried out in only ten minutes by a computerized device called a BTA S-1000. The device determines pH, resistivity, and redox values in blood, saliva, and urine. "Urine is a good indicator of the body's secretory ability and toxic load," says Dr. Greenberg. "Blood is a good indicator of toxicity and oxygen balance, while saliva offers insight into a person's digestive capacities."

For cancer patients, the test provides insight that can guide the physician in redirecting biochemical parameters in the patient, using nutrition, botanical medicines, exercise, and other approaches. "The goal is to move the body toward the optimal benchmark," says Dr. Greenberg. The therapeutic approach

A Primer on Cellular Terrain

The term **pH**, which means "potential hydrogen," represents a scale for the relative acidity or alkalinity of a solution. Acidity is measured as a pH of 0.1 to 6.9, alkalinity is 7.1 to 14, and neutral pH is 7.0. The numbers refer to how many hydrogen atoms are present compared to an ideal or standard solution. Normally, blood is slightly alkaline, at 7.35 to 7.45; urine pH can range from 4.8 to 7.5, although normal is closer to 7.0.

Acid-base metabolism refers to the metabolic processes that maintain the balance of acids and bases (alkalines) in body fluids. Acids release hydrogen ions, while bases accept them. The total number of these hydrogen ions present determines the pH of a fluid. Too many hydrogen ions (a pH below 7) produce an acidic state called acidosis, while too few hydrogen ions (a pH above 7) cause an alkaline excess called alkalosis; both can lead to illness.

Oxidation-reduction refers to a basic chemical mechanism in the cell by which energy is produced from foods. Electrons (negatively charged particles in an atom) are removed from one atom, resulting in "oxidation" of this first atom, and then are added or transferred to another atom, resulting in "reduction" of this second atom. This continual process of energy metabolism is actually a flow of electrons, or a minute electrical current within the cell.

indicated by BTA findings will vary greatly from one cancer patient to the next, and even for people with the same type and stage of cancer. "When the patient's body chemistry is balanced and maintained with a healthy diet, proper vitamin and mineral supplementation, adequate amounts of exercise and rest, the body can remain healthy and nourish a vibrant immune system to protect and sustain it."

The CBC Blood Test Report

The CBC Blood Test Report offers both doctors and patients user-friendly blood test analysis, opening "a therapeutic window" to one's unique biochemistry.

The Basic Status Report alphabetically lists the amounts detected of about 44 substances normally found in the blood. But it also ranks these items, such as cholesterol, lymphocytes, sodium, and bilirubin, by what percentage the client's readings are higher or lower than a statistical norm.

The analysis also offers a Panel Report. This groups the results according to 14 biochemical functions, such as electrolytes, kidney function, acid or alkaline pH, nitrogen, and protein. A particularly innovative feature is the Disease Indicators Report, in which the total blood status is compared with the known indicators of any of 140 diseases. The Drug Interactions Report identifies potentially aggravating effects if the patient were to use any of hundreds of conventional drugs. Finally, the Biochemical Pharmacology Report suggests which supplements are indicated for the given abnormal blood chemistry; the exact dosages are left to a physician to determine.

For more information about the **CBC Blood Test Report**, contact: Carbon Based Corporation, 153 Country Club Drive, Suite 5, Incline Village, NV 89451; tel: 702-832-8485; fax: 702-832-8488.

Tests for Heavy Metal Toxicity

Increasingly, practitioners of alternative medicine find that low-level but chronic exposure to a variety of toxic heavy metals poses serious health dangers if the metals are allowed to stay in the body. These toxins are now commonly found in our food, water, and air, as well as cooking utensils, cosmetics, auto exhaust, tobacco smoke, many of the building materials and fabrics in our work and living environments, pesticides in our foods, and dental materials in our teeth (mercury fillings).

Typical symptoms of heavy metal toxicity can include nervous system disorders, depression, fatigue, skin rashes, high blood pressure, hyperactivity, nausea, irritability, headaches, and more serious conditions including autism, intelligence deficits, and cancer. But before you can remove heavy metals from a person, you need first to determine which ones are present and in what amounts.

Maverick Monitoring Test

If you suspect toxicity as a contributing factor in cancer, first you must identify the toxins, explains Hildegarde A. Staninger, Ph.D., medical director of Sunstate Preventive Medicine Institute in Winter Park, Florida. Dr. Staninger is one of the country's experts in industrial toxicology, which uses a laboratory-based approach that enables physicians to quantify the level of dangerous toxic chemicals absorbed into a patient's bloodstream or tissues. Dr. Staninger relies on the Maverick Monitoring Test (MMT), an innovative protocol she developed to measure body levels of toxic agents that create harmful free radicals.

The Maverick Monitoring Test is actually a nontechnical name for a test to measure malondialdehyde (MDA) levels, the chemical end result of heightened free-radical activity and cellular damage, the oxidation of lipids (fats), and an irregular combination of fats and proteins. Maverick determines how much MDA is present in the patient's body by analyzing urine or a blood sample.

Maverick specifically looks at the compounds normally inside a cell that, when the cell wall is broken down and the compounds interact with substances outside the cell, will cause free-radical pathology. "This is what starts disease," Dr. Staninger explains. "It ends with the death of the cell." The amount of MDA tells the physician how much free-radical damage the body has sustained; it can also indicate how well the patient is responding to a nutritional antioxidant program, based on how much MDA levels decreased.

ToxMet Screen

The ToxMet screen from MetaMetrix Medical Laboratory provides a detailed analysis of the levels of specific heavy metals in a patient's system, based on a urine sample. ToxMet tests for levels of four highly toxic heavy metals—arsenic, cadmium, lead, and mercury; it also reports on levels for ten potentially toxic elements, such as aluminum, bismuth, boron, nickel, and strontium. Finally, information is gathered on a patient's status regarding 14 essential metals and minerals, such as copper, calcium, chromium, molybdenum, selenium, and vanadium. On the basis of this

For information on **Maverick**, contact: Sunstate Preventive Medicine Institute, 2699 Lee Road, Suite 303, Winter Park, FL 32789; tel: 407-695-1033. For **ToxMet**, contact: MetaMetrix Medical Laboratory, 5000 Peachtree Industrial Blvd., Suite 110, Norcross, GA 30071; tel: 770-446-5483 or 800-221-4640; fax: 770-441-2237.

For more on **detoxification**, see Chapter 9: Physical Support Therapies, pp. 254-297. For more on **antioxidants**, see Chapter 4: Nutrition as Cancer Medicine, pp. 130-159.

information, a physician is able to develop an individualized nutritional prescription and detoxification program to both eliminate the toxic metals from the system and to rebalance the amounts of essential nutrients.

Tests That Measure Antioxidant Protection

Individualized Optimal Nutrition–The comprehensive information provided by Metametrix's ION (Individualized Optimal Nutrition) Panel can be used preventively to catch imbalances and potential illness in their earliest stages. ION, which measures 150 biochemical components, is also highly useful for physicians who need detailed biochemical assessment, based on a blood and urine sample, of patients who might already have cancer.

ION checks for nutritional status in categories including vitamins, minerals, amino acids, fatty and organic acids, lipid peroxides, general blood chemistries (cholesterol, thyroid hormone, glucose), and antioxidants. Based on the individual's test results, ION can provide supplement recommendations. Finally, ION summarizes the test results into nine categories according to disease risk, such as cardiovascular, liver function, intestinal balance, energy, digestive disorders, and thyroid status.

Oxidative Protection Screen–The Oxidative Protection Screen from Antibody Assay Laboratories of Santa Ana, California, can provide your physician with a biochemical analysis of how well your body is handling free radicals. This information, in turn, is valuable for a physician in assessing a patient's overall health, the degree of antioxidant protection one has, and the possible need for further nutrient supplementation.

When lipids (fatty acids, steroids, and other organic compounds) are damaged by free radicals, they form lipid peroxides which circulate in the blood. Using a blood sample, the test determines the amount of lipid peroxides in the plasma. An elevated amount indicates a high production of free radicals. The Total Oxidative Protection Index™ will indicate your system's overall ability to withstand the "attack" of free radicals and thus your individual degree of oxidative protection.

The Pantox Antioxidant Profile–Based on a blood sample, this diagnostic screen measures the status of 20 factors determining the body's antioxidant defense system, in comparison with a database of 4,000 healthy profiles. On the basis of this precise biochemical information, both physicians and patients can take nutritional steps to prevent disease from developing. Specifically, the screen reports on the biochemical presence of lipoproteins (cholesterol, triglycerides), fat-soluble antioxidants (vitamins A and E, carotenoids, coenzyme Q10), water-soluble antioxidants (vitamin C, uric acid, bilirubin), and iron balance. The test helps determine if you are getting the right antioxidants in the correct amounts.

FORCYTE Cancer Prognostic System

Starting with a surgical or fine needle biopsy specimen of a tumor, the FORCYTE Cancer Prognostic System provides the oncologist with information useful in making predictions about treatment outcome. The FORCYTE system creates a subcellular portrait of a tumor by way of a three-dimensional multiparameter histogram. These parameters include information about cell subpopulations, their respective cell cycle phase, and DNA synthesis rate. FORCYTE provides objective indicators closely related to actual tumor cell activity with which a physician can decide what kind of treatment will be most effective.

For information about the **FORCYTE Cancer Prognostic System**, contact: Dianon Systems, 200 Watson Boulevard, Stratford, CT 06497; tel: 800-328-2666 or 203-381-4000.

For the **T/Tn Antigen Test**, contact: Heather Margaret Bligh Cancer Research Laboratories, Georg F. Springer, M.D., Director, Finch University of Health Sciences, The Chicago Medical School, 3333 Green Bay Road, North Chicago, IL 60064; tel: 847-578-3435; fax: 847-578-3432.

T/Tn Antigen Test

Georg Springer, M.D., an immunologist who founded the Heather Bligh Cancer Research Laboratories at the Chicago Medical School, uncovered evidence that certain proteins (antigens) on the surface of blood and skin cells can be identified by the immune system (antibodies). Dr. Springer recognized that the T and Tn antigens are specifically associated with cancers of all kinds and that the T and Tn antigens are found in places where cancer has spread, but not in benign breast tumors.[62]

The T and Tn antigens serve as specific markers for the presence of cancer; in the case of breast cancer, the more markers, the more advanced or aggressive the cancer. "What is unique about the T and Tn antibody test is that it enables detection of the majority of cancers before any biopsy can pick up the presence of cancer," says Dr. Springer. "We find that people without any previous cancer, who show positive test results, consistently develop cancer later on."

In general, the less aggressive cancers produce a higher proportion of T than Tn antigens, while Tn predominates in more aggressive primary cancers. The relative concentrations of these antigens, however, will vary depending on the cancer type and stage. The identification of these antigens enabled Dr. Springer to develop a skin-prick test to predict or indicate the likely future development of cancer. The test result, determined in 1-2 days, is positive when an area of skin greater than 4 mm turns reddish and hardens. Dr. Springer's skin-prick test depends on the body's "delayed hypersensitivity reaction" to the injected antigens, meaning it takes the body time to "decide" how it will react to these foreign proteins.

In a study of the T/Tn antigen test, positive test results occurred in the following: 94% of lung cancer patients (15 out of 16 people); 80% of breast cancer patients (20 out of 25 people); 7% of patients with benign (nonmalignant) tumors (26 out of 349 patients); 0% of healthy people (0 out of 148 people) in the control group.[63] A delayed skin reaction to T and Tn antigen does not occur in healthy people, but is usually found to be highly typical among cancer patients, where it indicates a sluggish or dysfunctional immune system. Dr. Springer's test can predict the onset of cancer, on average, six years in advance of other tests, and sometimes as much as ten years.

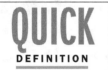

For more about **Dr. Govallo's approach**, contact: People Against Cancer, Box 10, Otho, IA 50569; tel: 515-972-4444. **Harris L. Coulter, Ph.D.**, Empirical Therapies, Inc., 4221 45th Street, N.W., Washington, D.C. 20016; tel: 202-364-0898.

Lymphocyte Size Analysis

Russian immunologist Valentin Govallo, M.D., recognized that lymphocytes (SEE QUICK DEFINITION) could be classified as either normal or enlarged. Lymphocytes tend to swell and increase in size among cancer patients compared to healthy people. Using a microscope, you can measure the diameters of lymphocytes and count the numbers of swollen versus normal cells in a sample of a patient's blood. Dr. Govallo calls this a "lymphocytogram." If the number of swollen lymphocytes is excessive, then cancer will most likely develop. The test's diagnostic accuracy for various types of cancer is 90%.[64]

QUICK DEFINITION

A **lymphocyte** is a form of white blood cell, representing 25%-33% of the total count, whose numbers increase during infection. Lymphocytes, produced in the bone marrow, come in two forms: T cells, which are matured in the thymus gland (behind the breastbone) and have many functions in the body's immune response; and B-cells, which produce antibodies to neutralize an antigen (foreign and potentially dangerous matter in the blood). Each B-cell produces a single and specific antibody.

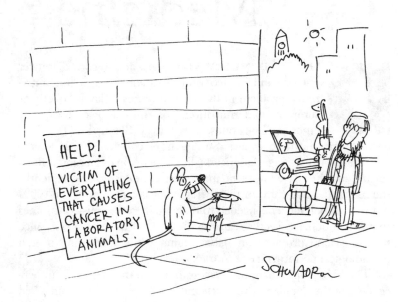

CHAPTER

Nutrition as Cancer Medicine

DIET AND NUTRITION are at the core of cancer etiology and its successful treatment. The leading nutritional problem in the United States today is "overconsumptive undernutrition," or the eating of too many empty-calorie foods, says Jeffrey Bland, Ph.D., a biochemist and nutrition expert. Studies have concluded that almost two-thirds of an average American's diet is made up of fats and refined sugars, and thus have low or no micronutrient density. Consequently, the remaining one-third of the average diet is counted on for 100% of the essential nutrients needed to maintain health. This contributes to nutrient deficiencies that can rob the body of its natural resistance to disease and promote premature aging while weakening overall physiological performance.

The U.S. Department of Agriculture found that a significant percentage of the population receives under 70% of the Recommended Daily Allowance (RDA) for vitamins A, C, and B-complex, and the essential minerals calcium, magnesium, and iron.[1] A separate study found that most diets contain less than 80% of the RDA for calcium, magnesium, iron, zinc, copper, and manganese, and that the people most at nutritional risk are young children and women from adolescence to old age.

While a cumulative lack of essential nutrients can contribute to illness, including cancer, the correct fortification with these nutrients can start reversing chronic conditions. However, it is important to appreciate that nutrients work together and act according to various biochemical relationships.

Vitamins and minerals help regulate the conversion of food to energy in the body, explains Dr. Bland. As such, they can be separated into two general categories: energy nutrients, which are principally involved in the conversion of food to energy; and protector nutrients, which help defend against damaging toxins derived from drugs, alcohol, radiation, environmental pollutants, or the body's own enzyme processes. "The B-complex vitamins and magnesium are examples of energy nutrients because they activate specific metabolic facilitators called enzymes, which control digestion and the absorption and use of proteins, fats, and carbohydrates."

In the process of converting food to energy, free radicals are produced that can damage the body and set the stage for degenerative diseases, including cancer, arthritis, heart disease, and premature aging. Protector nutrients such as vitamin E, beta carotene, vitamin C, and the minerals zinc, copper, manganese, and selenium, play a critical role in preventing or delaying these degenerative processes.

Vitamins and minerals "drive" the biochemical and electrical circuitry of the body. The body's functioning is therefore profoundly affected by how nutrients either work together or against each other. Nutrients taken simultaneously can inhibit each other. Iron, for example, is best absorbed when taken separately from pancreatic enzymes and should also not be taken with vitamin E. There are also nutrients that enhance the effects of other nutrients. For

Nutritional Substances and Therapies Covered in This Chapter

- *Acidophilus* (the *Lactobacilli* family)
- Amino acids
- Beta carotene
- Calcium
- Chromium
- Coenzyme Q10
- Copper
- Eicosapentaenoic acid (EPA fish oils)
- Flaxseed oil
- Gamma linolenic acid (GLA)
- Germanium
- Gerson Diet Therapy
- Inositol
- Iodine
- Kelley's Metabolic Therapy
- Manganese
- Molybdenum
- Orthomolecular Medicine
- Potassium
- Selenium
- Vitamin A
- Vitamin B complex
- Vitamin B3 (niacin)
- Vitamin B6 (pyridoxine)
- Vitamin C (ascorbic acid)
- Vitamin D
- Vitamin E
- Vitamin K
- Water
- Zinc

Nutritional Rating of Americans

A new Healthy Eating Index study of 4,000 Americans, conducted by the U.S. Department of Agriculture, reveals that 88% of the population does not get good grades for proper nutrition. More than 80% eat too much saturated fat and too little fruits, vegetables, and fiber-rich grains. The worst eaters are aged 15-39. Overall, the American diet achieves only 63% of what the USDA considers good nutrition.

example, vitamin C taken with iron facilitates the maximum absorption of the iron. Similarly, clinical studies have shown a relationship between low intakes of beta carotene, vitamin E, and vitamin C and higher incidences of cancer.[2]

In addition to disease control, specific nutrients can help people cope with specific lifestyle, environmental, and emotional/psychological factors. For example, when recovering from cancer surgery, a person may need higher levels of zinc;[3] individuals who are exposed to smog or other pollutants require higher levels of the protector nutrients such as selenium, vitamin E, and vitamin C;[4] and anyone under heavy emotional or physical stress, typical of the cancer experience, will need higher intakes of all the B vitamins.[5]

Benefits of a Whole-Foods, Mainly Vegetarian Diet

In light of this knowledge of nutrition and its specificity, there are two primary ways to gain the needed nutrients: through a carefully constructed diet or through an equally specific nutrient supplementation program.

A whole-foods diet promotes health by decreasing fat and sugar intake and by increasing the consumption of fiber and nutrients, particularly the numerous antioxidants and other phytochemicals (*phyto* means plant) that have been identified as beneficial anticancer nutrients. Fiber is found in plant foods, such as brown rice, broccoli, oatmeal, or almonds, but not in animal products like meat, cheese, milk, eggs, and butter. Fiber is the transport system of the digestive tract, "sweeping" food wastes out of the body before they have a chance to form potentially cancer-causing chemicals. These toxic chemicals can cause colon cancer or pass through the gastrointestinal membrane into the bloodstream and damage other cells.

A vegetable-based, whole-foods diet is typically much lower in fat. On a percentage-of-calories basis, most vegetables contain less than 10% fat and most grains contain 16%-20% fat; by comparison, whole milk and cheese contain 74% fat; a rib roast is 75% fat; eggs are 64% fat; a skinned, baked chicken breast still has 38% fat. A low-fat, whole-foods diet also means fewer calories: studies have shown that a diet containing fewer calories is associated with reduced DNA damage, thus lowering cancer risks and increasing longevity.[6]

Plant foods are richer sources of micronutrients than their animal counterparts. Compare wheat germ to round steak: ounce for ounce, wheat germ contains twice the vitamin B2, vitamin K, potassium, iron, and copper; three times the vitamin B6, molybdenum, and selenium; 15 times as much magnesium; and over 20 times the vitamin B1, folate, and inositol. The steak contains only three micronutrients in greater amounts: vitamin B12, chromium, and zinc.

Eating more nutrient-dense plant foods tends to decrease one's desire to consume processed sugars; lower sugar consumption decreases overall calorie intake. At the same time, the extra nutrients increase protection against cancer. A cup of broccoli, for example, provides 70 mg of vitamin C, more than any other vegetable except green peppers; vitamin C blocks the formation of cancer initiators and may keep cancer cells from growing into deadly tumors. Broccoli contains more fiber and calcium on a per gram basis than most vegetables, which may account for its protective effects against colon cancer. It is also a rich source of folate, a B vitamin that seems to protect against cervical cancer, and of beta carotene, the plant pigment that helps fight lung cancer. In a study of the diets of 1,200 people over 66 years old, those who consumed the most green vegetables had a significantly lower cancer risk than those who ate the least; people who ate broccoli less than once a week had increased their risk of developing cancer by 20%.[7]

There are compelling reasons for adopting a more plant-based diet. First, important antioxidant nutrients, including vitamin C, beta carotene, vitamin E, and many cancer-fighting substances known as phytochemicals, are found in fruits, vegetables, and grains. These antioxidant nutrients are considered the best protection against cancer. As mentioned above, the high-fiber content of plant foods helps keep the digestive tract clean by absorbing and eliminating many potentially dangerous toxins.

A Quick Review of Nutritional Factors in Reversing Cancer

Beta carotene—The precursor of vitamin A, beta carotene is found in carrots, sweet potatoes, spinach, and most leafy green vegetables. A diet high in carotenes, especially beta carotene, is protective against all cancers, but beta carotene is particularly important for women as a deterrent to cervical cancer.[8] Beta carotene has also been shown to protect the lungs against tobacco smoke and smog, thus inhibiting the development of lung cancer.[9] Ex-smokers who ate green and yellow vegetables high in beta carotene every day decreased their risk of stomach and lung cancer.[10]

Vitamin B6—Found in bananas, leafy green vegetables, carrots, apples, organ meats, and sweet potatoes, vitamin B6 is essential for optimal immune function and helps maintain the health of mucous membranes, which line the respiratory tract and provide a natural barrier to pollution and infection. Vitamin B6 also affords protection against cervical cancer.[11]

Vitamin C—Found in citrus fruits, cantaloupe, broccoli, green peppers, and many other fruits and vegetables, vitamin C is integrally involved in the maintenance of a healthy immune system, as well as protecting against a variety of cancers.[12]

Vitamin E—Found in dark green vegetables, eggs, wheat germ, liver, unrefined vegetable oils, and some herbs, vitamin E is a powerful antioxidant that can directly reduce the damage done by ozone smog. It can also help protect against bowel cancer.[13]

Selenium—An essential trace mineral found in fruits and vegetables, selenium helps the body produce glutathione, an enzyme essential for detoxification. Low dietary levels of selenium have been correlated with higher incidence of cancer; accordingly, supplementation of this nutrient acts as a deterrent against cancer in general.[14]

Folic Acid—This substance protects against cervical cancer and is necessary for proper synthesis of RNA and DNA. It is found in beets, cabbage, dark leafy vegetables, eggs, dairy products, citrus fruits, and most fish.[15]

Calcium—This mineral protects against colon cancer and is vital for proper bone formation, blood clotting, and cellular metabolism.[16] It is found in dark green vegetables, most nuts and seeds, milk products, sardines, and salmon.

Iodine—Available in seafood, sea vegetables such as kelp and dulse, and iodized salt, iodine protects against breast cancer and is needed for proper energy metabolism as well as the growth and repair of all tissues.[17]

Magnesium—Found in most nuts, fish, green vegetables, whole grains, and brown rice, magnesium protects against cancer and is necessary to maintain the pH balance of blood and tissues, as well as the synthesis of RNA and DNA.[18]

Zinc—This mineral protects against prostate cancer and is necessary for the formation of RNA and DNA, as well as for healthy immune function.[19] It is found in whole grains, most seafood, sunflower seeds, soybeans, and onions.

Garlic—Garlic or its components can help lower the risk of tumors in the stomach, colon, lung, and esophagus.[20] Research from China has reported that those who eat a great quantity of garlic have much lower rates of stomach cancer.[21]

Omega-3 Fatty Acids—These fats, essential for the proper functioning of all tissues and cells in the body, may inhibit cancer, especially breast cancer.[22] They're found in fish, such as salmon, mackerel, sardines, haddock, and cod, as well as flaxseed oil.

Fiber—Whole grains and other fiber-rich foods are essential to any anticancer diet, as fiber helps facilitate the prompt removal of toxins from the digestive tract. It is important to include a variety of whole grains in the diet because different whole-grain foods contain different kinds of fiber.[23] Consume at least 25-30 g of fiber a day, equivalent to six or more servings of grains and five or more servings of vegetables (including legumes) and fruits.[24]

Success Story: Reversing Prostate Cancer

Millard, 82, was a retired contractor who remained vigorous and active into his eighties. He had fathered 14 children and was still happily married to his wife. Millard came to James W. Forsythe, M.D., H.M.D., of Reno, Nevada, with prostate cancer; previously he had undergone surgery for prostate enlargement, but no signs of cancer were detected at that time. But two years later, a biopsy revealed poorly differentiated prostatic cancer. "This means that under the microscope, the cells look highly malignant as opposed to more benign in appearance," says Dr. Forsythe. Millard's prostate specific antigen (PSA, a prostate cancer marker) was 30, quite high compared to a normal of 0 to 4.

Millard's conventional oncologist offered him the treatment options of radiation therapy, radical prostatectomy, or castration, but he declined all three. By removing his testicles, the oncologist believed all androgen, a male hormone believed to be involved in prostate cancer, would be removed from Millard's body. "He came to me and said he wanted to take therapy he can live with, that won't be toxic to him, and that will meet his lifestyle. Millard is a pretty healthy, vigorous guy: he maintains a garden and every year he and his wife travel."

Even so, at the time of examination, Dr. Forsythe found that Millard's cancer was spreading to his right hip joint. Dr. Forsythe started Millard on anti-androgen therapy with an injection of Zolodex. "It's a conventional medication which he received once a month to 'turn off' the body's androgen," Dr. Forsythe explains. Androgen, or testosterone, is the primary male sex hormone; conventional oncologists believe that prostate cancer cells need testosterone to grow, so that removing or blocking its action, the prostate cancer should begin to shrink and reverse.

For **Dr. Forsythe's cancer protocols**, see *Alternative Medicine Definitive Guide to Cancer* (Future Medicine Publishing, 1997; ISBN 1-887299-01-7); to order, call 800-333-HEAL.

James W. Forsythe, M.D., H.M.D.: Cancer Screening and Treatment Center of Nevada, Hematology-Oncology, Ltd., 75 Pringle Way, Suite 909, Reno, NV 89502; tel: 702-329-5000; fax: 702-329-6219. Also: Century Wellness Center. 380 Brinkby Avenue, Reno, NV 89509; tel: 702-826-9500; fax: 702-329-6219.

In addition, Dr. Forsythe started Millard on a nutritional supplementation program including:
- Vitamin A (as beta carotene): 40,000 IU daily
- Vitamin C: 4 g daily (1 g taken four times)
- Vitamin E: 800 IU, in two divided daily doses
- Selenium: 200 mcg daily
- Calcium: 1 g daily
- Magnesium: 500 mg daily
- Zinc: 50 mg daily
- Flaxseed oil: two tablespoons daily
- Vitamin B complex: twice daily
- Pycnogenol grape seed extract: 200 mg, two times daily
- Echinacea: three capsules daily
- Barley grass: 500 mg, three times daily

Millard also started a vegetarian diet that emphasized fruit juices.

This program brought Millard's PSA down to 4 and, after only two months of treatment, the cancer was "under good control," says Dr. Forsythe. However, about four months after beginning treatment, Millard started having blood in his urine, which turned out to be a sign of bladder cancer that was obstructing his right kidney. Millard went on radiation therapy for three weeks and did a small dose of chemotherapy for four months for this large tumor, but he refused surgery.

The combined treatment was successful, says Dr. Forsythe. "The man today looks 12 years younger. He is without prostate or bladder cancer activity, and his chemistry panel is completely normal."

A Beginner's Guide to Nutritional Supplements

In addition to gaining needed nutrients through a carefully constructed whole-foods diet, the well-considered use of nutritional supplements can reliably fortify your body with the essential nutrients. Today, an estimated 46% of adult Americans take nutritional supplements, many on a daily basis, indicating that more people are taking a proactive approach to their own health care.[25] The annual U.S. expenditures for vitamins is an estimated $1.26 billion.[26]

Research has demonstrated that diet alone is usually not sufficient to supply the nutrients necessary for overall good health. While most experts agree that nutritional supplements are vital for a variety of illnesses, injuries, and age-related problems, vitamin and mineral supplements can also help to maintain optimal physical and psychological health, promote longevity, and prevent chronic disease.

Nutritionists Jeffrey Bland, Ph.D., and D. Lindsey Berkson, M.A., D.C., offer these recommendations for taking nutritional supplements:

■ Take supplements with meals to promote increased absorption. Take fat-soluble vitamins, such as vitamin A, beta carotene, vitamin E, vitamin D, and essential fatty acids with the one daily meal that contains the most fat.

■ Take amino acid supplements on an empty stomach at least an hour before or after a meal; take with fruit juice to help absorption. Whenever using an increased dosage of an isolated amino acid, be sure to supplement it with an amino acid blend.

■ If you become nauseated when you take tablet supplements, consider taking a liquid form, diluted in a beverage.

■ If you become nauseated or ill within an hour after taking nutritional supplements, consider a bowel cleanse or rejuvenation program prior to beginning your nutritional supplementation program.

Anyone currently under medical care, taking medications, or having a history of specific problems should always consult with a physician before making any changes in diet or lifestyle, including the use of supplements. To eliminate guesswork and frustration, consult a qualified health professional trained in nutritional biochemistry to help assess individual needs and develop an effective, personalized program.

The clinical use of nutritional therapies as part of a cancer treatment program should be further researched to validate and substantiate clinical results.

■ If you are taking high doses of supplements, do not take them all at one time; divide them into smaller doses and take throughout the day.

■ Take digestive enzymes with meals to assist digestion. If you are taking pancreatic or other enzymes for other than digesting food—for eliminating toxins, for example—be sure to take them on an empty stomach between meals.

■ Take mineral supplements at a different time than your highest fiber meal of the day, as fiber can decrease mineral absorption.

■ Whenever taking an increased dosage of an isolated B vitamin, be sure to supplement with a complete B complex.

■ When taking nutrients, be sure to drink adequate amounts of purified water or fresh vegetable or fruit juice to mix with digestive juices and prevent side effects.

Nutritional supplements are not a panacea, however, and it is important to be aware of certain potential risks. Prolonged intake of excessive doses of vitamins A, D, niacin, and possibly B6 may produce toxic effects. Other vitamins, minerals, and accessory nutrients can sometimes cause side effects when they interact with conventional drugs or interfere with a person's biochemical individuality. Nutritional supplements should never take the place of proper dietary habits or appropriate medical care when warranted.

Food Nutrients Can Complement Conventional Cancer Treatments

Research shows that nutrients and other biological response modifiers (BRMs) can directly impede tumor growth and metastases.[27] According to Keith I. Block, M.D., at least five lines of BRM research offer solid evidence that alternative therapies need to become integrated into conventional cancer care:

■ Natural killer (NK) cells can stop the spread of cancer cells. Research has shown that NK activity is amplified by supplementation with selenium,[28] germanium,[29] and ascorbic acid.[30] In fact, vegetarians may have double the NK activity of their meat-eating counterparts.[31]

■ Omega-3 fatty acids from fish oils, flaxseed, and certain plants tend to inhibit tumor-promoting substances. Women with high concentrations of omega-3 fatty acids in their breast tissues are five times less likely to develop deadly metastases than other women.[32] These "good fats" have recently been proposed as a standard addition to the treatment of liver cancer.[33]

■ Soybeans and other legumes contain daidzein and genistein, naturally occurring phytoestrogens that may block the action of estrogen, thus slowing the growth of hormonally dependent tumors.[34] Genistein can block the activity of certain oncogenes (SEE QUICK DEFINITION) and has antioxidant, anti-estrogenic, and antitumor activity.[35]

■ The essential oils of citrus fruits, spices, and herbs contain a substance called limonene, which stimulates liver detoxification. Limonene and its derivative, perillyl alcohol, may block both tumor promotion and progression by inhibiting a specific oncogene.[36]

■ The nutrients zinc, selenium, and folate have been shown to stimulate DNA repair enzymes.[37] A lack of these nutrients could be detrimental, since unrepaired mutated DNA in cancer-inhibiting (suppressor) genes can raise cancer risk.

More Antioxidants Mean Less Cancer

For an Italian study, the dietary habits of 2,569 women, aged 20-74, with breast cancer were compared to 2,588 women in the same age range without cancer. Researchers found that the women with cancer had significantly lower intakes of the antioxidants beta carotene, vitamin E, and calcium than the cancer-free women; to a lesser extent, lower intakes of riboflavin, iron, and potassium were also observed in the women with breast cancer, according to the *International Journal of Cancer* (1996).

The Future of Nutritional Medicine in Cancer Care

There is still some prejudice among conventional physicians regarding nutritional therapy for cancer and other diseases. Research has inadequately addressed the use of nutrition as an adjunctive treatment for cancer therapy. For this reason, the technical indications for using nutrition therapy adjunctively in cancer care remain controversial. Counterbalancing this situation, however, is the empirical fact that many physicians have used nutritional therapies successfully against cancer and other serious diseases and have the patient outcomes on record to prove their efficacy.

Increasingly, there is strong consensus regarding the preventive role of diet. This emphasis should be applied directly to the prevention of cancer recurrence after the initial tumor-killing therapies have been successfully employed. Many scientists have begun to outline a scientific rationale for dietary guidelines that may reduce the risk of some types of cancers, such as breast, colon, and prostate.[38] Among the more exciting trends in innovative cancer care is the growing interest in the use of nutritional supplements (primarily antioxidants) and in changing the quantity and quality of dietary fat as an adjunct to breast cancer treatment.

There is considerable evidence that antioxidants, by protecting against free radical–related tumor promotion, can help inhibit some forms of cancer from developing, as well as bolster the immune system.[39] One of the key insights is that the immune system itself, in mounting its response against cancer cells, toxins, and microbes, can produce highly potent and potentially harmful substances such as cytokines and oxidant molecules. Antioxidants are required in sufficient supply to protect the body against these "side effects" of the immune response.[40]

What's holding back greater acceptance of nutritional supplementation in cancer treatment? In most medical schools, students receive only a few hours of instruction on nutrition. As a result, most new doctors have little knowledge of the power of nutrition against disease. Without this knowledge, some feel threatened by patients who begin adopting nutritional strategies outside of their prescribed medical treatment. Further, since conventional medicine has a history of rejecting nutritional intervention, most doctors do not incorporate nutrition in their practices.

Richard P. Huemer, M.D., of Vancouver, Washington, a colleague of Dr. Linus Pauling and a pioneer in the field of orthomolecular medicine, forsees a change. "We need a paradigm shift, and I think it's beginning to occur. Nutrition needs to be looked at not as a means of preventing specific deficiency diseases, but as a means of contributing to the overall health of the person and their resistance to chronic diseases. We have to start looking for the optimum levels of nutrients necessary for optimum health instead of the minimum amount needed to prevent diseases."

A Glossary of Nutritional Supplements for Fighting Cancer

Acidophilus

Acidophilus is a generic term for the *Lactobacilli*, "friendly bacteria" (probiotics) that naturally inhabit the healthy intestine. These bacteria consist mainly of the species *L. acidophilus* or *L. bulgaricus* and *L. casei*; they can markedly enhance nutritional status and have specific and important therapeutic roles.[41] Among their many health-promoting functions, they:

(1) exert direct activity against tumors; (2) prevent cancer by detoxifying or preventing the formation of carcinogenic chemicals; (3) reduce the level of cholesterol, which indirectly aids in cancer resistance; (4) help produce important B vitamins that assist in immunocompetence; (5) curb or destroy potentially pathogenic bacteria and yeasts such as *Candida albicans*; and (6) through their production of lactic acid, preserve and enhance the digestibility of

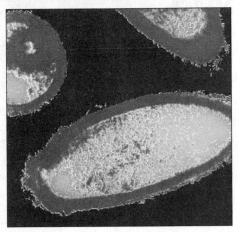

Lactobacilli or "friendly bacteria".

foods that are fermented with them, such as soy products (miso, tamari), sauerkraut, and pickles.[42]

A study of 138 patients with bladder cancer found that those given 1 g of *Lactobacillus* (specifically, *L. casei*) three times a day for 12 months were significantly less likely to develop a recurrence of bladder cancer than those patients receiving the placebo.[43] Other research showed that a derivative of *L. bulgaricus* improved survival among 100 advanced cancer patients.[44]

Amino Acids

Amino acids, the building blocks of protein, can have specific applications for cancer therapy. In humans, we find 22 amino acids that make up proteins (long chains of amino acids) and peptides (short chains of amino acids). Of these, eight are considered to be essential and cannot be made within the body and the rest are considered nonessential, as they can be synthesized within the body from the essential eight amino acids. Since amino acids work as a team, as do the other nutrients in the body, it is important not to be deficient in any of them. If any of the essential amino acids is found lacking, steps should be taken to correct the deficiency either with appropriate food or with amino acid supplementation. In addition, there are a few particular amino acids which play a special role in cancer treatment.

For sources of *acidophilus*, contact: Nature's Way Products, 10 Mountain Springs Parkway, Springville, UT 84663; tel: 800-962-8873 or 801-489-1500. Phillips Nutritional, 27071 Cabot Road #122, Laguna Hills, CA 92653; tel: 800-514-5115 or 702-898-8141. For a source of **amino acids**, contact: Bragg's Liquid Aminos, Live Food Products, Box 7, Santa Barbara, CA 93102; tel: 800-446-1990 or 805-968-1020.

For more about **probiotics as part of a detoxification program**, see Chapter 9: Physical Support Therapies, pp. 254-297.

The amino acid L-arginine may enhance the anticancer activity of cytotoxic T cells, NK cells, and other key immune components.[45] Animals fed a low-arginine diet showed an inability to increase their NK activity; however, when given arginine supplements, their NK activity increased.[46] Other types of white blood cells involved in the body's anticancer defenses are also stimulated by dietary arginine.[47]

Methionine, a sulfur-containing amino acid, when combined with choline, significantly increased the survival of mice with liver cancer.[48] Another sulfur-containing amino acid, cysteine (especially if given as N-acetyl-cysteine), assists in detoxification and reduces the side effects of chemotherapy and radiation treatments.[49] N-acetyl-cysteine is a precursor for the production of glutathione, which serves in the key antioxidant called glutathione peroxidase. Blood levels of glutathione peroxidase are typically lower in patients with malignant cancers.[50]

Reduced L-glutathione is often found in persons with mercury toxicity (such as those with amalgam dental fillings), which may increase cancer risk and progression.[51] Glutathione reduces free-radical damage and prevents depletion of other antioxidants, helps metabolize carcinogens, activates certain immune cells, helps synthesize and repair DNA, and may inhibit angiogenesis, a blood vessel-forming process required for tumor growth.[52] Glutathione supplements also diminish the toxic side effects of radiation and chemotherapy.[53]

Beta Carotene

Beta carotene is the pigment that accounts for much of the color in plants, including most fruits and vegetables. It is converted to vitamin A in concert with the body's needs for the vitamin. As an antioxidant and precursor to vitamin A, beta carotene can enhance the activity of natural killer (NK) cells and other immune cells against tumors.[54] A review of the scientific literature shows that beta carotene has antioxidant and immune-enhancing properties that are not found in vitamin A.[55] The immune system changes caused by beta carotene include a significant increase in T- and B-cell numbers, macrophage activity, interleukin production, and NK cell tumor-killing abilities.[56] There are over 500 naturally occurring carotenoids, of which a large number have been found to be pharmacologically active, such as phycopene, lycopene, and others. These carotenoids work together, so taking high doses of any one of them could offset the activities of the others. For this reason, it may be preferable to supplement with a natural carotenoid complex.

Calcium

Cancer patients may need to take a calcium supplement, particularly if they are suffering from a bone cancer that is causing bone-calcium losses. A 19-year prospective study found that calcium deficiency was associated with a higher risk of colorectal cancer.[57] Numerous animal studies have found that calcium may inhibit colon cancer, and human studies indicate that the mineral may reverse the rapid growth of colon cells.[58] Note that magnesium is involved in the body's uptake of both calcium and potassium, and a magnesium deficiency tends to promote deficiencies in these minerals. For this reason, when taking calcium supplements (which are best absorbed at bedtime), it is a good idea to also supplement with magnesium (which is better taken in the morning).

Chromium

Chromium supplements (either chromium picolinate or chromium polynicotinate) may help people regain normal thyroid function. Chromium forms part of the glucose tolerance factor (GTF), a molecule that assists in the control of blood sugar levels. Anything that helps better regulate blood sugar levels could substantially improve immune function and cancer resistance, since sugar promotes the "bad" eicosanoids, which in turn promote cancer growth.

The United States appears to be a chromium-deficient nation, probably due to overindulgence in refined grain products. Refined foods such as white sugar and white flour are extremely low in chromium since it is lost through refining processes. There is also an additive effect since our body's chromium needs increase in proportion to blood sugar levels; thus higher intakes of simple sugars tend to deplete the body of chromium.[59] Finally, excessive iron intake (either from red meat or iron supplements) can deplete chromium.[60]

Coenzyme Q10 (CoQ10)

CoQ10, also known as ubiquinone, is one of a family of brightly colored substances called quinones that are widely distributed in nature because they are essential for generating energy. The body produces its own coQ10, but usually produces less with aging; therefore dietary sources are important for this coenzyme, especially for older people. It is found in fairly high concentrations in fish (especially sardines), soybean and grapeseed oils, sesame seeds, pistachios, walnuts, and spinach.[61]

CoQ10 plays an important part in the body's antioxidant system. When combined with vitamin E, selenium, and beta carotene, coQ10 can significantly reduce free-radical damage in the liver, kidney, and heart tissues.[62] Another beneficial effect in cancer patients is to increase macrophage activity.[63]

In one study, 90 mg of coenzyme Q10 were given daily to 32 breast cancer patients for two years. All patients survived and six had partial remissions. One of the partial responders then received a high dose of 390 mg of coQ10 daily; within three months, the tumor had completely regressed. The researchers then gave 300 mg of coQ10 to a second breast cancer patient, who showed no evidence of tumor growth or metastasis after three months.[64] More recent findings substantiate the view that supplementation with coQ10 can cause complete regression of tumors in advanced breast cancer, including one patient with numerous metastases to the liver.[65]

Copper

This trace element is essential to proper functioning of a range of immune cells, including antibody-forming cells, T helper cells, and macrophages, all of which may help the body defend against cancer.[66] Copper functions as a cofactor for enzymes that speed up the body's energy-yielding reactions. It is intimately involved in healing processes, maintaining connective tissues, and formation of red blood cells. A deficiency of this element results in a lowered resistance to infections and a shortened life span following infection.[67] Copper also affects inflammation and bears a close relationship with zinc.

Eicosapentaenoic Acid (EPA Fish Oils)

Since copper and zinc are chemically antagonistic, their intake should be carefully controlled under medical supervision. Ingesting too much copper can readily reduce the body's zinc supply and vice versa.

Since EPA fish oil retards normal blood clotting, high doses (more than 5,000-6,000 mg daily) are contraindicated for people anticipating surgery. In addition, long-term supplementation with EPA may induce a deficiency of vitamin E, unless supplements of vitamin E are added.

Essential fatty acids, required for health and proper metabolism, include linoleic acid and alpha-linolenic acid (ALA). These essential fats are found in flaxseed oil and the oils of other seeds, nuts, and vegetables. They play an important role in reducing heart disease and in preventing and treating various cancers.[68]

Although most animal fats are harmful to human health, some, such as those found in fish, are actually helpful. Eicosapentaenoic acid, or EPA, is the primary fatty acid found in most fish oils. Classified as an omega-3 fatty acid, EPA helps maintain the proper levels of beneficial eicosanoids, hormone-like substances that mediate the body's response to cancer and other disease processes. There is evidence that EPA slows tumor growth[69] and reduces the invasiveness of human tumor cells in culture.[70] In addition, EPA improves the response of tumor cells to hyperthermia and chemotherapy.[71] Recent research suggests that EPA may have a beneficial role as an adjunctive treatment for breast cancer.[72]

Flaxseed Oil

About 58% of flaxseed oil (also known as linseed oil) is alpha-linolenic acid (ALA), one of the omega-3 fatty acids. This makes flaxseed the richest source of ALA. This particular omega-3 helps maintain the levels of health-promoting eicosanoids. ALA enhances immune function and cellular oxygen use, thereby helping to dissolve tumors.

A study involving 121 women with localized breast cancer found that those who had low levels of ALA were more likely to have their breast cancer spread to lymph nodes and to have tumors that exhibited an "invasive" quality. After a period of 31 months, researchers found that the 21 women in this group who developed postsurgical metastases into other body tissues were conspicuously low in ALA.[73]

Since flaxseed oil is highly unsaturated, it readily oxidizes when exposed to the open air. If the oil becomes highly oxidized and rancid, it can be dangerous for cancer patients. It has a short shelf life and must be purchased as fresh as possible and always kept tightly sealed in the refrigerator. Never heat or cook cold-pressed (unrefined) flaxseed oil under any circumstances.

Flaxseed oil exerts a strong anticancer effect because it is high in lignans. Once in the gastrointestinal tract, lignans are converted into enterolactone and enterodiol, which are believed to be the compounds in flaxseed with an anticancer effect. Studies showed that subjects receiving flaxseed oil experienced a significant reduction in tumor size and numbers after only 1-2 months. Researchers have found that lignans can bind to estrogen receptors in the body and obstruct the cancer-enhancing effects of estrogen on breast tissue.

ALA works best when mixed directly into sulfur-rich protein foods.[74] A typical recommended amount of pure cold-pressed flaxseed oil per day is 1-2 tablespoons.

Gamma-Linolenic Acid (GLA)

Gamma-linolenic acid, an omega-6 essential fatty acid, can stimulate the production of "good" eicosanoids, which can impede the growth of tumors. GLA can be converted into "good" or "bad" eicosanoids, depending on how much EPA, insulin, and sugar there is in the body at the time of conversion. One study found that GLA supplements provided both subjective and objective improvements in 21 cases of untreatable cancer.[75] When combined with vitamin C, GLA supplementation led to a doubling of the mean survival time for patients with liver cancer.[76] Combinations of GLA and EPA seemed to enhance the destruction of cancer cells.[77]

Under healthy conditions, the human body produces its own GLA through the body's conversion of linoleic acid to GLA. This essential conversion process is inhibited, however, by the following factors: (1) a diet containing high-cholesterol foods; (2) alcohol consumption; (3) zinc deficiency; (4) trans-fatty acids (from margarine, processed oils, and junk foods); (5) viral infections; and (6) the aging process.[78] High-sugar diets may also interfere with the mobilization of GLA from stored fats.[79]

The richest sources of GLA are borage oil, black currant oil, evening primrose oil, and mother's milk. The transformation of GLA into the good eicosanoids is promoted by zinc, vitamin C, and vitamins B3 and B6.

Germanium

This unusual trace element enhances the availability of oxygen to both healthy cells and cancer cells. The latter cannot thrive under oxygen-rich conditions. Germanium blocks or slows the growth of tumors and significantly lengthens survival times in laboratory animals.[80] A study in Japan found that people with inoperable lung cancer who were treated with germanium as well as chemotherapy and/or radiation showed a higher response rate and better survival times, particularly for small-cell lung carcinoma.[81] Not only were metastases reduced, but patients also reported an enhanced quality of life with fewer side effects from treatments.

Gerson Diet Therapy

Max Gerson, M.D. (1881-1959), emigrated from Germany to the United States in the 1930s. Shortly after graduating from the University of Freiburg in 1909, where he specialized in internal medicine and physiological chemistry, Dr. Gerson began to experience severe migraine headaches. By 1919, with his medical practice well established, Dr. Gerson had also found a cure for his migraines by reworking his diet to eliminate salt. After succeeding in this, he found that he was able to treat arthritis, pulmonary tuberculosis, and lupus patients with diet alone; then, in 1928, he took the next leap—treating cancer with diet. "The ideal task of cancer therapy is to restore the function of the oxidizing systems in the entire organism," Dr. Gerson explained. To accomplish this, three factors had to be addressed: first, detoxify the body; second, fortify the system with minerals from the potassium group; and third, continuously introduce oxidizing enzymes until the body's own ability to produce them is reactivated.

Dr. Gerson understood that cancer cells grow in conditions of limited or no oxygen and through fermentation. "The malignancies in human beings continuously fall back deeper and deeper into fermentation," he said. Regarding potassium, Dr. Gerson stated that in a sick body, and particularly in one that has cancer, potassium is inactive, and sodium and related minerals exist in an unfavorable chemical state.[82]

As he explained it, in chronic diseases such as cancer, sodium and calcium invade particular organs and cause their potassium to leach out. "From my own clinical experiments, I have learned that it is necessary to change the intake of proteins, enzymes, vitamins, etc., simultaneously to activate all natural healing forces which we need for our therapy."

Dr. Gerson further noted that cancer is not caused by a single deficiency. "Cancer is an accumulation of numerous damaging factors combined in deteriorating the whole metabolism, after the liver has been progressively impaired." Treatment must restore these functions so that the body's immune response, including the liver, can function appropriately again, Dr. Gerson said. Fundamental among these functions is the "production, activation, and reactivation of oxidizing enzymes" capable of raising the level of oxygen in the cells.[83]

Dr. Gerson believed that cancer would not occur in bodies with a properly balanced and functioning liver, pancreas, thyroid, and immune system. In his approach, thyroid extracts seem to enable the body to fight cancer more effectively by stimulating liver and thyroid function. Coffee enemas are used as needed for pain reduction, appetite stimulation, and liver detoxification; patients take 3-4 coffee enemas a day for detoxification and pain relief. Enemas of chamomile tea or castor oil are also used.

There is also supplementation with pepsin (an enzyme), potassium, iodine, niacin, pancreatin (a digestive enzyme culled from bovine pancreas), and vitamin C. The Gerson program includes salt and sodium restriction and potassium supplementation; high doses of micronutrients, especially through raw fruit and vegetable juices; severe restrictions on fat intake; and a reduction in protein intake by adopting a vegetarian diet. Dr. Gerson also restricted tobacco, sharp spices, tea, coffee, chocolate, alcohol, refined sugar and flour, all processed or canned foods, nuts, mushrooms, soybeans, pickles, cucumbers, pineapples, and all berries (except red currants).

Regarding potassium supplementation, Dr. Gerson recommended four teaspoons in juice ten times daily in a specific chemical formulation he developed. Dr. Gerson also recommended high doses of Lugol's solution (iodine plus potassium iodide) and thyroid extract, which he believed went directly to the tumor.

With his low-fat, nearly vegan dietary regime, Dr. Gerson found that he could reverse the majority of cancer in patients. Small amounts of dairy products are permitted on this diet. The caloric limit is 2,600–3,200 calories per day. Patients on the Gerson program supplement their main diet ten times a day with freshly cut fruit (primarily apples) and vegetable juices (primarily carrot), taken at hourly intervals. This inundates the body with the living nutrients from nearly 20 pounds of fresh, organic foods. In addition, there are large amounts of oranges, grapes, grapefruits, and tomatoes.

As mentioned previously, Dr. Gerson discovered that cancer patients had an excess of sodium far outweighing the potassium in their bodies; the two normally exist in a specific balance to each other. Sodium acts as a poison in the body because it is an enzyme inhibitor, whereas potassium is an enzyme activator. The fruits and vegetables in the Gerson diet help correct the sodium and potassium imbalance which, in turn, helps revitalize the liver so it can again rid the body of malignant cells.

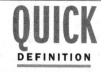

For more about **Gerson Therapy,** contact: The Gerson Research Organization, 7807 Artesian Road, San Diego, CA, 92127-2117, tel: 800-759-2966; fax: 619-759-2967. Max Gerson Memorial Cancer Center of CHIPSA, 670 Nubes, Playas de Tijuana, Mexico. The Gerson Institute, P.O. Box 430, Bonita, CA 91908-0430; tel: 619-585-7600; fax: 619-585-7610.

QUICK
DEFINITION

Staging in cancer terminology is a relative index of how much cancer exists in the body, its size, location, and containment or metastasis. Stage I, the earliest, most curable stage, shows only local tumor involvement. Stage II indicates some spreading of cancer to the surrounding tissues and perhaps to nearby lymph nodes. Stage III involves metastasis to distant lymph nodes. Stage IV, the most advanced and least easily cured, means the cancer has spread to distant organs.

Gar Hildenbrand of the Gerson Research Organization and Shirley Cavin from the University of California at San Diego's Cancer Prevention and Control Program compared five-year melanoma survival rates of Gerson therapy patients to rates found in comparable, conventionally treated groups. The study examined 153 cancer patients, 25 to 72 years old, in various stages of melanoma.[84] Here is a summary of the results:

■ Of patients with Stage I and II melanoma (localized), 100% of Gerson therapy patients survived for five years compared with 79% of patients receiving conventional treatment.

■ Of patients with Stage IIIa melanoma (regionally metastasized), 82% of Gerson therapy patients were still alive at five years compared with 39% of the conventionally treated patients.

■ Of patients with Stage IIIa and IIIb melanoma (regionally metastasized), 70% of Gerson therapy patients were still alive at five years compared with 41% of the conventionally treated patients.

■ Of patients with Stage IVa melanoma (a classification proposed by the authors to cover distant metastases), 39% of Gerson therapy patients survived for five years compared with 6% of patients treated by conventional medicine.[85]

Even considering possible weaknesses in the study's design, the substantial differences in survival between the Gerson patients and conventional patients is too great to be dismissed.

Inositol

This natural substance, an unofficial member of the B vitamin family, is found in virtually all body cells, where it plays important roles in sending signals between cells and their environment. Inositol hexaphosphate is a key phytochemical present in high-fiber foods and can be isolated from legumes, cereal grains, and citrus fruits. In the body, inositol helps the liver remove excess fat from tissues; this prevents liver stagnation from fat and bile buildup. John Potter, Ph.D., a researcher at Fred Hutchinson Cancer Research Center in Seattle, Washington, has identified inositol hexaphosphate as having shown anticancer activity.[86] It may be one of the key reasons why a high-fiber diet has a protective effect against cancer.[87]

For more on **Inositol**, see "IP-6—Can a Vitamin Help Reverse Cancer?" *Alternative Medicine* #26 (October/November 1998), pp. 79-83; www.alternativemedi-cine.com

Iodine

Iodine has anticarcinogenic properties[88] and may help protect against breast cancer.[89] Iodine may also lower one's cancer risk by fortifying the thyroid gland.[90] Iodine deficiency is the second most common malnutrition in the world, with about 400 million people suffering from this condition. Iodine is part of the structure of the thyroid hormones T3 and T4, which regulate the body's energy usage and numerous body functions.

Iodine's effects are far-reaching, since the metabolism of all the body's cells—except for brain cells—is influenced by thyroid hormones. White blood cells may use the conversion of iodide to iodine to produce free radicals, which help kill infectious organisms.[91] This is particularly important in advanced-cancer patients, many of whom die from infections because their immune systems are depressed.

Kelley's Metabolic Therapy

Individualized nutrition, detoxification, and the use of pancreatic enzymes make up the therapy advanced by William Donald Kelley, D.D.S. A dentist by training, Dr. Kelley developed his protocol in response to his own pancreatic cancer, which he reversed in the late 1960s. Dr. Kelley called his program "metabolic ecology" to indicate that the patient's entire way of life must be changed. "The person who has the disease should be treated, not the disease that has the person," he explained.

One of the main points of Dr. Kelley's therapy is that cancer is often caused by the body's inability to effectively metabolize protein;

The Ten Metabolic Types

Dr. Kelley classified patients into ten metabolic types, with slow-oxidizing vegetarians at one end and fast-oxidizing carnivores at the other, and, more precisely, according to the involvement and efficiency of the sympathetic or parasympathetic nervous system, and with respect to their relationship. These classifications may be generalized as follows:

- extreme sympathetic dominant, but efficient
- extreme parasympathetic dominant, but efficient
- balanced but inefficient
- balanced and efficient
- inefficient sympathetic
- inefficient parasympathetic
- requiring cooked foods
- average/healthy, requiring well-balanced meals
- sympathetic dominant (but less strongly so than earlier similar category)
- parasympathetic dominant (again, less strongly so than earlier similar category)

this inability can be linked to improper amounts of proteolytic enzymes. According to Dr. Kelley, these protein-digesting pancreatic enzymes, rather than the immune system, are the body's first defense against tumors. This led him to declare that, fundamentally, cancer is a deficiency of pancreatic enzymes; this deficiency then leads to a disordering of protein metabolism, and from there, to the proliferation of abnormal cells. He believed that excessive protein intake is the most significant cause of pancreatic enzyme deficiency.

His metabolic detoxification therapy calls for coffee enemas, restricting of protein intake, and emphasizing a diet of whole grains, fruits, and vegetables supplemented with proteolytic enzymes and raw juices. Dr. Kelley advised cancer patients to altogether avoid pasteurized milk, peanuts, white flour and sugar, chlorinated water, and all processed foods. He recommended that the diet consist of about 70% raw foods, such as fresh raw salads, to maximize the consumption of living enzymes. Dr. Kelley developed a line of 25 nutritional formulations for hard tumors (solid mass cancers) and 29 for soft tumors (leukemia, lymphoma, melanoma) which the patient takes until they are cancer free for two years.

Manganese

Manganese helps maintain the structural integrity of heart and kidney cell membranes and promotes tissue oxygen uptake, food absorption, neurotransmitter synthesis, insulin synthesis, fat and carbohydrate metabolism, and blood-clotting mechanisms.[92] It is part of the main antioxidant enzyme, superoxide dismutase, and there is some evidence that it may help to counteract the immune-suppressive effects of stress hormones. Manganese may increase the activities of white blood cells.[93]

Molybdenum
This trace element is required in tiny amounts for human health—the official recommended daily allowance (RDA) is 150-500 mcg daily. Molybdenum is an essential part of at least three key enzyme systems and supports the liver's detoxification of sulfites (in many preservatives), alcohol, aldehydes (a toxic by-product of metabolizing various chemicals), and copper-containing compounds.[94] A molybdenum deficiency is associated with cancer of the esophagus.[95]

Orthomolecular Medicine
In 1968, Nobel Prize–winner Linus Pauling, Ph.D., coined the term *orthomolecular* to describe an approach to medicine that uses naturally occurring substances normally present in the body. Orthomolecular physicians recognize that in many cases of physiological and psychological disorders, health can be reestablished by correcting the balance of vitamins, minerals, amino acids, and other such substances within the body.

Most conventional physicians still disregard the relationship of correct nutrition to health. The prevalent notion is that a "balanced" diet will provide the nutrients one needs, but what is overlooked is that most food is grown in nutritionally depleted soil, then highly processed. Orthomolecular physicians recognize these factors and know that biochemical individuality can play a crucial role in health.

The concept of biochemical individuality is based on the work of Roger J. Williams, Ph.D. Dr. Williams realized that each individual is nutritionally unique and requires variations in nutrient intake to function optimally. His concept of biochemical individuality relies on physiological data, as well as personal and family health history, dietary analysis, and biochemical screenings to determine a person's unique biochemical and nutritional status.

Although meeting RDAs for nutrients may prevent incidences of severe deficiency that lead to disease, orthomolecular physicians contend that these levels do not provide for optimal health, and people may need many more times the RDAs. Richard Kunin, M.D., of San Francisco, California, summarizes the principles of orthomolecular medicine in this way:[96]

■ Nutrition comes first in medical diagnosis and treatment, and nutrient-related disorders are usually curable once nutritional balance is achieved.

- Biochemical individuality is the norm in medical practice; therefore, universal RDA values are unreliable nutrient guides. Many people, because of genetic disposition and/or the environment in which they live, require certain nutrients far beyond the RDA (often called a megadose).
- Drug treatment is to be used only for specific indications and always mindful of potential adverse effects.
- Environmental pollution and food adulteration are inescapable facts of modern life, and avoiding them is a medical priority.
- Blood tests do not necessarily reflect tissue levels of nutrients.
- Hope is the indispensable ally of the physician and the absolute right of the patient.

The basis of orthomolecular medicine lies in creating a thoroughly healthy diet. Junk foods, refined sugar, and food additives are eliminated; every effort is made to eat nutritious whole foods, high in fiber and low in fat. Depending on the health condition, vitamins, minerals, and other nutrients are taken as supplements; the types and amounts of these nutrients are determined by blood tests, urine analysis, and nutrient-level assays. Supplementation is based not only on a patient's symptoms, but on results reported in medical journals and the clinical experience of the doctor.

Prescribed doses of vitamins are sometimes injected to speed the initial response, and follow-up treatment usually consists of vitamin pills several times a day until adequate dosage is achieved. Mentioned above, this dosage has often been called a "megadose" because the amounts of nutrients taken are often far greater than the levels needed to prevent deficiency. As a result, orthomolecular medicine has also been called "megavitamin therapy."

Potassium

As pioneering cancer doctor Max Gerson, M.D., found, raising the body's potassium supply seems to help counteract tumor growth. In addition, research shows that by controlling salt and water content at the cellular level, cellular function, energy production, and overall biological integrity can be improved or restored. Chinese studies indicate that high-potassium, low-sodium environments can partially return damaged cell proteins to their normal undamaged configuration.

Selenium

This trace element has a synergistic relationship with vitamin E, meaning that the two nutrients mutually reinforce the body's anti-cancer defenses. An integral part of the body's antioxidant enzyme system (glutathione peroxidase), selenium has key effects on DNA metabolism, cell membrane integrity, and optimal functioning of the liver and pancreas. As such, it can interfere with both the initiation and promotion phases of cancer development. Glutathione peroxidase protects tissues against free-radical damage, and its anti-cancer effects are dependent on the availability of selenium.[97]

According to biochemist Gerhard Schrauzer, Ph.D., selenium is often deficient in cancer patients.[98] This fact is significant, since even small doses of selenium have been found to greatly enhance the cancer-fighting activity of natural killer (NK) cells in laboratory animals.[99] Selenium supplements have been shown to impede the reappearance of tumors in animals whose tumors regressed following ovariectomy.[100] Many chemotherapeutic drugs and various heavy metals (lead, mercury, cadmium) tend to inactivate selenium, making it unavailable to the body.[101]

Antioxidants Stop Spread of Cancer

A Scottish study of 50 men, half of them cigarette smokers, demonstrated clearly that nutritional supplementation with antioxidants such as vitamins C, E, and beta carotene for up to 20 weeks had a "highly significant moderating effect" on DNA damage done by free radicals, according to *Cancer Research* (March 15, 1996). In particular, the antioxidants were able to stop the spread of cancer (metastasis) caused by the generation of free radicals. DNA taken from invasive, spreading cancer was shown to have twice as much free radical-caused DNA damage.

Vitamin A

This fat-soluble vitamin, which exists primarily in the form of retinol, has repeatedly been shown to enhance the activity of immune cells against tumor cells.[102] Research seems to indicate that vitamin A's greatest benefit is in preventing cancers or recurrences of cancer. Accutane (13-cis-retinoic acid) is a pharmaceutical derivative of vitamin A, and has proven effective "in preventing second primary tumors in patients who have been treated for squamous-cell carcinoma of the head and neck, although it does not prevent recurrence of the original [type of] tumor."[103]

In one study, nine men with an untreatable form of lung cancer (metastatic, squamous-cell lung carcinoma) were given vitamin A palmitate (a form of vitamin A) without other medical intervention. Fifteen months later, the men's immune function had improved and significant progress against the tumor had been made.[104]

Vitamin B Complex

This group of B vitamins, which includes B1, B2, B3, B6, folic acid, and pantothenic acid, acts as a biochemical team to help speed up chemical reactions and support overall energy metabolism. Deficiencies of any one of the B vitamins inhibit the immune system's ability to fight cancer.[105] Both pantothenic acid and vitamin B6 have been shown to inhibit the growth of tumors.[106] A B6 deficiency depresses numerous aspects of immune function, including T-cell activity and antibody responsiveness.[107] Cancer patients are frequently deficient in folic acid, which has been shown to inhibit the growth of tumors.[108] Vitamins B1 (thiamin) and B2 (riboflavin) are more indirect immune-system supporters and primarily serve in the maintenance of mucous membranes, formation of red blood cells, and metabolism of carbohydrates. The B-complex vitamins are typically used to maintain proper functioning of the immune and nervous systems and to reinforce the effects of B vitamins taken separately.

Vitamin B3 (Niacin)
There is growing evidence that vitamin B3, also known as niacin or nicotinic acid, may increase the efficacy of cancer treatment. This vitamin exists in nature primarily in the form of coenzymes NAD and NADP, which are required by more than 150 enzymes involved in respiration and the transfer of electrons. Without these enzymatic reactions, our body's energy production would shut down. Max Gerson, M.D., founder of the Gerson Therapy, successfully treated many cancer patients with a dietary regimen that included 50 mg of niacin 8-10 times per day.[109] Good dietary sources of niacin include brewer's yeast, fish, asparagus, and whole grains.

Vitamin B6 (Pyridoxine)
The immune and nervous systems are strongly influenced by the systemic supply of this B vitamin, which aids in DNA/RNA synthesis, metabolism, hemoglobin function, and tryptophan production (which affects mood and alertness).[110] Vitamin B6 has been shown to inhibit the growth of various tumors,[111] including liver cancer.[112] Vitamin B6 is also essential in the production of prostaglandin E1, which is necessary for normal thymus function and regulation of T cells. When vitamin B6 was given to 33 bladder cancer patients, there was a marked reduction in recurrence rates.[113] There is evidence that vitamin B6 helps protect against the toxic side effects of radiation treatment.[114]

Vitamin C (Ascorbic Acid)
Found in citrus fruits, broccoli, green peppers, and many other

fruits and vegetables, vitamin C is involved in the maintenance of a healthy immune system as well as protecting against a variety of cancers.[115] There is now solid evidence that this vitamin is essential for optimal functioning of the immune system.[116] Among immune components involved in fighting cancer are the natural killer (NK) cells, which are only active if they contain relatively large amounts of vitamin C.[117] Vitamin C also boosts the body's production of interferon, which has anticancer activity.[118]

Hugh Riordan, M.D., director of the Center for Human Functioning in Wichita, Kansas, notes that vitamin C increases intracellular peroxidases, enzymes that help protect the cell against free radicals.[119] Dr. Riordan also states that vitamin C is 20 to 30 times more toxic to cancer cells than to normal cells. Cancer patients taking vitamin C report an improved appetite and mental outlook, as well as a decrease in pain and the need for painkilling drugs.[120] Other research shows that vitamin C enhances the anticancer activity of some chemotherapy drugs, including Adriamycin;[121] the vitamin enhances the effects of radiation treatment and protects healthy tissues during such treatment.[122]

Vitamin C's Cancer Protection

Current studies lend strong support to the importance of vitamin C in slowing the development of cancer, cataracts, and heart disease. A recent study, conducted by James E. Enstrom, M.D., an epidemiologist at the University of California at Los Angeles, suggests that men who consume vitamin C every day, at levels that are 500%-666% of the U.S. RDA, live about six years longer than men who do not.[126]

A separate review by Gladys Block, Ph.D., an epidemiologist of the National Cancer Institute's Divison of Cancer Prevention and Control, found a statistically significant benefit in 33 of 46 studies.[127] She concluded that vitamin C affords added protection against cancers of the colon, rectum, pancreas, bladder, lung, larynx, oral cavity, esophagus, stomach, cervix, brain, endometrium, and breast.

Although vitamin C has extremely low toxicity even at high doses, certain side effects may occur.

This water-soluble vitamin has shown an ability to selectively kill tumor cells in a manner similar to chemotherapy drugs.[123] Vitamin C combined with various B vitamins may significantly limit tumor growth without harming the body's normal tissues.[124] A daily dose of 10 g (10,000 mg, spread throughout the day) of vitamin C significantly extended the survival and improved the quality of life in 100 cancer patients in Scotland.[125]

Vitamin C is usually started at between 4-6 g a day, in divided doses. This daily dosage is then increased until bowel tolerance is attained. The dosage is then reduced to just below that level and maintained for several months or preferably lifelong. On rare occasions, cancer patients with rapidly growing malignant tumors and a heavy tumor load taking vitamin C will show a sudden increase in tumor necrosis (the death of cancer cells causing toxic accumulation), a potentially fatal complication calling for careful treatment.[128] One study found that vitamin C enhanced leukemia development in some human leukemia cell lines, though it had the opposite effect in other leukemia cell lines.[129] Until more is known, patients with leukemia should be cautious about taking vitamin C, particularly in large doses.

Vitamin D

This vitamin, also classified as a hormone, appears to have cancer-killing properties.[130] Though research findings are still preliminary, vitamin D may inhibit the formation of new tumor blood vessels, induce the conversion of cancer cells back to normal cells (cell differentiation), and induce "cell suicide" (apoptosis) in cancer cells.[131] Researchers in Australia concluded that vitamin D may protect the body against prostate cancer, based on the fact that there are more cases of prostate cancer in northern areas such as Iceland, Denmark, and Sweden, where there is limited natural sunlight, compared to areas of more, sustained sunlight.[132]

CAUTION
In general, vitamin D should be reserved for cancer patients with low vitamin D levels; moreover, the patient must be carefully monitored to avoid toxicity.

Vitamin D may be given in the range of 400 IU to 1,000 IU daily. Note that vitamin D manufactured in the skin by the influence of sunlight will not cause toxicity, no matter how much sun exposure an individual receives. The body automatically shuts down its own vitamin D production once the requirement is reached, typically within 15 minutes of exposure to sunshine.

Vitamin E

This fat-soluble vitamin, one of the body's primary agents for protecting cell membranes, is also among the major nutrients required for strong immune responses to cancer and infection.[133] One study found that, for 43 patients with oral leukoplakia (a premalignant condition) who were given 400 IU of vitamin E twice daily for 24 weeks, nearly half (46%) showed significant clinical improvement.[134] In animal studies, the vitamin has reversed the development of chemically induced tumors[135] and has even been shown to prevent tumor development, suggesting a role in warding off recurrences of cancer.[136]

Vitamin E boosts the effectiveness of chemotherapy agents on tumors,[137] but lack of vitamin E increases the toxic effects of Adriamycin (a common chemotherapy agent) on heart tissue.[138] In addition, vitamin E helps protect against the toxic effects of radiation treatments.[139] Many physicians have begun to recommend the succinate form of vitamin E, which seems to enter cells more readily.

Vitamin K

This vitamin's primary function is as a coagulating factor, a nutrient that aids in blood clotting. There is some evidence that vitamin K, probably in the form of vitamin K3 (menadione), is effective as an anticancer agent. This form of the vitamin can be toxic, in contrast to the preferred nontoxic form, vitamin K1 (phylloquinone or phytonadione). A growing body of evidence indicates that vitamin K1 supplements enhance the antimetastatic effects of anticoagulant factors in the body.[140] In addition, severe vitamin K deficiency has been found in cancer patients receiving prescription antimicrobial antibiotics. A 1-mg-per-day oral dosage of vitamin K1 (phytonadione) should not represent any hazard to patients receiving anticoagulant therapy.

The injectable form of vitamin K that is administered to babies born in U.S. hospitals contains phenol, a known allergen and carcinogen. Unless you have a hereditary tendency toward blood coagulation problems, we do not recommend using injectable vitamin K, as there is some evidence that this may contribute to childhood cancers. Japanese doctors use the oral form of vitamin K, and many European physicians are increasingly following suit.

Water

Pure water is an integral part of anticancer nutrition. Determine the quality of water in your home by asking the water department for standards and analysis. Verify the condition of your home's water lines, because lead can leach out of the soldering on older water pipes into tap water. Drinking bottled water is a viable alternative, but be careful about the source—many waters are simply repackaged city supplies. Choose only those waters that provide a full analysis of their contents and sources, and look for waters that have been purified through deionization. Such brands are labeled "distilled" or "purified by reverse osmosis."

There are three basic types of water filtration systems:

■ **Solid block carbon filters**—appear to be much more effective in removing organic chemicals such as solvents and trihalomethanes than activated granular carbon filters. If you prefer to leave dissolved minerals in your water, carbon block filters are recommended because they do not remove these inorganic compounds.

■ **Reverse osmosis systems**—force water under pressure through a membrane. They are most effective against inorganic pollutants like nitrate and against metals like lead; deionization resins are also used to accomplish this purpose.

■ **Distillation**—purifies water by boiling and condensing it. Metals and inorganic compounds are effectively removed in this way because they are heavier and have a much higher boiling temperature, but some organic compounds may not be removed.

The best systems combine several methods of filtration for optimal pollutant removal, such as carbon block filtration combined with reverse osmosis, which is effective against organic and inorganic pollutants, as are carbon block and distillation combinations. Since it has been estimated that approximately 70% of all pollutants that enter the body from water come in through the skin during bathing or showering, it would be wise to use a good quality showerhead filter (with a combination carbon and KDF ion resin).

Microwater—This is a new water filtration system with potential therapeutic benefits, originally developed in Japan. Microwater uses a technology that filters and enhances the quality of water by making the size of water molecules smaller. The Microwater unit uses a carbon-activated filter to remove impurities from the water, then it injects a small electrical charge that separates the water into two kinds: acidic water (with positive ions) useful for topical, external uses; and alkaline water (with negative ions) for drinking.

Based on early reports from African and South American users, acidic Microwater acts as a "superoxidant" to disinfect and sterilize surfaces, skin, wounds, even surgical instruments. It can kill bacteria and viruses, it can promote the healing of acne, eczema, sore throats, and blisters, and it can improve skin quality. Acording to Hidemistu Hayashi, M.D., one of Japan's foremost Microwater researchers, alkaline Microwater can act as a powerful antioxidant in the body, destroying harmful free radicals. Dr. Hayashi reports that he and his colleagues have seen improvements in diabetes, constipation, ulcers, blood pressure, allergies, circulation, migraines, obesity, osteoporosis, and menstrual irregularities.

Zinc

This trace element is occasionally recommended as a temporary supplement (30-60 mg per day), but it should never be used routinely by itself. Zinc supports many aspects of the immune system and its deficiency can potentially make you more vulnerable to certain cancers.[141] Zinc is necessary for the free radical–quenching activity of superoxide dismutase (SOD), a powerful antioxidant enzyme. A deficiency of zinc can lead to depressed activity of NK cells and other white blood cells.[142]

Zinc has an antagonistic relationship with copper—an excess of one can cause a deficiency of the other. Both are essential to proper functioning of a wide range of immune cell types, including antibody-forming cells, T helper cells, and macrophages, which help the body defend against cancer.[143]

5 Herbs for Cancer

HERBS, OR BOTANICALS, contain a large number of naturally occurring chemicals that have biological activity. In the past 150 years, chemists and pharmacists have been isolating and purifying active compounds from plants in an attempt to produce safe and effective pharmaceutical drugs. Examples include digoxin (from foxglove, *Digitalis purpurea*), reserpine (from Indian snakeroot, *Rauwolfia serpentina*), colchicine (from autumn crocus, *Colchicum autumnale*), morphine (from the opium poppy, *Papaver somniafera*), and many more.

According to Andrew Weil, M.D., herb and plant derivatives reach the bloodstream and target organs by an indirect route, which means that their effects are usually slower and less dramatic than those of purified drugs. "Doctors and patients accustomed to the rapid, intense effects of synthetic medicines may become impatient with botanicals for this reason," Dr. Weil states.

But this delayed response is a relatively minor issue compared to what botanical medicine has to offer when used to facilitate healing in chronic health problems. Through skillful selection of an herb (or herbs in combination) targeted to the individual patient, major changes in health can be effected with less danger of the side effects inherent in drug-based medicine. However, the common assumption that herbs act slowly and mildly is not necessarily true; adverse effects can occur if an inadequate dose, a low-quality herb, or the wrong herb is prescribed.

In recent years, a great deal of pharmaceutical research has gone into analyzing the active ingredients of herbs to find out how and why they work—an effect referred to as the herb's action. Herbal actions indicate the ways in which the remedy affects human physiology. In some cases, the action is due to a specific chemical present in the herb or it may be due to complex synergistic interactions among various constituents of the plant. In the case of cancer, botanical agents work by:

- stimulating DNA repair mechanisms (via sulfur-containing compounds)

- producing antioxidant effects (via the quenching of free radicals by carotenoids and polyphenols)

- promoting induction of protective enzymes (e.g., proteases)

- inhibiting cancer-activating enzymes (via flavonols and tannins)

- inducing oxygenating effects (via flavonols and rare elements such as germanium).

The Herbal Foundation of Effective Cancer Therapy

Herbal medicine, also known as botanical medicine, phytotherapy, or phytomedicine, is the science of using plants medicinally. An herb can be the whole plant, leaf, flower, stem, seed, root, fruit, bark, or any other part deemed useful for its medicinal, food flavoring, or fragrant property. In many traditional medical systems, the different parts of each plant are known to have specific therapeutic properties, which were discovered only after many centuries of trial-and-error observation.

James A. Duke, Ph.D., notes that more than 25% of prescription drugs and other medications used today are derived from (or at least based on) substances naturally found in plants.[1] Out of an estimated 250,000 to 500,000 plants in existence today, only about 5,000 have been extensively studied for their medicinal applications. "[This] illustrates the need for modern medicine and science to turn its attention to the plant world once again to find new medicine that might cure

Herbs Covered in This Chapter

- Algae (chlorella, sea vegetables, green concentrates)
- Aloe vera
- Amygdalin/laetrile
- Astragalus
- Cat's claw
- Echinacea
- Essiac
- Flavonoids
- Garlic
- *Ginkgo biloba*
- Ginseng
- Grape seed extract/pycnogenols
- Green tea
- Haelan 851
- HANSI
- Hoxsey herbs
- Iscador (mistletoe)
- Larch arabinogalactan
- Maitake mushroom
- Pau d'arco
- Pectin, modified citrus
- Silymarin
- Turmeric

cancer and many other diseases," says Norman R. Farnsworth, Ph.D., Professor of Pharmacology at the University of Illinois at Chicago. "Considering that 121 prescription drugs come from only 90 species of plants, and that 74% of these were discovered following up native folklore claims," Farnsworth adds, "a logical person would have to say that there may still be more jackpots out there."

For example, the conventional anticancer drugs vincristine sulfate and vinblastine sulfate are alkaloids derived from the Madagascar periwinkle (*Catharanthus roseus*) traditionally used in whole, dried form by native healers of Madagascar. Though *Catharanthus* is not employed directly as herbal medicine for cancer, some physicians have begun to use it in homeopathic and "microdose" forms.

Another herb that has been incorporated into the chemotherapy arsenal is the dried root of the mayapple (*Podophyllum peltatum*) and Himalayan mayapple (*Podophyllum hexandrum*). A derivative of this plant has been administered intravenously in treating testicular and ovarian cancers, lymphomas, small-cell lung cancers, and certain forms of leukemia.[2] Sales of the drug, called podophyllotoxin, reached $100 million a year in 1990—the same year the plant was listed as an endangered species.

Among the more recent entries onto the anticancer herbal stage are the following:

Betulinic Acid from Birch Trees—This substance blocked the growth of human melanoma tumors that were transferred to mice, all without harming normal cells.[3] Tests in human cancer cell cultures indicated effectiveness against cancers of the lymph, lung, and liver as well.[4] Betulin, a compound that can be converted to betulinic acid, is a major constituent of white-barked birch trees, which are found in abundance throughout the northern hemisphere.

Some 3,000 or more plant species have been used in alternative and traditional treatments of cancer; the bulk of these remedies come from the rich history and practice of traditional Chinese medicine. Given the gross lack of funding for alternative medical research, however, it may be decades before these herbs are definitively tested as anticancer agents. In the meantime, people with cancer would stand to benefit from the seasoned advice and insights of doctors who are knowledgeable about the medicinal use of botanicals.

Thuja Tincture from "Tree of Life"—*Thuja occidentalis* (arbor vitae, or tree of life) has served as a successful adjunctive herbal therapy for many cancer cases. An 86-year-old woman had been suffering for 14 years from a large orange-sized tumor in her right breast. It had spread to the lymph nodes and doctors labeled it "inoperable, stage III breast carcinoma with lymph metastases." The tumor had never been treated. The woman was given tamoxifen, an estrogen blocker, as well as a tincture of *Thuja* herbal extract (20 drops, three times daily), echinacea (one tablet, three times daily), and various vitamins and minerals. She also applied *Thuja* cream locally and later took comfrey, passionflower, sweet violet, cleavers (bedstraw), and chickweed. After one month, the abnormal lymph nodules had disappeared and the tumor was softening; six months later the tumor had shrunk by 25%; after another six months, no sign of cancer remained.[5]

Bromelain from Pineapple—Bromelain, a mixture of proteases and other enzymes isolated from pineapple stems and fruit, has been used for centuries to treat inflammatory disease and other health problems. More recently, its anticancer activity has attracted the interest of scientists. Bromelain has been shown to induce differentiation of three leukemia cell lines (in culture) as well as to stimulate the anticancer defenses (monocyte and macrophage cell-killing activity) and to inhibit cancer cell growth.[6] The report cites these effects as a possible explanation for the observed tumor-killing potential of bromelain when combined with chemotherapy, and notes that such effects are seen even after oral administration. However, rectal administration of bromelain may be preferable for greatest effect.

> ## Low Cost of Herbs
>
> A major reason for the current government-level interest in herbs is to lower health-care costs, according to the *Medical Tribune* (January 1995). Botanicals can treat migraines at 10¢-25¢ per day compared to $2-$8 for conventional prescriptions. For lowering cholesterol, coated garlic tablets cost 15¢ per day compared to $4 for a prescription drug. Given that no new conventional anticancer therapy has emerged in over 20 years of dedicated research, looking to botanicals may "provide some light in the otherwise dark cancer tunnel."

Phenolic Antioxidants from Mint—Members of the mint family contain special antioxidant compounds that seem to be even more effective than vitamin E (perhaps the premier antioxidant) in helping to prevent recurrences of tumors. An example of these phenolic compounds is rosmarinic acid, which is found in high levels in some mints, including wild self-heal (*Prunella vulgaris*), long deemed by Native Americans and traditional Chinese doctors to be a major herbal medicine.[7]

Centella Extract from Gotu Kola (*Hydrocotyle centella*)—This nutrient-rich herb is said to neutralize and remove toxins, improve mental functioning, and help prevent a nervous breakdown.[8] Scientists at the

Amala Cancer Research Center in Kerala, India, found that gotu kola showed a strong ability to kill cultured cancer cells. They also showed that centella extract more than doubled the life span of mice with tumors and showed a remarkable lack of toxicity even in doses far in excess of those used for therapeutic benefit.[9]

Perillyl Alcohol from Lavender Flowers—The oil of lavender contains a cancer-fighting component called perillyl alcohol. This substance, which is also a derivative of the citrus oil limonene, has been shown in animal studies to inhibit more than 80% of all chemically induced breast cancers. It is thought that the compound blocks tumor growth by inhibiting the gene believed to initiate cancer.[10]

Pollen from Honeybees—Pollen is the male sex cell from a plant; bees pick up this substance when they enter flowers in search of nectar. Research dating back to 1948 found that animals whose diets were supplemented with bee pollen had a significantly lower tumor incidence.[11] A study in *Nature* reported that royal jelly (derived from pollen) protected all mice injected with cancer cells for longer than 12 months, in contrast to those in the control group, injected with the same number of cancer cells, all of which died within 12 days.[12] In studies of women suffering from inoperable uterine cancer, those given bee pollen were found to maintain strong immune systems and to suffer less from nausea, hair loss, and fatigue. Similar results have been reported in studies of cancer patients undergoing radiation treatment.[13]

Other Herbs—Other herbal medicines have been identified as potentially useful adjuncts to cancer treatment. These include: pearl barley (*Hordeum vulgare*); reishi mushroom (*Ganoderma lucidum*); shiitake mushroom (*Lentinula edodes*); cauliflower (*Brassica oleracea*); wax gourd (*Benincasa hispida*); calendula (*Calendula officinalis*); chaparral (*Larrea divaricata* and *Larrea tridentata*); white mulberry (*Morus alba*); Japanese pepper (*Piper futokadsura*); thyme (*Thymus serpyllum*); Chinese cucumber (*Trichosanthes kirilowii*); and stinging nettle (*Urtica dioica*).[14]

Rather than consider herbal treatments as alternatives for early or follow-up cancer care, cancer researchers are more likely to investigate the use of herbs as an adjunct conventional treatment. Botanicals have been shown to directly counteract the dangerous effects of chemotherapy and radiation, which are toxic to the body, suppress the immune system, and can cause serious damage to cells. Certain botanicals enhance immunity whereas others stimulate the body's detoxification and antioxidant systems. Still others may block the activity of tumor-stimulating hormones, such as estrogen and prolactin. The use of botanical agents in tandem with conventional treatment may not necessarily be the optimal strategy in every case. Combining these two divergent approaches affords a way for conventional medicine to begin making the transition to a more sensible and ultimately more effective way of treating cancer.

Traditional Chinese Medicine and Herbal Cancer Treatment

Traditional Chinese medicine (TCM) is an ancient system of medicine that combines the use of herbs with acupuncture, food therapy, massage, and therapeutic exercise. TCM regards energy imbalances as causing the patterns of disharmony in the body that lead to disease. Viewing each patient as unique, the goal of all treatment is to restore balance to the whole person. Dr. Pan Chen-lian of the Zhejiang Research Institute of Traditional Chinese Medicine, states: "The clinical anticancer therapies are based on principles such as clearing away heat and toxic materials, treating toxifying diseases, activating blood to remove stasis, softening and resolving hard lumps, and invigorating *qi* [life energy]."[15]

Research has shown that TCM can effectively complement conventional medicine when used in concert against cancer.[16] In China, a combination of TCM and Western medicine has been shown to be more effective for treating liver cancer than conventional Western medicine alone.[17] TCM can also reduce or minimize the toxic side effects of chemotherapy and radiation while reinforcing their cancer-killing effects. Conventional oncologists who use herbs have been surprised to find that their patients not only suffer far less from nausea, hair loss, and depressed immunity, but also that their rate of recovery increases.

Fu Zhen **Therapy**—Among the better-studied Chinese anticancer herbal treatments, *Fu Zhen* features the following herbs: ginseng, ligustrum, astragalus, codonopsis, atracylodes, and ganoderma. *Fu Zhen* helps restore energy levels, enhances digestion, and strengthens the immune system by increasing the activity of macrophages and T cells, both integral parts of the body's anticancer defenses.[18] The *Journal of the American Medical Association* reported that life expectancy doubled for patients with rapidly advancing cancers when *Fu Zhen* was added to their treatment plan: "Patients who received *Fu Zhen* therapy survived longer and tolerated their treatment better than those patients who were treated by Western medicine alone." In addition, the five-year survival rate was twice as high among patients with nasopharyngeal (nasal passage and pharynx) cancer (53% versus 24%).[19]

Liu Wei Di Huang ("Six Flavor Tea")—Those diagnosed with small-cell lung cancer may enhance the benefits of conventional treatment by taking a traditional Chinese kidney tonic known as Six Flavor Tea or *Jin Gui Shen Qi* (Gold Book Tea). Researchers at the Beijing Institute for Cancer Research found a significantly higher incidence of tumor reduction and survival among cancer patients taking the teas.[20] Median survival for the group receiving both treatments was 16 months compared to ten months for the conventionally treated group.

Rabdosia rubescens—A study of 115 patients with inoperable cancer of the esophagus showed that patients taking *Rabdosia rubescens* in combination with chemotherapy showed a three-fold increase (41.3%) in survival rates compared to those receiving only conventional treatment (13.6%).[21]

Other Chinese Anticancer Herbs—A Chinese herb called *jian-pi yi-qi li-shui* was shown to reverse chemotherapy-caused kidney failure by 93%.[22] A commonly used herb, Chuling (*Polyporus umbellatus*), stimulated immune activity around tumor sites and increased the life span of tumor-bearing test animals by 72%.[23] The anticancer drug cyclophosphamide resulted in significantly improved antitumor activity and reduced toxicity when combined with *Buzhong Yiai* or Central Qi Pill.[24] Chinese doctors often recommend using actinidia root in cancer treatment; this root contains a complex sugar that has immune-enhancing and antitumor properties.[25]

Researchers at Longhua Hospital of Shanghai Traditional Chinese Medical College selected 60 patients with advanced squamous (oral and lung) cancer and randomly divided them into two groups. One group was treated with traditional medicinal herbs and the other with chemotherapy. The average length of survival for the herbal group was 465 days while that of the chemotherapy group was only 204 days.[26] The survival rates after 12 and 24 months were 67% and 13% for the herbal group, and 33% and 3%, respectively, for the chemotherapy group.

Kampo—No discussion of TCM approaches to cancer therapy would be complete without some mention of kampo, the Japanese version of

Chinese herbal medicine. Though there are over 140 different kampo preparations, most of the research has focused on *Shi-un-hou*, *Juzen-taiho-to*, and *Sho-saiko-to*. *Shi-un-hou* has been particularly effective in blocking the formation of skin tumors in animals.[27] *Juzen-taiho-to*, which consists of astragalus, angelica, cinnamon, foxglove, ginseng, licorice, nettle, peony root, and other herbs, may dramatically boost the anticancer activity of natural killer cells.[28] *Sho-saiko-to* is composed of the following traditional Chinese herbs: *Bupleurum* root, pinellia tuber, scutellaria, jujube fruit, ginseng, licorice, and ginger. This kampo medicine appears to override the inhibition of macrophage immune cells, enabling macrophages to more effectively fight cancer.[29]

Ayurvedic Medicine's Herbs for Cancer Treatment

Practiced in India for the past 5,000 years, Ayurvedic medicine is a comprehensive medical system that combines natural therapies with a highly personalized approach to the treatment of disease. Ayurvedic medicine places equal emphasis on body, mind, and spirit and strives to restore the innate harmony of the individual.

Herbs Can Complement Low-Dose Chemotherapy

When chemotherapy must be employed, the strategic use of certain herbs known to Chinese medicine can mitigate its effects.

- For stomach cancer patients receiving Chinese herbs, there is improved natural killer cell activity and a significant improvement in the ability to tolerate chemotherapy compared to patients not receiving herbs (95% vs. 79%). The herb-treated patients reported higher energy levels, improved weight gain, and better overall quality of life.[30]

- Survival rates are improved for patients with lung, breast, throat, and nasopharyngeal cancers who used Chinese herbs in combination with chemotherapy or radiation, versus conventional treatment alone.[31]

- Despite several cycles of chemotherapy, there was no significant drop in immune cell counts in a group of breast cancer patients using Chinese herbs.[32]

Ayurvedic physicians regard cancer as a product of internal disharmony caused by the interaction between a person's constitutional tendencies and various dietary and environmental factors that lead to an accumulation of toxins, which eventually weaken the body's ability to defend against cancer. A person's constitution, how a specific individual's mind/body is designed to function, is the touchstone of Ayurvedic medicine. It refers to the overall health profile of the individual including strengths and susceptibilities. To determine an individual's constitution, Ayurvedic doctors first identify the patient's metabolic body type or *dosha*, which may be one of three types: *vata*, *pitta*, and *kapha*. The *dosha* is akin to a blueprint that outlines all of the innate tendencies built into a person's system.

The Ayurvedic herbs that may offer the most promise for treating cancer are called *rasayana* or rejuvenation herbs. Ayurvedic physicians say that *rasayana* extends longevity by slowing down the biological clock and retarding the aging process—a process associated with the development of cancers. The herbal formulations of choice for cancer therapy include Maharishi-4 (M-4) and Maharishi-5 (M-5). Both M-4 and M-5 were found to reduce the incidence of chemically induced breast cancer in up to 88% of laboratory animals. In the animals that did not receive the *rasayanas* prior to the chemical induction of breast cancer, subsequent administration of the herbal medicines caused up to 60% of fully formed tumors to regress.[33]

Researchers at the Institute of Medical Sciences at Banaras Hindu University in Varanasi, India, reported on over 400 cases of cancer patients undergoing Ayurvedic treatments alone or in combination with conventional treatment. The patients who received Ayurvedic medicines alone, such as *Amora rohitica*, *Glycerriza glabra*, and *Semecarpus anacardium*, achieved the most favorable results. These formulas were effective in bringing about remissions, in controlling the growth of malignant cells, and in improving the quality of life.[34] Those receiving chemotherapy alone had poor survival rates during a ten-year follow-up. When the Ayurvedic formula was combined with chemotherapy, however, the survival span increased significantly.

Success Story: Controlling Prostate Cancer with Herbal Medicine

At age 60, Lou received a diagnosis of prostate cancer, based on a biopsy which revealed a Gleason (SEE QUICK DEFINITION) 7 adenocarcinoma (moderately malignant). The urologist advised surgical removal of the prostate. A second biopsy, conducted at another institution, came back with a Gleason score of 8, indicating severe malignancy. His urologist recommended either surgery or radiation for his condition. One radiation oncologist recommended placement of radioactive needles in Lou's prostate. Another thought the cancer was too advanced and that external beam radiation therapy was the appropriate treatment.

When Lou decided to undergo treatments with Michael B. Schachter, M.D., instead of the conventional approach, his urologist wrote a formal letter to Lou strongly criticizing this decision and repeating his recommendation to have either a radical prostatectomy or radiation treatment.

Unfortunately, Lou's insurance would not cover Dr. Schachter's injectable program (although they would pay for prostate surgery or radiation), so Lou had to forgo injections. Instead, he began an intensive program of oral supplements along with proteolytic enzyme and shark cartilage rectal retention enemas. The oral supplements included vitamin C, beta carotene, shark cartilage, amygdalin, sodium selenite, flaxseed oil, Vitae Elixxir, cod liver oil, maitake mushrooms, FlorEssence (a form of Essiac herbs), coenzyme Q10, pycnogenol, apricot kernels, hydrazine sulfate, and a multivitamin/mineral formula. The modalities were introduced over a six-week period.

Within a month, Lou's energy levels improved and he reported feeling well. His prostate symptoms, which included occasional bed-wetting, were much reduced. Over the next year, Lou's prostate specific antigen (PSA) counts fluctuated considerably, but eventually showed a continual downward trend, dropping from a high of 17.8 to stabilize at 8.23, which is a moderate count (normal being 0 to 4).

According to Dr. Schachter, Lou continues to feel well and remains physically active. His only symptoms are waking once nightly for urination and occasional bed-wetting, which had begun prior to his first consultation. Some 28 months after his diagnosis, Lou's PSA was 9.79, still within the moderate range, his prostatic acid phosphatase was 1.4, which is normal. (This blood test, known as the male PAP, is less sensitive than the PSA in monitoring prostate cancer. Usually when it is elevated, there are metastases to the bones.) Lou continues to feel well, working full time and playing racketball for three hours at a stretch several days each week, reports Dr. Schachter.

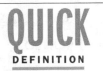

DEFINITION

The **Gleason score** is a way of grading the microscopic appearance of prostate cancer. First, different areas of the slide are rated from 1 to 5 with 1 appearing most benign and 5 appearing most malignant. Then the two most predominant patterns are added together for a Gleason score, with 2-4 being mildly malignant, 5-7 moderately malignant, and 8-10 severely malignant. The higher the score, the worse the prognosis.

Michael B. Schachter, M.D.: Schachter Center for Complementary Medicine, Two Executive Boulevard, Suite 202, Suffern, NY 10901; tel: 914-368-4700; fax: 914-368-4727.

For **Dr. Schachter's cancer protocols,** see *Alternative Medicine Definitive Guide to Cancer* (Future Medicine Publishing, 1997; ISBN 1-887299-01-7); to order, call 800-333-HEAL.

A Glossary of Herbs, Biological Response Modifiers, and Nontoxic Pharmacological Agents

Numerous herbs can be used to intervene therapeutically at various stages of the development of cancer. In addition to traditional botanicals, we examine the biological response modifiers (BRMs) as well as nontoxic pharmacologic anticancer agents currently in use among innovative cancer physicians. BRMs are substances derived from both plants and animals that have biological activity in the human body. Many of these have also been called phytochemicals, which means "chemicals made by plants." Some BRMs stimulate immune function directly, while others modulate the activities of hormones, enzymes, and other biological components that can alter the course of cancer.

Algae (Chlorella, Sea Vegetables, Green Concentrates)

Algae are simple microscopic organisms that grow in masses in water and contain an abundance of nutrients.

Chlorella—In Japan, *Chlorella pyrenoidosa*, a freshwater single-celled green algae, is more popular as a regular supplement than vitamin C. An estimated five million people use this medicinal algae every day. Chlorella contains 60% protein, including all the essential amino acids, and high levels of vitamin A and chlorophyll. It is chlorella's high chlorophyll content to which many researchers attribute its health benefits, but new research from Japan suggests that chlorella's secret might lie elsewhere—in its albumin. Continually secreted by the liver, albumin is the most abundant protein found in the blood, where it acts as a natural antioxidant, contributing an estimated 80% of all neutralizing activity against free radicals.

At least 38 scientific studies have demonstrated the strong relationship between high blood levels of albumin and a longer cell life span. This research, says Tim Sara, president of Nature's Balance, a major U.S. supplier of chlorella, "has confirmed that levels of albumin are extremely accurate indicators of overall health status and that low albumin levels exist at the onset of virtually every nonhereditary, degenerative disease, including cancer and heart disease."

A series of studies with rats demonstrated that chlorella supplementation increases albumin levels by 16%-21%. Both scientific documentation and reliable anecdotal reports indicate that chlorella is effective in helping to reduce the symptoms of numerous types of cancer, diabetes, low blood sugar, arthritis, AIDS, pancreatitis, liver cirrhosis, hepatitis, peptic ulcers, infections, anemia, and multiple sclerosis.

Chlorella contains more than 20 different vitamins and minerals and 19 amino acids, including large concentrations of lysine, which is helpful against viruses associated with leukemia and cervical cancer. Extensive research on the antitumor activity of chlorella has shown strong promise for the treatment of leukemia and breast cancer.[36] Researchers in India recently fed spirulina, a type of blue-green algae, to 44 people who had precancerous mouth lesions from chewing tobacco; after one year, the patches disappeared in 20 of those who ate the algae and five others showed significant improvements.[37]

Chlorella as a Detoxifier

Chlorella is considered a first-string detoxifying agent, capable of removing alcohol from the liver and heavy metals (such as cadmium and possibly mercury) as well as certain pesticides, insecticides, and polychlorbiphenyls (PCBs) from the body's tissues. A Japanese study showed that taking 4-6 grams of chlorella before consuming alcohol can prevent hangovers 96% of the time—even after a night of heavy drinking. Chlorella can also absorb toxins from the intestines, help relieve constipation, favorably alter the bacteria flora of the bowel, and eliminate intestinal gas. It is also effective in healing wounds, both mild and severe.[35]

Sea Vegetables—Also known as marine algae or seaweeds, sea vegetables have strong anticancer activity. Tumor growth in mice was inhibited in the range of 89% to 95% when mice were fed with a seaweed called kombu.[38] Overall, tumors underwent complete regression in more than half of the mice.[39] Other animal research found that a diet containing 5% kombu significantly delayed the inducement of breast cancer.[40] Scientists at McGill University in Canada have found that the most common edible seaweeds, such as kelp and kombu, contain a substance called sodium alginate, which can reduce the amount of radioactive strontium absorbed through the intestine by 50%-80%.[41] The researchers stated that marine algae may aid in preventing absorption of radioactive products and could possibly be used as a natural decontaminator.[42]

For **ProGreens**, contact: Nutricology, Inc., Allergy Research Group, P.O. Box 489, 400 Preda Street, San Leandro, CA 94577; tel: 510-639-4572 or 800-545-9960; fax: 510-635-6730. For **Green Magic**, contact: New Spirit Naturals, Inc., P.O. Box 3300, San Dimas, CA 91773; tel: 800-922-2766 or 909-592-4445; fax: 909-599-4035. For **chlorella**, contact: New Chapter, 22 High Street, Brattleboro, VT 05301; tel: 800-543-7279 or 802-257-9345. Shoko's Natural Products, 3402 Edgemont Avenue, #373, Brookhaven, PA 19015; tel: 800-654-4394 or 610-876-9850. For **Green Vibrance**, contact: TAAG, Vibrant Health, 432 Lime Rock Road, Lakeville, CT 06039; tel: 800-242-1835 or 860-435-3506; fax: 860-435-3576. For **Pure Synergy**, contact: Synergy Company, P.O. Box 2901, Castle Valley, UT 84532; tel: 800-723-0277 or 801-259-5366; fax: 435-259-2328.

Green Concentrates—Green concentrates typically include combinations of chlorella, wheat and barley grass, spirulina, blue-green algae, and other nutrients. Green grasses such as wheat, barley, alfalfa, and oat provide complete proteins.

One green concentrate product, ProGreens, is a dry powder containing 33 nutritional substances. It is taken in water or juice, 1-2 times daily, on an empty stomach. The benefits of the ingredients in ProGreens, according to company president Stephen Levine, Ph.D., include immune system support, antioxidant protection, gastrointestional fortification, energy boosting, and overall nutrient supplementation. Among the four algae in the product, chlorella is known as the "unpoisoner" because it can detoxify the body of heavy metals such as cadmium and lead and of uranium radiation. The "probiotic" or friendly bacterial cultures (about five billion organisms from eight dairy-free sources) regulate and balance the intestines. The product also contains natural fibers (flaxseed meal), bioflavonoid extracts (milk thistle, bilberry), herbs (ginseng, echinacea, licorice root), and other high-nutrient foods (lecithin, bee pollen, beet juice powder).[43]

Another product, Green Magic, is a drinkable green superfood containing 16 ingredients. Its benefits include nourishing the body, strengthening the immune system, and detoxifying the blood. In addition to chlorella, spirulina, and wheat, barley, and kamut grasses, the product contains coenzyme Q10 (benefits the cardiovascular system and increases cellular energy), superoxide dismutase (neutralizes toxins), and Jerusalem artichoke flour (stabilizes blood sugar and supports colon health). Green Magic comes in powder form and can be used daily (1-3 tablespoons) as a source of multiple nutrients.[44]

Aloe Vera

Aloe is a garden succulent that has long been used medicinally for symptom relief and healing of cuts, burns, and skin problems, as well as for infections and constipation. Certain aloe-containing seeds contain a chemical called aloe emodin, which shows significant pharma-

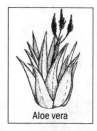

Aloe vera

cologic activity against leukemia.[45] Some studies indicate that aloe bolsters the tumor-fighting activity of macrophages.[46] Recent research shows that aloe juice reduces new tumor mass and the frequency of metastases at different stages of the cancer's development.[47] Acemannan, a water-soluble compound found in aloe, is a potent stimulator of immune function. While the therapeutic efficacy of acemannnan for human cancer remains to be proven, the compound has demonstrated anticancer activity in animals.[48]

For more on **aloe**, contact: International Aloe Science Council, P.O. Box 141837, Irving, TX 75014; tel: 972-258-8772; fax: 972-258-8777. Carrington Laboratories, 2001 Walnut Hill Lane, Irving, TX 75038; tel: 800-444-2563 or 214-518-1300; fax: 800-358-5233 or 214-550-7556.

Amygdalin/Laetrile (Vitamin B17)

This substance, highly concentrated in the pits of apricots and other fruits, allegedly was used some 3,500 years ago by Chinese doctors for the treatment of tumors. The noted biochemist Ernest Krebs, Jr., Ph.D., first identified amygdalin as an anticancer agent. Amygdalin has been found to have strong cancer-fighting potential, particularly with regard to secondary cancers, including a 60% reduction in lung metastases.[49] Epidemiologic studies, animal studies, and clinical studies show evidence of amygdalin efficacy. Research indicates that it can extend the lives of both breast and bone cancer patients.[50]

Amygdalin is one of many nitrilosides, which are natural cyanide-containing substances found in numerous foods, including the seeds of the prunasin family (apricots, apples, cherries, plums, and peaches), buckwheat, millet, and cassava melons. Amygdalin consists of two sugar molecules, a benzaldehyde and a cyanide radical. In the body, the sugar molecules are split off in the liver and replaced by glucuronic acid. This results in a selective toxicity to cancer cells because the enzyme glucuronidase, which splits off the glucuronic acid, is high in cancer cells and low in normal cells. Prolonged survival among those with advanced inoperable cancers has been observed following intravenous benzaldehyde treatment,[51] and antitumor responses were seen in patients with various forms of advanced metastatic cancers (lung, liver, stomach, prostate, and bone.)[52]

Astragalus

In recent years, astragalus has captured the interest of conventional doctors because of its ability to reduce the toxic effects of conventional cancer treatment. Astragalus appears to protect the liver against the toxic effects of chemotherapy and may be effective in treating terminally ill liver cancer patients.[53] In a study conducted at the Peking Cancer Institute, researchers observed a much higher survival rate among advanced liver cancer patients when they were treated with both radiation and astragalus compared to those treated with radiation alone.[54]

Clinical research in Japan indicates that a ginseng-astragalus combination (GAC) may have a regulatory effect on natural killer (NK) cell function, increasing it if NK activity is low and decreasing it

Herbs Can Be Used in Many Forms

Whole Herbs: dried plants or plant parts that are cut or powdered. Depending on their source, whole herbs can have varying degrees of potency and contamination. Buy whole herbs from reputable manufacturers.

Teas: loose or teabag form; steeping in boiled water for a few minutes, releases the fragrance, aromatic flavor, and the herb's medicinal properties.

Capsules and Tablets: convenient and popular form of herbs; some herbs, such as goldenseal, have repulsive flavors which are hidden in a capsule or tablet.

Extracts and Tinctures: high concentrations of an herb that are more quickly assimilated by the body than tablets; Alcohol (or sometimes glycerin) is used as a solvent to extract non-water-soluble compounds from the herb and as a preservative. Tinctures usually contain more alcohol than extracts (sometimes 70% to 80% alcohol). Herbal tinctures and extracts should look and taste like the herb or plant it was derived from.

Essential Oils: distilled from various parts of medicinal and aromatic plants except oils of citrus fruits, which come directly from the fruit peel. Essential oils are highly concentrated and should be used sparingly for internal purposes. Dilute essential oils in water or in fatty oils if using topically except eucalyptus and tea tree oils, which can be applied directly to the skin without concern of irritation.

Salves, Balms, and Ointments: used for muscle aches, insect bites, or wounds; usually available in a vegetable oil or petroleum jelly base.

slightly if excessive.[55] When GAC was used in laboratory animals as an adjunct to chemotherapy, various immune cell counts and the usually observed chemotherapy-induced decreases in key blood measures were significantly prevented and toxic side effects were reduced.[56]

In China, physicians frequently combine astragalus with another Chinese herb called ligustrum. Research at Loma Linda University in California found that astragalus and ligustrum when taken together enhance each other's immune-stimulating properties; ligustrum has been shown to increase the number and activity of various immune cells, whereas astragalus helps increase NK activity and interferon levels.[57]

Cat's Claw (*Uña de Gato*)

The indigenous peoples of Peru have traditionally used this rain forest vine as a tribal medicine for cancer, arthritis, and other diseases. The name, cat's claw, derives from the fact that the thorns found on this vine resemble the claws of a cat. Recent studies indicate that the plant, *Uncaria tomentosa*, contains substances that have immune- and digestion-enhancing properties.[58] These beneficial constituents include polyphenols, triterpines, and plant steroids,[59] which may account for the antioxidant and antitumor properties of cat's claw.[60]

Echinacea

This herb has well-known immune-enhancing abilities. Echinacea was found to increase NK cell activity by 221% in patients with inoperable metastatic esophageal or colorectal cancer.[61] Patients with advanced liver cancer showed a 90% increase in their NK activity when echinacea was combined with a thymus-stimulating agent.[62] In addition, a natural chemical substance in echinacea, arabinogalactan, stimulates the tumor-killing activity of macrophages.[63] The primary role of echinacea is to provide protection against infection, a common and sometimes deadly complication in advanced-stage cancers.

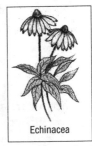

Echinacea

Essiac

In the 1920s, a Canadian nurse named Rene Caisse introduced a nontoxic herbal tea for treating cancer. The tea was originally named Lasagen by the Ojibway, a Native American tribe based in Ontario, Canada. Caisse obtained the formula for this natural herbal combination from a breast cancer patient who had been healed by an Ojibway medicine man; she renamed it Essiac (which is Caisse spelled backwards) and used it to treat thousands of cancer patients. Although Essiac has never undergone randomized clinical trials, Caisse and her associates recorded many impressive case histories attesting to its efficacy. The recoveries encompass cancers of the pancreas, breast, ovaries, esophagus, bladder, bones, and bile ducts, as well as lymphoma and malignant melanoma.

Essiac's Anticancer Benefits

According to a recent report, Essiac tea: (1) strengthens the immune system; (2) reduces the toxic side effects of many drugs; (3) increases energy levels; and (4) diminishes inflammatory processes.[64] Studies of some of Essiac's main components—burdock, Indian rhubarb, sheep sorrel, slippery elm—have each demonstrated a significant amount of anticancer activity.[65] Emodin, one of the main constituents in rhubarb, has been shown to inhibit various cancer cell lines[66] and to reduce tumor cell numbers and increase survival time in leukemic mice.[67] Japanese researchers have identified a potent factor in burdock that can block cell mutation."[68]

In 1937, Caisse was introduced to Dr. John Wolfer, then director of the cancer clinic at Northwestern University Medical School. Wolfer arranged for Caisse to treat 30 terminal cancer patients with Essiac under the supervision of five doctors. After 18 months, the

For information about **Essiac**, contact: Essiac Products Services, P.O. Box 6013, Pompano Beach, FL 33060; tel: 954-786-5220; fax: 954-786-1110.

doctors concluded that Essiac had relieved pain, shrunk tumors, and improved the survival odds of these patients. Also in 1937, Emma Carson, M.D., spent 24 days inspecting the Bracebridge Clinic in Ottawa, Canada, where Caisse had done most of her work. Dr. Carson reviewed over 400 cases of cancer patients who had been treated with Essiac and recorded indisputable improvements. She declared: "The vast majority of Miss Caisse's patients are brought to her for treatment after [conventional treatment] has failed and the patients are pronounced incurable. The actual results from Essiac treatments and the rapidity of repair were absolutely marvelous and must be seen to convincingly confirm belief."[69]

Flavonoids

This class of phytochemicals is responsible for many of the bright colors in fruits and vegetables, and they are also among the most beneficial substances found in cancer-fighting foods. Among the better-known flavonoids are citrin, hesperidin, rutin, and quercetin; other flavonoids include the proanthocyanins and anthocyanins. Studies indicate that quercetin dramatically inhibits the growth of cancer cells in the stomach.[70] Anthocyanins and other flavonoids extracted from citrus and grape seeds are highly effective "scavengers" of free radicals—highly reactive and unstable molecules that promote tumor growth.[71]

Garlic

Long appreciated as a folk remedy, scientific research now highlights garlic's ability to work as a cancer inhibitor and as a valuable adjunct to cancer therapy. Studies of eating habits in China and Italy, where garlic consumption is high, established that the risk of stomach cancer declined by about 50% among those people with a high raw garlic intake. Residents of Cangshan County in China regularly ate 20 g of garlic daily and had the lowest death rate due to stomach cancer in

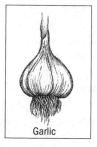

Garlic

China, while residents in Qixia County, where garlic consumption was minimal, had a death rate from stomach cancer that was 13 times higher.

Animal studies have shown that aged garlic extract appears to stop the growth of cancers of the breast, bladder, skin, and colon, and the initial development of malignant tumors of the esophagus, stomach, and lungs. One study involving mice who received 20 once-weekly injections of diallyl sulfide, a garlic constituent,

showed reduced frequency of colon and rectal cancer by
74%. Research involving human cell cultures indicates that
garlic may inhibit the proliferation of breast, skin, and nerve
cancer cells. A study at the National Medical Center
Hospital in Japan showed that garlic extract (with vitamins
B1 and B12 and liver extract) produced a "moderately effective" response in 70% of patients. Garlic helped reduce
anorexia and fatigue, side effects of radiation and
chemotherapy.

For more about
**Kyolic® Aged Garlic
Extract™**, contact:
Wakunaga of America
Co., Ltd., 23501
Madero, Mission Viejo,
CA 92691;
tel: 714-855-2776;
fax: 714-458-2764.

Garlic may produce these anticancer benefits by speeding up the
excretion of chemical carcinogens from the cells, protecting DNA
from damage, enhancing the activity of enzymes that detoxify poisons, and boosting the immune system. Components of garlic inhibit the initiation and promotion phases of oncogenesis; in addition,
garlic seems to strengthen the immune system's response to tumors.[72]
More specifically, garlic extract appears able to enhance natural killer
cell activity, improve the ratio between helper/suppressor T cells,
stimulate macrophages, and enable lymphocytes to become more
cytotoxic (cell-killing) against tumors. Garlic may also block the
adhesion of cancer cells to the surface of blood vessels, thereby helping to prevent metastases.[73]

Ginkgo Biloba

For thousands of years, ginkgo has been a staple of Chinese herbal
medicine, recommended for coughs, asthma, and acute allergic
inflammations. Ginkgolide B, one of the active compounds in ginkgo,
apparently works by interfering with a chemical in the body known as
PAF (platelet-activating factor); PAF may act as a tumor-promoting
agent by stimulating inflammation and inducing angiogenesis.[74] PAF
levels tend to be higher in patients with malignant breast tumors compared to those with benign breast tumors.[75]

British research has shown that ginkgolide B is effective in treating kidney disorders and counteracting a number of
toxins.[76] A study at Loma Linda University found that
Ginkgo biloba extract (GBE) is a highly effective antioxidant that may greatly curtail the free-radical damage
that naturally accompanies the anticancer activity of
macrophages.[77] Other studies have found that GBE
can dramatically lessen the damage to normal cells
that is typically associated with the chemotherapy
drug Adriamycin.[78]

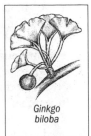

Ginkgo
biloba

Ginseng (*Panax*)

For over 2,000 years, Chinese doctors have prescribed ginseng, either in powder or extract form, as a general tonic to promote strength, vitality, appetite, emotional stability, and "wisdom."[79] *Panax ginseng*, a small perennial woodlands plant is different but related to Siberian ginseng (*Eleutherococcus senticosus*), a medium-sized shrub that is more widely distributed in Nature. Ginseng contains a number of active constituents, including saponins, essential oils, phytosterol, amino acids, peptides, vitamins, and minerals.

All forms of ginseng should be taken in moderate doses based on the product's gin- senoside content. As a general rule of thumb, a standard dose is 4 g to 6 g daily; be careful of doses larger than this as they may inhibit immunity.

Over a dozen saponins have been identified as the most active therapeutic constituents in ginseng.[80] Ginseng saponins have been shown to stimulate macrophage and NK cell activity, as well as to promote antibody production.[81] *Panax ginseng* has a wide range of beneficial actions, including antiaging, immune enhancement, antistress, and antitumor effects,[82] which may be attributed to ginseng's ability to protect against free radicals.[83]

In one study, those animals receiving ginseng had a 75% lower rate of liver cancer and a 29% lower rate of lung cancer compared to animals that did not receive ginseng.[84] Japanese scientists have observed strong inhibitory effects of ginseng on human ovarian cancer cell growth in test animals.[85] Regular use of *Panax ginseng* can cut one's cancer risk in half, according to Korean researchers who conducted a survey of 1,987 pairs of individuals, each pair including a person with cancer, age- and sex-matched to a person without cancer. People who had used ginseng for one year had a 36% lower cancer rate than nonusers; those who used ginseng for five years or more had a 69% lower cancer rate.[86] Siberian ginseng stimulates the anticancer activity of NK cells and may also help regenerate NK cells destroyed by conventional treatments.[87]

Grape Seed Extract/Pycnogenols

Grape seed extract contains various phytochemicals, including a variety of bioflavonoids such as the proanthocyanins and anthocyanins. Anthocyanins and other flavonoids are highly effective in curbing free-radical damage, which can alter fats circulating in the bloodstream and embedded in cell membranes.[88] Pycnogenols have been shown to be up to 50 times more effective than vitamin E and 20 times stronger than vitamin C in free radical–neutralizing power. Many researchers contend that pycnogenols might be the most powerful antioxidants yet discovered. Among the benefits claimed for grape seed extract, is its ability to:

- improve blood and lymph circulation
- reduce thickening of the arteries
- dramatically improve peripheral circulation
- protect central nervous system tissues
- block the release of enzymes that produce histamines (the culprit in allergy attacks)
- help tone skin and restore flexibility to joints, arteries, capillaries, and other body tissues.

For grape seed extract, contact: Carotec, Inc., P.O. Box 9919, Naples, FL 34101; tel: 800-522-4279 or 941-353-2348; fax: 941-353-2365. Prolongevity Ltd., P.O. Box 229120, Hollywood, FL 33022; tel: 800-544-4440 or 954-766-8433; fax: 954-761-9199.

Grape seed extract is now widely prescribed in France and Italy, where grapes are abundant, for improving blood flow to the brain and heart, treating varicose veins, bleeding gums, glaucoma, hemorrhoids, excessive menstrual bleeding, and hardening of the arteries. Researchers suggest saturating the body tissues with a dosage in the range of 200-300 mg a day for 5-10 days, followed by a daily maintenance dose of 60-150 mg.

Green Tea

Green tea (*Camellia sinensis*) is a highly popular beverage among the Chinese and Japanese, who consume, on average, 2-10 cups daily. Green tea contains a substance called epigallocatechin gallate, which inhibits the growth of cancers and lowers cholesterol.[89] This is one of a number of chemical compounds known as catechins, which are many times stronger than vitamin E in defending the body against free radicals.[90] The catechins found in green tea support the immune system's responsiveness and have demonstrated powerful anticarcinogenic effects.[91] Studies indicate that green tea consumption can reduce the risk of cancers of the liver and throat.[92] Green tea flavonols (the active bioflavonoids in the tea) may offer substantial cancer protection if consumed on a regular basis.

Haelan 851

This liquid soybean concentrate is rich in zinc, selenium, vitamins A, B1, B2, B12, C, D, E and K, as well a variety of amino acids. The soybeans used to make Haelan 851 are grown in special, mineral-rich soils, and harvested at the peak of ripeness to ensure maximal nutrition. A fermentation process then splits the soybean proteins into amino acids, compounds that are rich in nitrogen, by-products (through fermentation) of naturally occurring substances called isoflavones, protease inhibitors, saponins, and other compounds.

Studies indicate that when Haelan is combined with chemotherapy in laboratory animals with liver cancer, survival is significantly increased.[93]

For **Haelan 851**, contact: Haelan Products, Inc., 18568 142nd Avenue NE, Bldg. F, Woodinville, WA98072; tel: 425-482-2645 or 800-542-3526. Beso® Biological Research, Inc., 21660 E. Copley Drive, #180, Diamond Bar, CA 91765; tel: 800-898-2376. ecoNugenics, Inc., 3060 Kerner Blvd., Suite 5, San Rafael, CA 94901; tel: 800-308-5518; fax: 415-451-6277; website: www.econugenics.com. For **Genista**, or soy protein isolate, contact: Cartilage, USA, 9 Commerce Road, Fairfield, NJ 07004; tel: 800-700-REAL or 973-808-1400; fax: 973-276-0639.

Haelan has demonstrated effectiveness against gastric cancer, immune dysfunction, and free-radical damage.[94] Chinese researchers conducted a clinical study of Haelan in combination with other treatments on 239 people who had been diagnosed with various cancers—lung, stomach, esophagus, intestines, and lymphatic system. Haelan greatly improved the patients' physical functioning and quality of life, helped resolve "vital energy deficiencies," strengthened the immune system, improved appetite, and "by means of supporting healthy energy and lowering toxicity," relieved side effects caused by conventional treatments.[95]

The apparent efficacy of Haelan 851 underscores the nutritional, even therapeutic, benefits of soybeans and soy products. To illustrate how important this can be, Michael Schachter, M.D., cites recent research on isoflavones, the most studied of which is genistein, found in high concentrations in soy products. As Dr. Schachter explains, these products may help to fight cancer in several ways:

First, they can induce apoptosis, or programmed cell death, which speeds up the death of unwanted cancer cells. Second, genistein is a tyrosine kinase inhibitor. Tyrosine kinase is an enzyme that helps platelets to aggregate or cluster together. Excessive platelet aggregation can lead to clot formation and heart attacks and help cancer gain a foothold.

Third, genistein inhibits another enzyme known as DNA topoisomerase II, which slows down the synthesis of DNA and cell division. The result is a slowing down of the growth of cancer, whose cells are multiplying too quickly. Fourth, genistein and other isoflavones inhibit angiogenesis, or new blood vessel formation. Solid cancers, such as breast, prostate, lung, and colon, require new blood vessel formation in order to grow. Without angiogenesis, a cancer will not grow any larger than the size of a pencil point.

Fifth, under conditions of excessive sex hormone stimulation, genistein appears to inhibit the availability of the hormones, thus helping women with hormone-sensitive breast cancer and men with hormone-sensitive prostate cancer. Sixth, isoflavones appear to induce differentiation of cancer cells, which means they help to move cancer cells back toward normalcy.[96]

HANSI

The name HANSI refers to a series of homeopathically prepared herbs that have been proven effective in the treatment of cancer and chronic fatigue. The product was developed by Argentinian biologist Juan Jose Hirschmann. The initials stand for Homeopathic Activator of the Natural Immune System, which concisely describes the product. When Hirschmann first introduced HANSI in Buenos Aires, Argentina, in July 1990, so great was the demand for this alternative cancer formula that even with 40 physicians on staff, his clinic reached operating capacity in its first week, registering 1,200 patients a day. Since then, an estimated 100,000 cancer patients have used HANSI with good results, indicated most notably in dramatic increases in levels and activity of natural killer cells, central to the immune response to cancer, says David C. Christner, managing director of Hansi International, Ltd., in Sarasota, Florida.

For more about **HANSI**, contact: Hansi International, Ltd., 1941 Northgate Blvd., Sarasota, FL 34234; tel: 941-358-8500; fax: 941-358-8522.

The basic product starts with about ten components, then is adjusted according to whether it is to address cancer, chronic fatigue, AIDS, asthma, or other conditions. For example, the basic HANSI contains low-potency homeopathic dilutions of mostly rain forest and desert plants such as cactus, aloe, arnica, lachesis, licopodium, and others. HANSI variations include these plus *Colocinthis*, *Pulmonaria reticulosa*, *Berberis vulgaris*, and silica.

In a study in 1992 involving 87 patients with advanced pancreatic cancer (which is usually fatal within 3-6 months), 60 of the patients taking HANSI daily remained alive one year after the study began. Two years later, more than 50% of the patients were still alive and well. Further, appetite remained stable in 57% of the cases and increased in 7%, 73% had no pain or only mild pain, 56% reported no nausea or vomiting, and 36% experienced a reduction in these symptoms. HANSI was able to stop weight loss (which is typical of advanced cancer) for 34% and 11% gained some weight. Patients receiving HANSI did not have chemotherapy or radiation during this treatment. Several studies have shown conclusively that HANSI has no toxicity or secondary effects for patients. Subsequent studies indicate that HANSI produces a greater tolerance for radiation and chemotherapy.

Hoxsey Herbs

Harry Hoxsey was an herbal folk healer who eventually attracted a devoted following of cancer survivors after he developed an herbal therapy that originated with his great-grandfather. Hoxsey formula comes in a potassium iodide solution and contains the following herbs: red clover (*Trifolium pratense*), buckthorn bark (*Rhamnus purshianus*),

Individuals taking the Hoxsey tonic are cautioned to avoid tomatoes, alcohol, processed flour, and vinegar because they can negate the tonic's effects.

For more on **Hoxsey Herbs**, contact: Bio-Medical Center, P.O. Box 727, 615 General Ferreira, Colonia Juarez, Tijuana, Tijuana, B.C., Mexico; tel: 52-814-9011 or 52-814-9132.

burdock root (*Arctium lappa*), stillingia root (*Stillingia sylvatica*), barberry bark (*Berberis vulgaris*), chaparral (*Larrea tridentata*), licorice root (*Glycyrrhiza glabra*), Cascara amarga (*Picramnia antidesma*), and prickly ash bark (*Zanthoxylum americanum*). The Hoxsey therapy consists of a mix of herbal preparations for internal and external use, and an emphasis on diet, vitamin and mineral supplements, and personal counseling. The external formula (but not the internal one) includes *Sanguinaria canadensis*, also known as bloodroot, which has been used by Lake Superior Native Americans to treat cancer.

Wide-ranging laboratory research has found definite biological activity in the various ingredients of the Hoxsey herbal formula. Studies have shown antitumor effects with components of prickly ash and stillingia,[97] burdock,[98] and extracts of barberry.[99] In addition, the genistein found in red clover may be responsible for a wide range of anticancer activities, including antioxidant activity, anti-estrogen activity (slowing tumor growth in some cancers), and inhibition of new blood vessel formation (blocks tumor growth).[100] Licorice (*Glycyrrhiza uralensis*) has a variety of immune-stimulating properties and direct antitumor effects;[101] it also demonstrates a unique ability to block estrogen's cancer-stimulating effects.[102] Not all studies have been able to demonstrate anticancer effects for these ingredients, however, and different types of cancers react differently to the formula.

Cancers that have responded favorably to the Hoxsey combination include lymphoma, melanoma, and skin cancer. A five-year preliminary study followed patients with advanced cancer who were treated at three alternative cancer clinics. Six of 16 patients treated at the Hoxsey clinic remained alive and were reported to be disease free after five years. Two of these patients had cancers that are normally considered incurable or "terminal." In contrast, all patients from the other two clinics, where Hoxsey herbs were not used, had died at the end of five years.[103]

The Hoxsey approach includes a psychological component, whose objective is to encourage patients to maintain a strong fighting spirit toward their cancer. Generally, patients take the herbal tonic daily and begin to feel more energetic and vital within a few weeks. Typically, they will continue the treatment for several years, at which point they usually feel their health has been restored.

Iscador (Mistletoe)

Iscador is the trade name for a mistletoe preparation that has been used by European physicians since 1920. Iscador consists of fermented extracts of European mistletoe (*Viscum album*), some forms of which are combined with small amounts of metals to produce anticancer effects.[104] Originally conceived by Rudolf Steiner (1864-1925), Austrian scientist and founder of anthroposophic medicine, the therapeutic success of Iscador has been reported in nearly 5,000 case studies. In animal experiments, Iscador has been found to kill cancer cells, stimulate the immune system, and significantly inhibit tumor formation.[105]

The activity of various immune cells, including NK cells, increases significantly within 24 hours of injecting Iscador.[106] These effects might explain various findings that Iscador selectively inhibits the growth of different types of tumor cells.[107] Two reviews of the clinical research have concluded that treatment with Iscador increases both the length and quality of life, stabilizes the cancer, causes tumors to shrink, and improves the overall condition of the patient.[108]

Iscador's potential as a cancer therapy is strongly supported by the following findings: (1) significantly more breast cancer patients treated with Iscador were alive after ten years compared to patients who received no Iscador; (2) people with cervical cancer who had a combination of surgery, Iscador, and radiotherapy showed an 83% survival rate after five years compared to a 69% survival rate for those who received radiation alone; (3) normally 50% of bladder papillomas become malignant in three years, but with Iscador, only three out of 14 did; (4) among bronchial cancer patients, 75% of those given Iscador were still alive after four years compared to only 35% of those without Iscador; and (5) the survival rate after three years for skin cancer patients on Iscador was 80% compared to 65% for those without it.[109] In addition, Iscador has successfully extended the lives of individuals with cancers of the lung, breast, stomach, colon, ovaries, and cervix.[110]

Despite the wealth of clinical and research data demonstrating the benefits of Iscador, it is not currently licensed by the FDA for sale in the United States.

Iscador is available in the U.S. in liquid form (*Viscum compositum*) to qualified health-care practitioners. Contact: Biological Homeopathic Industries (BHI), 11600 Cochite SE, P.O. Box 11280, Albuquerque, NM 87123; tel: 505-293-3843; fax: 505-275-1672. Weleda, 175 North Route 9W, Congers, NY 10920; tel: 800-241-1030 or 914-268-8572; fax: 914-268-8574; M.D.s and D.O.s may order from Weleda.

Larch Arabinogalactan

This immune enhancer is a sweet-tasting medicinal powder, highly concentrated in complex carbohydrates or long-chain sugars, derived from the Western Larch tree (*Larix occidentalis*). It was first identified and developed by naturopathic physician Peter D'Adamo in 1992. Dr. D'Adamo holds exclusive rights for the use of larch (as pharmaceuti-

For **Larix** (available to qualified physicians only), contact: North American Pharmacal, 17 High Street, Norwalk, CT 06851; tel: 203-866-7664.

cal grade Larix) as a "nutraceutical," that is, as a plant-derived therapeutic agent.

The large size of the sugars in Larix is thought to account for its special properties, including its ability to stimulate the activity of various immune cells. Larix readily dissolves in water and maintains its chemical stability over a wide range of concentrations, pH, and temperature changes. According to Dr. D'Adamo, Larix enhances the delivery of other medicinal agents, including chemotherapy drugs. It is presumed to make capillaries more permeable for microabsorption and to stimulate the liver to produce antibodies.

The role of Larix as a modulator of immune system activity is not surprising since several major immune-enhancing herbs are known to contain significant amounts of arabinogalactans, such as *Echinacea purpurea*,[111] *Baptisia tinctoria*,[112] *Thuja occidentalis*,[113] *Angelica acutiloa*,[114] and *Curcuma longa*.[115] In addition, many edible plants are rich sources of arabinogalactans, including carrots, radishes, tomatoes, wheat, maize, pears, coconuts, and many other foods.[116]

At least two animal studies have demonstrated that Larix can inhibit liver metastases and prolong survival times.[117] In a third animal experiment, arabinogalactans blocked highly metastatic lymphoma cells from colonizing the liver.[118] The immune-related effects of Larix include stimulation of NK cells and macrophages. In one study, the enhanced tumor cell–killing of NK cells was not a direct effect of Larix, but was due to stimulation of other immune cells (monocytes); these cells increased their production of various immune-enhancing chemicals known as cytokines, including gamma-interferon and interleukin-2.[119] This research is still preliminary, however, and wide variations were seen in Larix's ability to stimulate NK activity.[120] Larix appears to be totally safe for regular daily use.

Maitake Mushroom (*Grifola*)

According to researchers at the National Cancer Center in Japan, complete tumor elimination was experienced in about 80% of cancer-induced animals fed extracts from maitake, shiitake, and reishi mushrooms.[121] Compounds in each of these mushrooms increase the tumor-fighting activity of NK cells and improve antibody responses, but maitake seems to have the strongest and most consistent effect.

Maitake exhibits potent activity against cancer, inhibiting both carcinogenesis and metastasis, according to researchers. Animal research suggests that maitake supplements increase the body's ability to kill tumors.[122] When maitake was compared to a common form of chemotherapy, maitake demonstrated superior ability to inhibit the growth of tumors (80% versus 45%).[123] Maitake increases immune cells' production of interleukin-1, a protein that aids in defense against cancer and viruses.[124]

For a source of **maltake mushroom**, contact: Shoko's Natural Products, 3402 Edgemont Avenue, #373, Brookhaven, PA 19015; tel: 800-654-4394 or 610-876-9850. For **pau d'arco**, contact: Frontier Cooperative Herbs, 3021 78th Street, Norway, IA 52318; tel: 800-669-3275 or 319-227-7996.

Pau d'Arco

This herbal extract from the inner bark of trees of the *Tabebuia* genus, found in South American rain forests, offers another herbal option in treating cancer. The main active ingredient is a substance called lapachol, which can induce strong biological activity against cancer.[125] Nine patients with various cancers were given pure lapachol (250 mg) with meals. All nine patients showed a shrinkage of tumors and reductions in tumor-related pain; three patients experienced complete remissions, and there were no adverse side effects.[126] In studies of mice injected with leukemia cells, the life span of animals given lapachol was 80% greater than that of the control group.[127] Lapachol is well tolerated and causes no severe side effects; nausea, vomiting, and slow clotting have occurred only at very high oral doses.[128]

Pectin, Modified Citrus

This substance is a special pH-altered form of citrus pectin, a type of fiber that lowers blood cholesterol levels. Research indicates that its therapeutic potential for helping to prevent cancer metastases is quite strong. A compound called rhamnogalacturonan found in modified citrus pectin enhances the cell-killing ability of T cells, which play a critical role in the body's immune response to cancer.[129] Another study indicates that NK cell and macrophage cytotoxic activity are also enhanced by modified citrus pectin.[130]

For **modified citrus pectin**, contact: ecoNugenics, Inc., 3060 Kerner Blvd., Suite 5, San Rafael, CA 94901; tel: 800-308-5518; fax: 415-451-6277; website: www.econugenics.com. Allergy Research Group, 400 Preda Street, P.O. Box 489, San Leandro, CA 94577; tel: 800-545-9960 or 510-639-4572; fax: 510-635-6730.

A specially modified form of citrus pectin has provisionally been shown to be effective in halting the spread of cancer cells in rats with prostate cancer. This study demonstrated that modified citrus pectin, when administered at the rate of up to 1% (weight/volume) in the rodents' drinking water for three weeks, significantly reduced the spread of cancer from the prostate to the lungs and lymph nodes.[131] Six other clinical studies suggest that the substance also enhances the anticancer effect of certain immune system cells. Human studies are under way to see whether modified citrus pectin can similarly act to stop the spread of cancer in the human body.

Silymarin (Milk Thistle)

The liver is our primary filter for poisons circulating in the blood-stream, converting potentially toxic substances into excretable substances. Highly toxic chemicals can overwhelm the liver, resulting in dysfunction, which is why, for centuries, European herbalists have used silymarin for restoring liver function. The herb has served as a 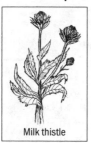 supportive treatment for cirrhosis (associated with liver cancer) and hepatitis, as well as fatty degeneration of the liver caused by alcohol and other chemicals.[132] A review of double-blind studies concluded that silymarin accelerates the process of regeneration of damaged liver tissue.[133] Rich in antioxidants and bioflavonoids, silymarin appears to reduce the levels of various liver enzymes found in patients with chronic liver disease, suggesting a liver protective effect.[134]

Milk thistle

Turmeric

This East Indian herb of the ginger family, a major ingredient of curry powder, appears to exert powerful antioxidant effects, sufficient to reduce carcinogenesis. Research indicates that turmeric can inhibit cancer at various stages of development.[135] After one month, smokers who took two tablets containing 750 mg of turmeric daily had a significant reduction in the level of urinary mutagens (indicating damage from cigarette smoking), whereas the control group's level remained unchanged.[136] In another study, turmeric was shown to decrease the formation of abnormal DNA after exposure to a carcinogen.[137]

The main active component of turmeric is a yellow pigment called curcumin, which possesses both anti-inflammatory and antioxidant properties. Recent animal studies indicate that curcumin inhibits skin cancer.[138] One study of 62 patients focused on those with skin cancer or ulcerating oral cancers that had not responded to conventional therapies. After topical treatment with a gel containing 9.5% curcumin, all 62 patients showed significant reductions in the size of their cancerous lesions, as well as decreased itching, pain, odor, and drainage.[139] In addition, dietary curcumin suppresses colon tumor size and may inhibit the progression of the cancer.[140]

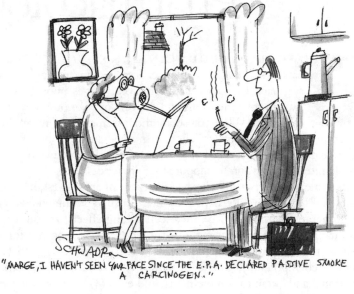

"MARGE, I HAVEN'T SEEN YOUR FACE SINCE THE E.P.A. DECLARED PASSIVE SMOKE A CARCINOGEN."

The New Cancer Pharmacology

BEFORE INTRODUCING INNOVATIVE anticancer substances used by cancer doctors forging a new approach to nontoxic pharmacology, it is important to explain the limitations and dangers of chemotherapy and radiation. While these methods remain the norm for conventional cancer treatment, there is no conclusive body of evidence or data demonstrating long-term successful outcomes or reasonable rates of remission to support these practices.

As some oncologists and alternative practitioners suggest, however, perhaps less is more. Perhaps a highly weakened or diluted dose of chemotherapy might produce cancer cell–killing effects without creating dangerous toxicity throughout the body. In fact, on the forefront of this new approach, physicians are experimenting with (1) low-dose chemotherapy, (2) chemotherapy combined with protective nutritional and botanical supplements, and even (3) homeopathically prepared chemotherapy.

Chemotherapy may be clinically necessary to control tumor mass (as opposed to being routinely prescribed) in some patients. Low-dose chemotherapy is preferable to what is presently regarded as today's normal dose and can be useful when used with alternative modalities in the hands of an experienced physician. What needs to be strongly challenged is the prevailing concept that only chemotherapy in full strength is a viable way to treat cancer.

There are techniques, such as darkfield microscopy and electrodermal screening, that enable the trained physician or oncologist to assess the appropriateness of chemotherapy, in whatever dose or combination, based on specific indications from an individual patient. Surely this approach is preferable to the "one-drug-fits-all" approach of high-dose chemotherapy routinely prescribed by today's oncologists.

The physician and the patient must always remember that the decision to use chemotherapy or to employ the alternatives, or to do both, is patient driven. Responsible physicians should help guide the individual patient to an informed choice of treatment.

A Toxic Treatment Feared Almost as Much as Cancer Itself

Today's conventional cancer treatment will be remembered as a crude and often inhumane technique that causes extensive damage to the body. Surgery excises normal tissue along with malignant tissue and often compromises the lymphatic and other systems vital to the body's resistance to disease. Surgery is generally the lesser of three evils, for the damage caused by radiation and chemotherapy may be far more grievous, given that both destroy normal cells as much as cancer cells and actually increase one's risk of eventually dying from cancer. All chemotherapeutic agents are cytotoxic, or poisonous to cells,[1] and their cell-killing ability is not specific.

When technicians drop the chemotherapy "bomb" inside a living human body, a great deal of "collateral damage" results. The body's rapidly dividing cells found in the bone marrow (the source of all immune cells), the lining of the gastrointestinal tract, and the hair follicles bear the brunt of chemotherapy-induced damage, giving rise to side effects such as diarrhea, nausea, hair loss, anemia, and suppressed immunity.

Other common side effects include mouth sores, infections, nervous system problems, skin rashes, and problems with the lungs, kidneys, and liver—the body's primary detoxification organs. So morbid are people's associations with this sickening form of treatment that the

Anticancer Substances Covered in This Chapter

- Alkylglycerols
- Antineoplastons
- Carnivora®
- Cartilage, bovine
- Cartilage, shark
- Cesium
- DMSO
- Glutathione and N-acetyl-cysteine
- Hydrazine sulfate
- Indocin
- Mellitin
- Nucleic acids
- 714X
- Sodium butyrate
- Staphage lysate
- Tagamet®
- Ukrain
- Urea

Radiation Therapy Speeds Up Prostate Cancer Doubling Time—Media Ignores Facts

According to the *Cancer Communication Newsletter*, mainstream media are dangerously misrepresenting conventional medical procedures for prostate cancer, including radiation, by not disclosing the serious side effects.

Radiation therapy—implanting radiation seeds in the prostate gland—routinely given for early signs of prostate cancer can actually hasten the development of that cancer. Prostate cancer cells can double in as little as 1.2 months after radiation treatment, while unradiated prostate cancer cells may take an average of four years to double. Similarly, it will take up to 20 years for the average untreated prostate cell to double five times, but if treated with radiation therapy, it can double five times in only six months—40 times faster, said *Cancer Communication Newsletter*.

Meanwhile, despite these facts or perhaps unaware of them, urologists send thousands of patients with suspected prostate cancer to radiation therapists every year. According to medical statistics culled from *Urological Nursing, Family Urology*, and other sources, and published in the *Cancer Communication Newsletter*, about 30%-40% of men in their fifties have signs of prostate cancer, but only about 8% will ever feel the effect of this disease in their lifetime and less than 3% will die from it.

Yet if a man in his fifties has an elevated prostate specific antigen (PSA, a standard prostate cancer marker) and undergoes prostate surgery, he has a 20% risk of the following scenario happening: The surgery can actually release cancer cells into the blood, and from six months to five years later, he will again have an elevated PSA, indicating cancer.

The man who initially had a 92% likelihood of having no ill effects from latent prostate cancer, now, as a result of surgery or radiation treatment, is likely to become incontinent or impotent and have to deal with a rapidly growing cancer. In light of this evidence, men should seriously consider all their medical options before undertaking radiation therapy for prostate cancer. Men are further encouraged to demand of their conventional physicians that they investigate these research results and take them into consideration in designing a treatment program.

SOURCES—*Cancer Communication Newsletter* 12:4 (September 1996), 15-16. *Family Urology* (Spring 1996), 11. *Journal of American Medical Association* 275:4 (January 24/31, 1996), 289. *Urological Nursing* (March 1994), 14.

mere thought of having another "chemo" treatment can trigger anticipatory vomiting.[2] Victims of the chemical assault feel sick and tired on a regular basis—probably much sicker than they would have felt had they been left untreated.

It is this long list of toxic effects, which may in fact become life-threatening, that makes chemotherapy a highly questionable method.

According to Howard Greenwald, M.D., "The patient may become exhausted because loss of appetite has led to malnutrition; bone marrow poisoning may undermine resistance to infectious disease; lung damage, kidney dysfunction, and hemorrhage may occur."[3] The rationale for chemotherapy and radiation is that cancer is an enemy that must be killed or destroyed, even when the treatment causes the person great discomfort, perhaps even death. Chemotherapy drugs originated out of mustard gas, designed as a poison for use in warfare. No wonder chemotherapy is feared almost as much as cancer itself.

Virtually all the FDA-approved anticancer drugs are markedly immunosuppressive, because they ruin a person's natural resistance to disease, including cancer. Ulrich Abel, Ph.D., of the Heidelberg Tumor Center in Germany, conducted a comprehensive review of the world literature on survival among cancer patients receiving chemotherapy. He found that chemotherapy can help only about 3% of the patients with epithelial cancers (breast, lung, prostate, and colon).[4] These cancers account for about 80% of all cancer deaths. In a study of chemotherapy-treated breast cancer patients, the researchers concluded, "Survival may even have been shortened in some [breast cancer] patients given chemotherapy."[5] In general, chemotherapy's effectiveness is seen only with small, early tumors, not with large tumors.

One of the ironic "side effects" of chemotherapy or radiation is an increased likelihood that cancer will reappear later on as secondary tumors or that it will eventually spread to other parts of the body.[6] When chemotherapy and radiation are used at the same time, secondary tumors occur about 25 times more than the expected rate.[7]

Despite the aggressive, even militaristic "kill-or-cure" zeal of today's oncologists, chemotherapy's success record is dismal. It can achieve remissions in about 7% of all human cancers;[8] for an additional 15% of cases, survival can be "prolonged" beyond the point at which death would be expected without treatment. This kind of survival is not the same as a cure or even restored quality of life. The statistics show that chemotherapy is useless in treating about 80% of malignant tumors, in particular those that occur most frequently, such as cancers of the lungs, breast, colon, pancreas, and bladder.[9] Chemotherapy's 7% "cure" rate is all the more pathetic when you consider that it typically refers to survival for only five years and thus overlooks the risk of "secondary cancers" or recurrences.

On September 15, 1993, the *Journal of the National Cancer Institute* published the results of a major study examining the effectiveness of chemotherapy for all types of cancer. The results were dismal: chemotherapy provided a "durable response" in only 3% of cases, while another 4% of the patients had "a significantly long survival period." In other words, at best, only 7% of patients benefited from chemotherapy in any way.[10]

A search for clinical trials testing the effectiveness of chemotherapy agents over the past decade did not find even one double-blind, placebo-controlled trial. The only such trials were those designed to study which supportive agents could help prevent or minimize chemotherapy-associated nausea and vomiting. Ironically, among the most recent "agents" to have proven efficacy is ginger.[11] How can the cancer establishment get away with claiming that most herbal medicines (as well as other alternative therapies, for that matter) are "unproven" when the effectiveness of their own chemotherapy drugs are unsubstantiated by the very clinical trials they regard as standards?

Why Chemotherapy Kills More Patients Than It Cures

Researchers at Stanford University recently gained an insight into why chemotherapy is such a dismal failure.[12] Aside from burdening the body's detoxification system and suppressing the immune system, chemotherapy can cause a mutation in the gene that is supposed to protect the body against cancer. This "tumor suppressor gene" (also known as the p53 gene) normally codes for a protein that stops the growth of potential cancer cells by binding to the cells' DNA and blocking cell division.

Here is where chemotherapy wreaks even worse damage than is commonly understood. Chemotherapy kills cells by damaging their DNA. All malignant tissues harbor some cells that have a natural resistance to many chemotherapy agents, just as bacteria exposed to antibiotics develop resistance to those drugs. Although the chemotherapy agents initially affect most cancer cells, those that are resistant survive and eventually they develop into an even more dangerous tumor. This process is accelerated by the tendency of cancer cells to mutate with ever greater frequency as the tumor develops.[13]

To make matters worse, some of the cells develop mutations in their p53 genes, and the defective p53 protein can no longer do its job. These mutated cells have an enormous competitive advantage and eventually dominate the tumor. When the p53 gene mutates, the tumor's growth spins out of control. Since their p53 is no longer effective, the mutated cancer cells refuse to die and continue to multiply, while the rest of the body suffers from the poisons of chemotherapy. This biological scenario helps explain why most cancer patients treated with standard chemotherapy are worse off than they would have been without the drugs.

This is why many now claim that the so-called success of conventional cancer treatment is often illusory. Dr. Abel observes that the temporary shrinking of a tumor mass—defined as either a partial or complete remission—is not necessarily a good sign, because the remaining tumor cells often grow much faster and more virulently after the first series of chemotherapy treatments.[14] Highly aggressive chemotherapy actually shortens survival times compared with patients in whom chemotherapy was delayed or administered less aggressively, according to Dr. Abel. Paradoxically, patients whose tumors showed no response to chemotherapy actually survived longer than patients who did respond.[15]

A related insight is that free-radical damage to DNA increases the risk of cancer cells spreading. It is the metastases that typically kill cancer patients. Human DNA from invasive, spreading cancer contains twice as much damage due to free radicals as DNA from noninvasive tumors.[16] This fact explains why patients who manage to survive chemotherapy and radiation tend to develop more deadly cancers later on, because both chemotherapy and radiation generate free radicals in abundance. On the basis of this research, there are strong grounds for advising that, with rare exceptions, chemotherapy should be avoided or its use minimized to keep your DNA intact and your immune system functioning optimally.

If you have already received conventional chemotherapy and radiation, you can start mitigating the damage by boosting your body's antioxidant supply. Studies have shown that supplementation with antioxidants can bring about a significant increase in survival for breast cancer patients[17] and prevent recurrences of bladder cancer;[18] in addition, decreasing the consumption of dietary fat, another common source of free radicals, increases the survival rates of breast cancer patients.[19]

Biological Response Modifiers and Low-Dose Chemotherapy

Nutrients and numerous other "biological response modifiers" (BRMs) can directly impede tumor growth and metastases.[20] BRM research offers solid evidence that alternative therapies need to become integrated into sensible cancer care:

■ A number of herbs have proven to be effective when used in complement with fractionated chemotherapy, a form of low-dose chemotherapy (LDC) that entails very small doses spread out over a longer period of time.

Chemotherapy Breeds More Cancer

Patients who take chemotherapy for Hodgkin's disease are 14 times more likely to develop leukemia as a result, according to experts from 14 cancer centers who studied 10,000 cases. Use of chemotherapy also increased the risk of bone, joint, and soft-tissue cancer by six times, according to the *Journal of the National Cancer Institute* (May 1995). Radiation therapy increased the risk of developing respiratory cancer by 2.7 times and female genital cancers of the uterus and ovaries by 2.4 times.[24]

■ For stomach cancer patients receiving Chinese herbs, NK cell activity increased and the ability to tolerate chemotherapy improved significantly compared to patients not receiving herbs (95% vs. 79%). The herb-treated patients reported higher energy levels, improved weight gain, and better overall quality of life.[21]

■ Survival rates improved in patients with lung, breast, throat, and nasopharyngeal cancers who used Chinese herbs in combination with chemotherapy or radiation, versus those who relied on conventional treatment alone.[22]

■ No significant drop in immune cell counts was observed after several cycles of chemotherapy in a group of breast cancer patients using Chinese herbs.[23]

For more on **herbs helpful in cancer treatment**, see Chapter 5: Herbs for Cancer, pp. 160-186.

Combining the LDC approach with strategic use of Chinese botanicals, nutraceuticals (food-derived BRMs), and phytochemicals (plant-derived BRMs), reduces the toxic potential of chemotherapy to the point where adverse side effects are entirely avoided.

Making Chemotherapy Use Rational

Conventional cancer treatment routinely administers powerful and toxic chemotherapy drugs to cancer patients based on statistical probabilities that these drugs will have some effect. Yet often patients find that particular cancer drugs are ineffective for them only after taking them and enduring their toxic side effects. As mentioned earlier, a new lab test takes the guesswork out of conventional and alternative cancer treatments. It is called the Ex Vivo Apoptotic Assay and was developed by Robert A. Nagourney, M.D. Dr. Nagourney, a board-certified oncologist, hematologist, and pharmacology professor, is founder and medical director of Rational Therapeutics of Long Beach, California, which provides the test.

Apoptosis is a clinical term that means "programmed cell death." The concept of apoptosis underscores an important fact about cancer, says Dr. Nagourney. "In terms of what defines cancer, it is not that cancer cells grow too much; it is that they die too little. The entire hypothesis of modern cancer research has been largely focused on cancer as a disease of cell proliferation and cancer treatment as a mechanism for inhibiting this proliferation. In simplistic terms, cancer drugs were designed as birth control pills for cancers. More correctly understood, what you need to do in a patient is not stop the cells from growing as much, as to actually stop the cancer cells from living. Instead, you must arrest their viability, stop them in their tracks, and make them die as they are programmed to do."

Dr. Nagourney's test is a short-term measure of the ability of a substance to produce cancer cell death. "Our role is to inject some logic and sense into a rather hectic and haphazard administration of therapies," says Dr. Nagourney. "We call our approach 'rational therapeutics' because we think it is a very intelligent way to deal with cancer."

Let's say your physician tells you that the use of Adriamycin (a chemotherapy drug) induces remissions in 38% of women with breast cancer. How can you tell in advance if you're part of the 38% for whom it works or the 62% for whom it has no effect? "We can now painlessly determine things in a test tube for a patient that they would only be able to find out if they went through the treatments," Dr. Nagourney says. "This is crucial since I've never seen a correctly administered chemotherapy for an 'average' patient."

Based on their cumulative results, Dr. Nagourney's team has compiled data that shows the range of sensitivity and resistance to different drugs among individuals with the same kinds of cancer. His test can determine the likely effect on human cancer tissue from any of about 70 chemotherapy drugs, given singly or in combination. It can also test botanical substances such as betulinic acid (from white birch bark), antineoplastons, interferons, or, theoretically, any substance capable of killing cancer cells. All that is required is a living tissue sample of cancer cells obtained from the patient by biopsy or a blood sample in the case of leukemia. The goal is to see which substances produce cancer cell death during a 72-96 hour process in which the cancer is grown in a test tube. The result objectively indicates the likely human response of an individual patient to a specific drug, says Dr. Nagourney. On this basis, the physician can then tailor a customized treatment plan with a fair measure of assurance that it will be effective.

On the average, Dr. Nagourney says, a patient that is found "sensitive" (responsive) to an identified drug or substance is 2-3 times more likely to respond favorably when that drug is given clinically.

This also means that the test can produce 2-3 times better outcomes in patients than the national averages, Dr. Nagourney notes. Generally, the assay's ability to predict outcomes was scored at 19 out of 21 in a test published in the *Journal of Hematology Blood Transfusion* in 1990, while between 85% to 95% of specimens submitted provide successful studies.

While Rational Therapeutics does not prescribe medicines for cancer, as a complement to the test results, clinicians will suggest "a carefully developed antioxidant and nutrition program designed to aid in the patient's recovery and minimize the toxic side effects of chemotherapy treatments," says Dr. Nagourney. It is a holistic approach in that "we make a global or 'whole person' assessment of each patient," so that treatment can be individualized.

Preventing Breast Cancer Recurrences

A high degree of success in preventing recurrences or metastases of breast cancer is possible, says Wolfgang Kostler, M.D., when you correct the inner environment of the body, strengthen the immune system, detoxify the cells, and neutralize the negative effect of free radicals. If you change the cellular terrain and its biochemical conditions, breast cancer will not recur. Dr. Kostler bases his perspective on cancer on the premise that it is not the primary tumor that kills the patient, but the recurrences and metastases. "There are body conditions that favor the cancer's ability to thrive. This means we have a cancer-prone environment inside the body. If you don't focus on this internal environment, you can't effectively treat cancer because the cancerous internal milieu still elicits the creation of the tumor."

President of the Austrian Society of Oncology, Dr. Kostler studied medicine at the University of Vienna and continued his studies in oncology at Lainz Hospital in Vienna, Austria. In 1977, he opened a private practice in Vienna, where he continues to treat patients and conduct research. In 1986, he cofounded a modern cancer treatment clinic in Vienna called the Sanatorium Dobling, where he is chief of the ambulatory care unit.

For the **Ex Vivo Apoptotic Assay**, contact: Rational Therapeutics Cancer Evaluation Center, 750 East 29th Street, Long Beach, CA 90806; tel: 562-989-6455; fax: 562-989-8160; website: www. Rational-T.com.

Prevention of metastases and cancer recurrences is the area of oncology that affords the greatest opportunity for winning the war against cancer, says Dr. Kostler. He and his colleagues have demonstrated that if strong immune function is maintained and free-radical damage is minimized, then the cancer patient will not relapse and new tumors will not form.

If a person receives the appropriate measures at the right time, the chances of recurrences after surgery are greatly minimized. Making dietary and lifestyle changes before surgery gives the body a head start and prepares it for the stress unavoidably caused by surgery. "The operation is only the removal of a symptom," says Dr. Kostler. "It is just the end product of a very toxic situation." In principle, any tumor's growth can be halted and effectively reversed if the right treatment choices are made at the right time, Dr. Kostler contends. Dr. Kostler is dismayed that many oncologists adopt a passive, anti-prevention attitude toward the cancer patient's prognosis. "The key is to take an active stance against the possibility of recurrences and metastases, not to succumb to the old wait-and-see policy which allows these processes to take place and push the cancer out of control."

Working Against Tumor-Causing Factors

The goal of Dr. Kostler's Oncological Basic Therapy (OBT) is to prevent recurrences and metastases by identifying and compensating for all known tumor-causing factors. This large, multifaceted program includes the following components:

■ Antioxidant Therapy: Free radicals damage the membranes of the mitochondria inside cells. "The mitochondria are the energy generators or power plants of the cell," says Dr. Kostler. "If the energy of the cell is decreased, then disorganized processes will follow. This means that the suppressor genes will not work and will not block the oncogenes that form cancer." Free radicals are unavoidable, but the body's main radical-scavenging mechanisms are supported by vitamins C and E, beta carotene, copper, zinc, manganese, and selenium.

■ Biological Dentistry: Biological dentistry (SEE QUICK DEFINITION) calls for the removal of infected teeth and mercury amalgams to restore healthy functioning of soft tissues.

■ Regulation of Intestinal Balance: The use of probiotics or friendly bacteria (SEE QUICK DEFINITION) helps create an optimal balance of intestinal microbes.

■ Detoxification of Heavy Metals: In addition to dental mercury amalgam removal, selenium

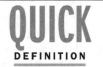
QUICK
DEFINITION

Biological dentistry stresses the use of nontoxic restoration materials for dental work and focuses on the unrecognized impact that dental toxins and hidden dental infections can have on overall health. Typically, a biological dentist will emphasize the safe removal of mercury amalgams; in many cases, either the avoidance or removal of root canals; the investigation of possible jawbone infections (cavitations) as a "dental focus" or source of bodywide illness centered in the teeth; and the health-injuring role of misalignment of teeth and jaw structures.

Friendly bacteria, or probiotics, refer to beneficial microbes inhabiting the human gastrointestinal tract where they are essential for proper nutrient assimilation. The human body contains an estimated several thousand billion beneficial bacteria comprising over 400 species, all necessary for health. Among the more well known of these are *Lactobacillus acidophilus* and *Bifidobacterium bifidum*. Overly acidic bodily conditions, chronic constipation or diarrhea, dietary imbalances, overly processed foods, and the excessive use of antibiotics and hormonal drugs can interfere with probiotic function and even reduce their numbers, setting up conditions for illness.

supplementation, chelation, heat therapy, and other techniques can aid in this process.

■ Nutritional Therapy: Supplementation with minerals, trace elements and vitamins, as well as dietary adjustments, may be needed.

■ Immune Modulation: Imbalances in various types of immune cells can be rectified through nutritional, botanical, and BRM supplementation.

■ Hormone Therapy: The use of tamoxifen and other hormone blockers can help curb tumor growth.

■ Antiviral and Antimycotic Therapies: Viral and fungal infections can be sources of free radicals and contribute to cancer, so they need to be effectively countered.

■ Psychotherapy: Music, meditation, relaxation techniques, and activities that create pleasure and happiness can help activate the immune system.

■ Physical Therapy: Massage and other aspects of physical therapy are helpful for patients whose condition has deteriorated. Physical training and exercise strengthen the anticancer defenses.

Dr. Kostler's therapies work best when they can be started before surgical removal of the tumor (he recommends surgery in most cases). The initial goals of his therapies are to detoxify the body, stimulate the immune system, and block estrogen activity. The use of tumor-killing therapies such as chemotherapy and radiotherapy are in most cases ineffective in helping the cancer patient, because the elimination of the tumor does nothing to change the environment that allowed the tumor to grow. If such therapies are employed, it is crucial to have an aggressive OBT program before, during, and after treatments, Dr. Kostler emphasizes.

Wolfgang Kostler, M.D.:
Sofienalpanstrasse 17,
A-1140 Wien, Austria.

For more about **colon detoxification** and **biological dentistry**, see Chapter 9: Physical Support Therapies, pp. 254-297.

Dr. Kostler prefers to work with people who have not undergone conventional measures, including lumpectomy. "Breast cancer can be easily treated if you do the right things at the right time. This means that you improve the environment inside the patient—the same environment that once allowed the cancer to grow—before the body is subjected to a surgical procedure of any kind." If you change the internal environment—the cellular terrain, its biochemical conditions—breast cancer will not recur.

High Post-Surgical Survival Rates for Breast Cancer Cases

Few doctors can claim the therapeutic success rate Dr. Kostler has achieved with prevention of breast cancer recurrences and metastases. Based on his experience with 250 women who have received his protocols for breast cancer since the early 1980s, Dr. Kostler is confident in claiming that recurrences can be prevented with his approach.

However, there is no way to guarantee the prevention of recurrence or metastasis if the tumor diameter is greater than 4 mm; that is because angiogenic factors (which promote formation and growth of new blood vessels critical to a tumor's survival) are produced in cancers of this size, and they enable cancer cells to spread through the blood and lymph. In addition, the breast cancer patient must receive OBT before the surgery to prevent recurrences or metastases.

If the hormonal factors are blocked and the immune system is stimulated, the body has a much stronger chance of fighting off any further development of cancer. To block hormonal estrogen activity, Dr. Kostler uses tamoxifen and has not observed any adverse effects of this treatment, despite evidence linking tamoxifen use for breast cancer to the later appearance of endometrial cancer. Tamoxifen is typically prescribed after breast cancer surgery to block the regrowth of remaining cancer cells (the drug blocks the activity of estrogen).

Though the use of radiation following lumpectomy has recently been touted to prevent recurrences, Dr. Kostler disagrees with this practice. Radiation is a source of free radicals that can damage DNA and predispose the body to later cancers. "It may eliminate the cancer initially, but not in the long run." This is true even if a person receives a great many antioxidants prior to the radiation. Dr. Kostler has compared his data with published research findings on lumpectomy with radiation, examining incidence for both recurrences and metastases. His breast cancer patients have shown much better survival rates than patients who have undergone lumpectomy or mastectomy followed by radiation.[25] Among those breast cancer patients who have attended Dr. Kostler's clinic, those with the longest survival have been free of cancer for 13 years; the median survival is 5-6 years without any recurrences.[26]

Success Story: Reversing Prostate Cancer

After Bob, 67, was diagnosed with prostate cancer, he underwent surgical removal of his prostate, a procedure called radical prostatectomy. For the next decade, Bob lived with the hope that the oncologists had removed all the malignant prostate cells and that his life could return to normal. But in the tenth year after the operation, Bob began to experience severe bone pain.

Laboratory tests revealed high levels of prostate specific antigen (PSA, a cancer marker), indicating the presence of a prostatic tumor.

Martin Milner, N.D.:
Center for Natural
Medicine, Inc., 1330
SE 39th Avenue,
Portland OR 97214;
tel: 503-232-1100;
fax: 503-232-7751.

For **Dr. Milner's can-
cer protocols**, see
*Alternative Medicine
Definitive Guide to
Cancer* (Future
Medicine Publishing,
1997; ISBN 1-887299-
01-7); to order, call
800-333-HEAL.

Four months later, bone scans revealed that the prostate cancer had metastasized to the bone; six months later, Bob underwent surgical removal of his testes (bilateral orchiectomy) in an effort to halt hormonal stimulation of the cancer. But one week before the surgery, Bob started taking shark cartilage at the rate of 5 g daily, on the recommendation of Martin Milner, N.D., of Portland, Oregon.

By the time of the surgery, the excruciating pain in his bones had disappeared. However, the cancer had spread to his shoulders, sacrum (tailbone), left thigh bone, and right hip bone. With the cancer spreading so rapidly through his bones, Bob's doctors did not expect him to live more than a few months.

After the surgery, Bob increased his shark cartilage intake gradually from 5 g to 60 g. Two months later, he doubled this dosage, and after another five months, it was up to 150 g per day. Bob was also taking 250 mg of grape seed extract, twice daily. Within three months of beginning this program of intensive supplementation, bone scans revealed that the metastasis had stopped and was beginning to reverse itself. About nine months later, Bob's oncologist noted that the previously identified sites of metastasis were less diseased or active and that no new lesions were present. All the bone scans indicated general improvement and his PSA levels were 17 times lower than before, a highly encouraging sign.

"By this time, Bob's metastatic prostate cancer had clearly improved according to standard medical tests," says Dr. Milner. "In addition, he was now pain free. We attribute this success to the combination of shark cartilage and orchiectomy, since such results are virtually unheard of with orchiectomy alone." Today more than 3½ years since the metastasis was diagnosed, Bob has survived well beyond what his conventional doctors "expected."

A Glossary of New Pharmacological Substances for Treating Cancer

Alkylglycerols

A group of compounds called alkylglycerols can bolster anticancer defenses and protect the body against the harmful effects of radiation-induced injury.[27] The richest source of these special fats is shark liver oil,[28] but these fats are found to a lesser extent in mother's milk and cow's milk.[29]

Animal studies have indicated that alkylglycerols have antitumor activity, probably mediated through macrophages in the form of selective destruction to cancer cells.[30] Cell-culture studies have shown that this "selection" seems to be affected by the cholesterol concentration of the cancer cell; as the cholesterol level drops, the cancer cells die more rapidly.[31]

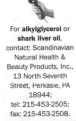

For **alkylglycerol** or **shark liver oil**, contact: Scandinavian Natural Health & Beauty Products, Inc., 13 North Seventh Street, Perkasie, PA 18944; tel: 215-453-2505; fax: 215-453-2508.

Extracts of shark liver oil may help people tolerate both chemotherapy and radiation. The administration of alkylglycerols prior to radiation treatment was found to cause advanced tumors to regress toward less advanced stages;[32] alkylglycerols also caused reversal of tumor growth in animal studies.[33] A possible explanation for these findings is that this substance can inhibit a variety of tumor-promoting substances. One potential area of concern, however, is contamination of shark liver oil by ocean pollutants. No published research, to our knowledge, has yet addressed this issue nor have the potential toxicities at normal doses been adequately studied.

Antineoplastons

Beginning in the 1960s, Stanislaw Burzynski, M.D., isolated several peptides (chains of amino acids, the building blocks of protein) from human urine and found them to be effective in controlling the growth of certain types of cancer. Dr. Burzynski originally identified five antineoplastons (meaning substances that work against a neoplasm or an abnormal growth of new tissue, such as a tumor). He determined that these molecules have a strong anticancer effect at a genetic level: specifically, they appear to stimulate the activity of tumor suppressor genes, genes that literally turn off the activity of certain oncogenes (SEE QUICK DEFINITION).[34] By this action, antineoplastons can actually stop cells from multiplying out of control, said Dr. Burzynski.

Dr. Burzynski has successfully used antineoplastons, which he produces himself in an FDA-approved manufacturing facility in his Houston, Texas, clinic. As part of a study, he used antineoplastons to treat 20 patients who had advanced astrocytoma, a particularly fast-growing type of brain tumor. Nearly 80% of them responded favorably, and a number of them were tumor free four years later.[35] Animal studies in Japan indicate that low doses of an orally administered synthetic antineoplaston help prevent cancers of the breast, lung, and liver.[36]

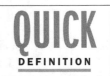

QUICK

DEFINITION

An **oncogene** is a gene believed to transform normal cells into cancer cells, thus initiating the development of cancer. Some of these genes have reportedly been identified in cancer-causing viruses. Proto-oncogenes are genes in a neutral, inactive stage that under certain conditions become oncogenes.

For more about **antineoplastons and Dr. Burzynski**, contact: Burzynski Research Institute, Inc., Stanislaw Burzynski, M.D., 9432 Old Katy Road, Suite 200, Houston, TX 77055; tel: 713-335-5697; fax: 713-935-0649.

According to scientific reports presented at the 86th Annual Meeting of the American Association for Cancer Research in March of 1995, Dr. Burzynski's antineoplastons increase the activity of tumor suppressor genes.[37] At this time, there is no other treatment available that is directed to this critical mechanism in the development of cancer. Ironically, instead of being acknowledged for this discovery, Dr. Burzynski has been repeatedly harassed by the FDA and the Texas medical board.

Carnivora®

This extract of the Venus' flytrap (*Dinoea muscipula*) plant was introduced into cancer therapy by German oncologist Helmut Keller, medical director of the Chronic Disease Control and Treatment Center in Bad Steben, Germany. Dr. Keller has treated over 2,000 cancer patients with Carnivora, so named in honor of the plant's well-known insect-eating ability. One of the active ingredients appears to be a chemical called plumbagin, which has anticancer properties;[38] when topically applied, it can lead to a total reversal of skin cancer.[39]

Although Dr. Keller's work has not been published in peer-reviewed journals, his laboratory studies indicate that Carnivora directly inhibits the metabolic activity of cancer cells. In a clinical study of 210 cancer patients for whom conventional treatments had failed, each received 50-60 drops of Carnivora orally five times a day plus one intravenous infusion daily. The results were excellent: 16% of patients showed tumor remission and 40% had no further tumor progression; in the remaining 44% no improvement was noted, although about one-quarter of these patients experienced a palliative effect. The study showed that more than half, or 56%, experienced either a tumor remission or their cancer development became stable and did not worsen.

Known side effects from Carnivora® are minimal: taken orally without dilution, it can sometimes produce nausea or vomiting; when injected, it can produce a temporary increase in body temperature. Ninety-day studies with rats, in which the rodents received doses 30-60 times higher than the recommended human dose, showed no toxic reactions.

Carnivora is an immunomodulator, which means it stimulates the activity of T helper cells. This enables the body to wage a more vigorous defense against the illness, explains Dr. Keller. Carnivora appears to target tumor cells and bolster the immune system. People should not attempt to produce their own Carnivora, however, since it first must be purified of naturally occurring plant toxins that would otherwise cause adverse reactions.

For more about **Carnivora®**, contact: Carnivora-Forschungs-Gmbh, Postfach 6, Lobensteiner Strasse 3, D-96365 Nordhalben, Germany.

Cartilage, Bovine

In 1954, John F. Prudden, M.D., discovered that bovine cartilage had a remarkable ability to help wounds heal faster. Today, bovine cartilage is one of the few substances proven to accelerate wound healing, which is why most surgical textbooks mention it. But Dr. Prudden became deeply intrigued with the wider therapeutic potential of this obscure substance. When he watched it dramatically shrink a breast tumor and reduce the malignant ulceration of the chest wall of a desperate patient, he was hooked for life.

The development of new blood vessels (angiogenesis) is a prerequisite for tumor growth, yet this process can be stopped by cartilage from either cows or sharks. Bovine tracheal cartilage (BTC) causes a general activation of the body's anticancer defenses and has demonstrated effectiveness against cancers of the ovary, pancreas, colon, and testes.[40] Since 1972, Dr. Prudden has used bovine cartilage to successfully treat 110 cases of advanced cancer; the partial and complete response rate, taken overall, is approximately 30% within a seven-month treatment period.[41]

In 1985, Dr. Prudden reported on the results of a trial with 31 cancer patients who had failed to respond to conventional therapies or had a cancer that was not treatable at all. After starting a regimen of cartilage—typically 9 g daily, taken orally in 3-gram installments three times daily—90% of the patients had a partial or complete response. Dr. Prudden also reports success in causing a large rectal tumor to disappear, leaving the patient cancer free for 18 years. Bovine cartilage produced a complete healing of breast cancer after all other therapies had failed; and a man with prostatic cancer that had spread to the bones had a complete remission.

As impressive as these early results sound, bovine tracheal cartilage is not a cancer cure but a very successful palliation. It is not, strictly speaking, a cure because patients who respond to it must continue taking it at the rate of 9 g daily for the rest of their lives. It also takes up to four months for the initial positive effects to appear, Dr. Prudden advises. In more than 25 years, he has never observed any toxic side effects from using bovine cartilage.

Bovine cartilage contains large sugar molecules called mucopolysaccharides that appear to block cell division in the cancerous cells. Bovine cartilage also seems to stimulate the activity of macrophages, immune cells that "eat" all foreign materials in the body, including cancerous cells. In addition, the cartilage works to decrease the size and population of malignant cells, thus normalizing the renegade cancer cells.

Cartilage, Shark

The popularity of shark cartilage is largely due to William Lane, Ph.D., an agricultural biochemist who published two popular books, *Why Sharks Don't Get Cancer* (1992) and *Why Sharks Still Don't Get Cancer* (1996). Researchers at Massachusetts Institute of Technology put cartilage on the treatment map in the mid-1970s when they demonstrated in rabbits and mice that an infusion of cartilage stopped tumor growth with no sign of toxicity.

In a Cuban study, 14 out of 29 "terminal" cancer patients survived after receiving shark cartilage; of those who died, nine actually died of cancer and six others died of other causes. At 23 months, which was four times the expected life span, half (14) of the original group of 29 patients were still alive, doing well, and enjoying completely normal lives. After 33 months of receiving no treatment other than a modest dose of shark cartilage daily, no new deaths had been reported.[42]

According to Dr. Lane, ovarian cancer responds the most consistently to shark cartilage, while uterine, cervical, and central nervous system cancers respond positively. Further, Dr. Lane reports that shark cartilage is highly effective against advanced prostate tumors, achieving tumor reduction rates of 15% to 67%. It is also capable of significantly lowering PSA counts in 12-16 weeks. Generally, shark cartilage works best against solid tumors; pancreatic cancers, provided they are not too advanced, also respond well.[43]

In 1990, T. Oikawa further confirmed the clinical benefit of shark cartilage by finding a "significant inhibition of angiogenesis."[44] One substance found in sharks, called squalamine, has recently demonstrated the ability to attack tumors via anti-angiogenesis. According to researchers at Johns Hopkins University, animal studies of squalamine suggest a potential therapeutic benefit for patients with brain cancer.[45]

Cesium

This nonradioactive form of cesium, a rare alkali metal widely distributed in the Earth's crust, has been used with some success as an alternative cancer therapy. Interest in cesium therapy began when scientists observed that areas with low cancer rates had high concentrations of alkali metals in the soils.[46] As early as 1927, Japanese researchers identified cesium as having antitumor activity. It was then suggested that alkalinizing the body fluids could push the normally acidic (low) pH of the cancer cell toward a weakly alkaline (high) pH (SEE QUICK DEFIN-

For **bovine tracheal cartilage**, contact: Phoenix BioLogics, 2794 Loker Avenue West, #104, Carlsbad, CA 92008; tel: 800-947-8482 or 760-631-7729. Source Naturals, 23 Janis Way, Scotts Valley, CA 95066; tel: 800-777-5677 or 831-438-1144. For information on **shark cartilage**, contact: BioTherapies, Inc., 9 Commerce Road, Fairfield, NJ 07004; tel: 973-808-1400. For Benefin™ and Immunofin™ (organically processed shark cartilage products), contact: Lane Labs USA, Inc., 110 Commerce Drive, Allendale, NJ 07401; tel: 800-526-3005 or 201-236-9090.

ITION), promoting the cancer's demise.[47] Thus cesium emerged as a high pH–inducing therapy.

A study reported that cesium chloride, when combined with chelation therapy and nutritional supplements, led to significant improvement in about half of all "terminal" cancers of the breast, colon, gallbladder, liver, lung, lymphoma, pancreas, prostate, and pelvis, most of which had not responded to conventional therapy. The cesium treatment consistently resulted in the disappearance of pain within three days; autopsies revealed the absence of cancer cells in most cases, which is why the doctors involved in this study called this "a remarkably successful outcome of treatment."[48]

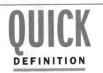

QUICK DEFINITION

The term **pH**, which means "potential hydrogen," represents a scale for the relative acidity or alkalinity of a solution. Acidity is measured as a pH of 0.1 to 6.9, alkalinity is 7.1 to 14, and neutral pH is 7.0. The numbers refer to how many hydrogen atoms are present compared to an ideal or standard solution. Normally, blood is slightly alkaline, at 7.35 to 7.45; urine pH can range from 4.8 to 7.5, although normal is closer to 7.0.

There appears to be an intracellular relationship between cesium and potassium that promotes the destruction of cancer cells.[49] Cesium is similar to potassium, which may explain why it is taken up so easily by cancer cells;[50] this uptake is enhanced when supported by vitamins A and C, and the minerals zinc and selenium.[51] These supplements, along with a high-potassium diet, may also help eliminate the potential toxicity of cesium.[52] Ironically, cesium has been used in cancer therapy for many years, but in the form of radioactive isotopes or "seeds" implanted in cancer patients as part of radiation therapy.

DMSO (Dimethylsulfoxide)

This substance is present in small quantities in grains, fruits, and vegetables and is naturally present in the human body.[53] It is more commonly known as a solvent derived from coal, oil, and lignan, a structural material in plants. Although the primary clinical use of DMSO has been to treat inflammation, it is also known to induce the differentiation of malignant cells—that is, it causes them to become benign.[54]

Some researchers propose that DMSO may be particularly beneficial to cancer patients who require bone marrow transplantation, since it causes differentiation of malignant bone marrow cells.[55] DMSO has demonstrated effectiveness in slowing or halting the progress of cancers of the bladder, colon, ovary, breast, and skin.[56] Malignant leukemia cells have been observed to revert to normal cells following DMSO treatment.[57] One of the most exciting aspects of DMSO is its apparent ability to help deliver anticancer substances to the site of the cancer,[58] where it seems to enhance the effects of various cell-killing agents while simultaneously reducing the toxicity of conventional treatments.[59]

DMSO stimulates various parts of the immune system and scavenges free radicals.[60] Since free radicals promote tumor growth, this may be one of the mechanisms by which DMSO interferes with the development of cancer. It may also explain why patients who receive DMSO while undergoing either chemotherapy or radiation—both of which generate free radicals in order to kill cancer cells—are far less prone to such side effects as hair loss, nausea, and dry mouth.[61]

Glutathione and N-Acetyl-Cysteine (NAC)

Glutathione is a protein that contains the amino acids cysteine, glycine, and glutamic acid; NAC, a derivative of cysteine, is an amino acid precursor for the body's production of glutathione. Cysteine accounts for glutathione's antioxidant activity and its role in the key antioxidant enzyme, glutathione peroxidase. Blood levels of glutathione peroxidase tend to decrease after the sixth decade of life and are typically lower in patients with malignant cancers.[62] Supplementing regularly with a combination of glutathione and NAC may be especially important for older people who have been exposed to numerous toxins in their diet and environment.

Glutathione reduces free-radical damage to DNA and prevents depletion of other antioxidants. It also helps metabolize carcinogens, activates certain immune cells, helps repair DNA, and may inhibit angiogenesis.[63] Glutathione is also a component of an enzyme that assists in the liver's metabolism of drugs and toxic chemicals. Glutathione and NAC supplements have been found to diminish the toxic side effects of chemotherapy and other conventional treatments.[64]

Glutathione is most effective if absorbed under the tongue (at a typical dose of 100-500 mg daily) rather than being swallowed; this is because stomach acid and digestive enzymes can degrade it. Typical NAC dosage is 1,200 mg every other day for a 150-pound person, and less for people under that weight.

Hydrazine Sulfate

This experimental synthetic chemical developed by Joseph Gold, M.D., seems to inhibit the loss of body mass caused by cancer, while at the same time exerting indirect antitumor effects. A study of 740 cancer patients (200 with lung cancer, 138 with stomach cancer, 66 with breast cancer, 63 with Hodgkin's disease, 31 with melanoma, and others) reported tumor stabilization or regression in 51% of patients, while 46.6% of the patients reported symptomatic improvements, such as fewer respiratory problems and a decrease in fever.[65] Decreased pain was noted even in cases of metastatic bone cancer, and some patients improved so markedly that they were once again able to walk and care for themselves. In one study, the compound significantly improved the nutritional status and survival of lung cancer patients;[66] it may also aid in treating cancers of the breast, lung and larynx, as well as Hodgkin's disease, desmosarcoma, and neuroblastoma."[67]

Hydrazine sulfate improves appetite, increases a patient's sense of well-being, results in weight gain in those who have lost weight, and may contribute to a shrinkage of tumors. It seems to work by interfering with the liver's ability to produce glucose from lactic acid, a process known as gluconeogenesis. Cancer cells thrive on glucose, which allows the cancer to grow quickly while normal cells in the body break down. This destructive cycle may continue, resulting in a wasting away of the lean mass of the patient. By interfering with gluconeogenesis, hydrazine sulfate inhibits the cancer while allowing normal cells to thrive, thus reversing the vicious cycle. Although the substance is inexpensive and nonpatentable, the FDA has made it illegal for chemical companies to sell hydrazine sulfate to the public.

For information about **hydrazine sulfate**, contact: Syracuse Research Institute, Joseph Gold, M.D., 600 East Genesee Street, Syracuse, NY 13202; tel: 315-472-6616. The general public may obtain hydrazine sulfate from: Great Lakes Metabolics, 1724 Hiawatha Court N.E., Rochester, MN 55906; tel: 507-288-2348; fax: 507-285-4475.

Indocin (Indomethacin)

By inhibiting the production of the "bad" eicosanoid, prostaglandin E2, indocin effectively slows tumor growth, permitting more macrophages to enter the tumor.[68] A growing body of research indicates that indocin may be effective against various cancers.[69] This substance, a member of the family of nonsteroidal medications, has about the same contraindications as aspirin, the worst of which is bleeding or perforated ulcers; however, either can be a surgical emergency.

Mellitin

This substance is derived from the "sting" of honeybees. Increasingly used as a folk remedy for rheumatoid arthritis and multiple sclerosis, the honeybee's venom has recently shown promise as an anticancer agent as well. Immunologist and pathologist Robert Raison, Ph.D., of the University of Technology in Sydney, Australia, found that bee venom can be combined with certain antibodies to target cancer cells without damaging normal cells. The venom's main poison, mellitin, killed tumor cells by damaging their outer membrane, causing them to break open.[70]

Nucleic Acids

The use of homeopathically potentized nucleic acids is based on the collaborative work of Maurice Janaer, M.D., president of the Belgian Homeopathic Medicine Federation, and Bernard Marichal, M.D., honorary president of the Italian Medical Association for Immunotherapy. These physicians discovered novel homeopathic strategies for helping cancer patients.

Dr. Janaer has long asserted that toxicity was the main factor limiting the use of nucleic acids and various biological response modifiers (BRMs) in conventional treatment protocols. To prevent toxic side effects, Dr. Janaer applied the homeopathic principles of dilution and potency. In so doing, he was able to demonstrate their effectiveness in "re-balancing" the immune systems of large numbers of patients.[71] Drs. Janaer and Marichal investigated the clinical usefulness of homeopathic nucleic acids and have observed consistently strong benefits with the use of two homeopathic blends, called 2LC1 and 2LCL1.

For homeopathic nucleic acids 2LC1 and 2LCL1, contact: Labo-Life Espana SA, Ctra Palma-Inca, Km 17.8, 07330 Consell (Majorca), Espana; tel: 34-71-14-20-17; fax: 34-71-14-20-69. Labo-Life, La Rambourgere Sainte-Marie, 79160 La Chapelle-Thireuil, France; tel: 011-33-49-0422-12; fax: 011-33-49-0422-13.

This innovative approach is based on three fundamental principles: (1) perilingual absorption, which helps bypass the disadvantages posed by the action of digestive juices and slow assimilation; (2) infinitesimal dilutions, which bypass toxic side effects; and (3) sequential treatment, which means spreading treatment over a period of time instead of prescribing the same substance each day. Using this approach, Dr. Marc Patte, director of medical communications for LaboLife in Spain, has documented numerous recoveries from a wide variety of advanced cancers, including metastatic liver cancer, breast cancer, leukemias, and others.[72]

714X

This unique compound, discovered by French Canadian biologist Gaston Naessens, consists of nitrogen-rich camphor and organic salts. Dr. Naessens discovered that tumor cells produce a substance, cocancerogenic K factor (CKF), that paralyzes the immune system. 714X seems to neutralize CKF, thereby enabling the immune system to more readily identify and destroy cancer cells. In animal studies, 714X was effective against bone cancers and breast cancer. In humans, researchers reported a shrinking of the tumors, weight gain or weight stabilization, reduction or elimination of pain, and extended survival.[73] Dr. Naessens has collected hundreds of case histories in which 714X was effective against melanomas, carcinomas, lymphomas, and other types of cancer.[74]

For more about **Dr. Naessens**, see Chapter 3: Early Detection and Prevention, pp. 94-128.

The usual treatment course involves three consecutive series of injections of 714X directly into the lymph nodes of the groin. The injections are given once daily for periods of 21 consecutive days, followed by a break of two days while the natural defenses of the body are restored. 714X has no harmful side effects, other than burning sensations at or around the site of injection.

To obtain **714X** within Canada, a physician must request permission from the Emergency Drug Release Program in Ottawa for authorization. To contact them: Emergency Drug Release Program, Bureau of Pharmaceutical Assessment, Holland Cross, Tower B, 1600 Scott Street, Ottawa, Ontario, Canada K18 1B8; tel: 613-941-2108; fax: 613-941-3194. To obtain 714X outside of Canada, contact: Cerbe, Inc., 5270 Mills Street, Rock Forest, Quebec, Canada J1N 3B6; tel: 819-564-7883; fax: 819-564-4668.

Sodium Butyrate

Butyrate is another term for butyric acid, an oily substance present in cow's butter; technically, it is a short-chain fatty acid produced by bacteria in the colon. Widely used as an artificial flavoring in liqueurs, syrups, and candies, sodium butyrate has also been investigated as a treatment for various forms of cancer, notably colon cancer.[75] The primary effects seem to include an ability to convert malignant cells to benign cells and to trigger cancer cell death. Since butyric acid degrades quickly, however, some researchers believe its usefulness is limited.[76] Caution should be exercised, since sodium butyrate actually seemed to promote the development of colon cancer in laboratory animals;[77] to counterbalance the effects, potassium, magnesium, or calcium supplements may be needed. The paradox of the use of this substance is that in other contexts, as an artificial flavoring, sodium butyrate is considered a potential carcinogen; yet here, it demonstrates therapeutic merit.

Staphage Lysate

This vaccine consists of remnants of a common bacterium called *Staphylococcus aureus* as well as viruses which attack the bacterium and appears to be useful as a general immune booster, a stimulator of macrophage production, and an inducer of interferon.[78] Robert E. Lincoln, M.D., of Medford, Massachusetts, first pioneered the use of staphage lysate in the 1940s. By 1952, the use of this substance had become so controversial and politicized—not, apparently, from any therapeutic shortcomings—that Dr. Lincoln was expelled from the Massachusetts Medical Society and staphage lysate was listed with the American Cancer Society (ACS) as an "unproven" method. In 1975, staphage lysate was quietly reinstated by ACS.

In 1987, Dr. Cecil E. Pitard of the University of Tennessee School of Medicine proposed making staphage lysate a standard adjunctive treatment for cancer.[79] The basic principle of its operation is that the immune system is "tricked" into producing cells that would target and eliminate not only these foreign substances found in the *Staphylococcus aureus* vaccine, but also any cancer cells in the system. Staphage lysate increases delayed cellular immunity and other immune functions that play a role in cancer resistance.[80] Staphage lysate is not currently available in the United States owing to FDA obstruction.

Tagamet® (Cimetidine)

This common prescription drug is best known for its ability to inhibit the formation of stomach acid, thereby aiding in the treatment of duodenal ulcers. Since the side effects (diarrhea, headaches, and occasional allergic reactions) are generally mild or quite rare, Tagamet seems worthy of consideration. As early as 1978, scientists noted that tumor cell growth could be inhibited with Tagamet.[81] Tagamet seems to bolster the cancer-fighting activity of natural killer cells[82] and increase the number of T helper lymphocytes.[83] At the same time, it helps reduce the activity of suppressor T cells (which suppress other immune functions).[84]

However, since Tagamet reduces gastric acid production, it likely impairs absorption of essential minerals and amino acids and, secondarily, impairs the formation of important hormones, enzymes, neurotransmitters, antibodies, and structural proteins. It may also increase toxic undigested protein in the bowel and blood.

Ukrain

This substance is derived from a combination of a common plant called celandine (*Chelidonium majus*) and thiophosphoric acid (also called thiotepa, one of the original chemotherapeutic agents). The combination appears to neutralize the toxic effect of the alkaloids contained in thiophosphoric acid; by this method, Ukrain has been rendered almost completely nontoxic. Ukrain does not harm the body's healthy tissues and anticancer defenses but actually fortifies them.[85]

Clinical research has shown that Ukrain improves the overall condition and extends the survival of "terminal" cancer patients by giving their immune systems a boost and by blocking tumor growth.[86] In two studies of Ukrain treatment, significant clinical benefits (tumor regression) occurred for both lung cancer[87] and cervical cancer patients.[88] Ukrain helps fortify the immune system in people with a variety of cancers;[89] it consistently increases the number of T helper cells, which coordinate key immune-related activities. At the same time, Ukrain increases the oxygen (O_2) in both normal and malignant cells. In normal cells, the O_2 then stabilizes; in cancer cells, however, O_2 consumption drops down to zero.[90] Since the cancer cells stop "breathing" at this point, after 15 minutes of Ukrain treatment, they die.

Ukrain also inhibits the synthesis of genetic material and protein in cancer cells, but not in normal, healthy cells.[91] This may account for the findings supporting Ukrain's ability to completely inhibit growth in 57 of 60 human cell lines representing cancers of the lung, colon, kidney, ovary, breast, and brain, as well as melanoma and leukemia.[92]

Cancer Remissions with Ukrain

Scientists at the Ukrainian Anticancer Institute in Vienna, Austria, have carried out clinical studies of Ukrain over a ten-year period on 206 patients with cancers at various stages of development. Total remissions were achieved even in cases of advanced metastatic cancer; the best success rate with Ukrain (93%) was achieved with cancer patients starting treatment at the earliest stage of tumor development (no metastasis). For those starting therapy in Stage II (minimal metastasis), the success rate was 72%, and for those in Stage III (advanced, metastatic cancer), the success rate was 30%.[94]

Only two leukemia cell lines and one brain cancer cell line were not inhibited by Ukrain. At high concentrations (100 mcg per ml), however, Ukrain causes "100% growth inhibition" in all 60 human cancer lines. Finally, Ukrain possesses a strong selectivity for cancer cells, and when exposed to ultraviolet light, it glows. For these reasons, it can be used to determine whether a suspicious growth is malignant.[93]

Urea

One of the natural by-products of protein digestion (nitrogen) is urea, a natural diuretic (which means it induces urination) compound that also shows strong antioxidant activity. Approximately one ounce of urea is excreted daily in human urine. Urine-derived products have been used in cancer treatment since the 1940s, although they remain controversial. When given orally, urea reaches high enough concentrations in the liver to inhibit cancer growth. Specifically, urea appears to work against solid tumors by destabilizing components called fibrin stroma; it also works against the formation of new blood vessels in tumors.

Observations made over an 11-year period by Evangelos Danopoulos, professor at the Medical School of Athens University in Athens, Greece, indicate substantial clinical benefits from using urea

Urea is available in powder form (in a formula with creatine monohydrate) from: Innovative Therapeutics, 2020 Franklin Street, Carlyle, IL 62231; tel: 888-688-9922 or 618-594-8244; fax: 618-594-7712.

to treat liver cancer.[95] Significant healing responses were reported in 15 of 22 patients diagnosed with cancer that had metastasized to the liver.[96] Since the liver is the only organ that shows high concentrations of urea after oral administration, this therapy may not be effective against cancers other than those of the liver. Dr. Danapoulos found that injections of a 50% urea solution directly into a mass of large, fast-growing tumors was effective and that injections around the tumor site were even more effective.[97] The theory behind urea therapy is that it alters the chemical properties of the cellular surfaces around malignant tumor cells, and thereby disrupts the processes necessary for uncontrolled cellular growth.[98]

Dr. Danapoulos then found, in the 1970s, that oral administration of urea was effective against liver cancer. In a study of 18 patients who were given 2.0-2.5 g of urea orally 4-6 times per day, the patients survived an average of 26.5 months—five times longer than expected. In a separate study, 11 patients with primary liver cancer and 17 with metastatic liver cancer were treated with 10-15 g of urea daily. Again, survival among this group was superb, averaging nearly 26 months.[99] Dr. Danopoulos stated that as urea goes directly to the liver when introduced into the human body, if the liver is more than 30% involved in the cancer, urea treatment will not work, but if liver involvement is less than this, it is likely to be effective.

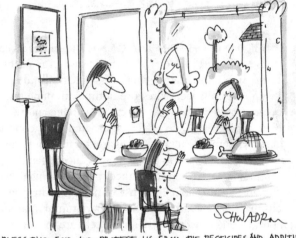

"BLESS THIS FOOD, AND PROTECT US FROM THE PESTICIDES AND ADDITIVES THEREIN."

Boosting the Immune System

ANY DISCUSSION OF CANCER, either its cause or reversal, must include the immune system as a central factor. Immunotherapy—therapies specifically designed to support, enhance, or restore optimal immune function—can enable the body to effectively subdue and reverse the cancer without the adverse side effects associated with conventional therapies. In short, immunotherapy enlists the human immune system itself and its system of defenses as a potent anticancer agent.

A strong immune system can stop cancer by identifying cancer cells and mounting an effective attack against tumors and small groups of renegade cells that have spread from the primary tumor. Natural killer cells, macrophages, and cancer cell–killing T cells are the main types of immune cells involved in the body's protection against cancer. Their anticancer effects are particularly strong in the early stages of disease. The body's lymphatic system (thymus, spleen, and lymph nodes) is the primary route, along with arteries and veins, whereby these immune cells travel to and identify cancer cells for destruction and removal.

Surgery, radiation, and chemotherapy strongly suppress and weaken the immune system, sometimes producing irreversible damage. Blood transfusions, which often accompany surgery, will markedly suppress the immune system for 1-2 months on average and may actually elevate the risk of contracting cancer later. When the immune-suppressing effects of these toxic treatments are placed upon an immune system already weakened by chronic stress, pollution, faulty nutrition, and aging, it is easy to see why many cancer patients have a difficult time surviving orthodox treatments.

In conventional medicine, if immunotherapies are used, it is typically only after surgery, radiation, or chemotherapy, and little or no effort is made to reduce the toxic effects produced by these therapies. Administering these conventional treatments without detoxifying the body and protecting the immune system, is, we believe, negligent medical practice.

Success Story: Strengthening the Immune System and Avoiding Mastectomy

A strong focus of alternative medicine's approach to cancer treatment is to strengthen the immune system and thus allow the body's natural cancer-fighting abilities to resume full functioning. When she was 49, Rebecca, a switchboard supervisor, noted a lump in her left breast. When a needle-guided excision biopsy indicated a tumor was present, Rebecca's doctor planned a mastectomy for her. When she insisted that he perform a simple excision instead and he refused, Rebecca started looking for an alternative. She found it in Douglas Brodie, M.D., of Reno, Nevada.

This was bold on Rebecca's part because, first, the breast cancer was highly malignant and, second, both her mother and a cousin had died of breast cancer at an early age. Rebecca told Dr. Brodie that if she must have conventional treatment she wanted to at least build herself up in preparation. Along with the small cancerous mass in her breast, her immune function was very poor, based on an analysis of her live blood cells with darkfield microscopy (SEE QUICK DEFINITION).

Dr. Brodie started Rebecca on his program of immune system augmentation, using intravenous infusions of high doses of numerous nutritional sub-

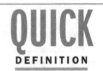

QUICK DEFINITION

Darkfield microscopy is a way of studying living whole blood cells under a specially adapted microscope that projects the dynamic image, magnified 1,400 times, onto a video screen. With a darkfield light condenser, images of high contrast are projected, so that the object appears bright against a dark background. The skilled physician can detect early signs of illness in the form of microorganisms in the blood known to produce disease. Relevant technical features in the blood include color, variously shaped components such as spicules, long tubules, and roulous, and the size of certain immune cells. The amount of time the blood cell stays viable and alive indicates the overall health of the individual. Specifically, darkfield microscopy reveals distortions of red blood cells (which indicate nutritional status), possible undesirable bacterial or fungal life forms, and blood ecology patterns indicative of health or illness.

The Major Players in Your Immune System

The immune system guards the body against foreign, disease-producing substances. Its "workers" are various white blood cells including one trillion lymphocytes and 100 million trillion antibodies produced and secreted by the lymphocytes. Lymphocytes are found in high numbers in the lymph nodes, bone marrow, spleen, and thymus gland.

Lymph Nodes: Lymph fluid flows in the lymphatic vessels throughout the body, helping to maintain the fluid level of cells and carrying various substances from the tissues to the blood. The human body has 1-2 quarts of lymph fluid. Lymph nodes are clusters of immune tissue that work as filters or "inspection stations" for detecting foreign and potentially harmful substances in the lymph fluid. Acting like spongy filter bags, lymph nodes are part of the lymphatic system, which is the body's master drain. While the body has many dozens of lymph nodes, they are mostly clustered in the neck, armpits, chest, groin, and abdomen.

Thymus and Spleen: The thymus, located behind the breastbone, secretes thymosin, a hormone that strengthens immune response. It also instructs certain lymphocytes to specialize their function.

Leukocytes: Leukocytes are white blood cells divided into six types (neutrophils, basophils, eosinophils, monocytes, B-lymphocytes, T-lymphocytes) and two groups, according to the shape of the nucleus and the presence of granules within the cells; one group includes primarily neutrophils, the other includes lymphocytes. The princi-

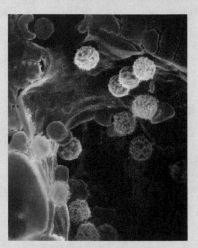

pal activity of the neutrophil is to ingest foreign particles, especially virulent bacteria and fungi.

Lymphocyte: A lymphocyte is a form of white blood cell, representing 25%-40% of the total count, whose numbers increase during infection. Lymphocytes, produced in the bone marrow and found in lymph nodes, come in two forms: T cells, which are matured in the thymus gland and have many functions in the body's immune response; and B cells, which produce antibodies to neutralize an antigen.

Antibodies: An antibody is a protein molecule made by B lymphocyte cells in the lymph tissue and set in motion by the immune system against a specific antigen (foreign and potentially dangerous protein). An antibody is also referred to as an immunoglobulin and may be found in the blood, lymph, saliva, and the gastrointestinal and urinary tracts, usually within four days after the first encounter with an antigen. The antibody binds tightly with the antigen as a preliminary for removing it from the system or destroying it. There are five main types of immunoglobulins: IgG, IgA, IgM, IgD, and IgE.

T Cells: T cells specialize their immune function to become helper, suppressor, or natural killer cells. Helper cells facilitate the production of antibodies by the B cells. Suppressor cells suppress B-cell and immune activity.

Natural Killer Cells: Natural killer (NK) cells are a type of nonspecific, free-ranging immune cell produced in the bone marrow and matured in the thymus gland. NK cells can recognize and quickly destroy virus and cancer cells. "Armed" with an estimated 100 different biochemical poisons, they can kill target cells without having encountered them previously. As with antibodies, their role is surveillance, to rid the body of aberrant or foreign cells before they can grow and produce cancer. Decreased numbers of NK cells have been linked to the development and progression of cancer, as well as chronic and acute viral infections.

Macrophages: Macrophages are a form of white blood cell (originally produced in the bone marrow and called monocytes) that can "swallow" germs and foreign proteins, then release an enzyme that chemically neutralizes whatever is ingested. The name means "big" (*macro*) "swallower" or "eater" (*phage*). Macrophages are the vacuum cleaners of the immune system, ingesting everything that is not normal healthy tissue, even old body cells or cancer cells.

Interferon: Interferon, familiar to many as a cancer treatment, is a natural protein produced by cells in response to a virus or other foreign substance. Vitamin C and certain herbs can also stimulate its production.

Interleukin: Interleukin is a class of proteins with various immune functions, including T-cell activation.

---

stances, along with injections into the muscles of thymus peptides (several amino acids joined together). To complement the injections, Rebecca took oral supplements and glandular extracts. This phase took three weeks. During this time, Rebecca's immune system vitality improved from 20% of normal to 100%, as evidenced by white blood cell activity viewed through darkfield microscopy. Dr. Brodie sent her home with a self-care supplement program.

For more information on the **AMAS test**, see Chapter 3: Early Detection and Prevention, pp. 94-128. For more on **glandular extracts**, see Chapter 8: Enhancing Metabolism, pp. 232-253.

Rebecca managed to persuade her surgeon to perform a lumpectomy (surgery to remove just the tumor in the breast), in which he removed only 25% of her left breast where the tumor resided. He had wanted to cut the whole breast off and excise the lymph nodes as well. The surgical pathology indicated that this 25% portion actually

Douglas Brodie. M.D.: 309 Kirman Avenue #2, Reno, NV 89502; tel: 775-329-5000.

contained no cancer at all. About ten weeks later, an AMAS test, which quite accurately measures levels of antibodies to cancer cells, came back normal, indicating no trace of cancer.

For **Dr. Brodie's cancer protocols**, see *Alternative Medicine Definitive Guide to Cancer* (Future Medicine Publishing, 1997; ISBN 1-887299-01-7); to order, call 800-333-HEAL.

Eight months later, Rebecca saw Dr. Brodie again, reporting that stress from obstacles she was facing in her life had weakened her system. Tests indicated she had no return of cancer but that her immune system had dropped in vitality. Dr. Brodie put her on a seven-day intravenous supplementation program and gave her stress-management counseling. In one week, her immune system had regained its vitality. Back home, once she dealt with the personal stress in her life, her mood, energy level, and sense of well-being rapidly improved. Two years after her initial visit with Dr. Brodie, Rebecca told him that all her cancer markers were normal and that she was in an "excellent state of mind and health."

Coley's Toxins

In the 1920s, New York physician William B. Coley, M.D., found that certain infectious diseases—notably, from bacteria—might stimulate a therapeutic effect against malignancies when introduced into the body in the form of a sterilized vaccine (SEE QUICK DEFINITION). Dr. Coley found his "toxins" could give the body's anticancer defenses a nonspecific "kick" against the cancer cells by mobilizing them against an easier opponent.

Dr. Coley was a surgeon at Memorial Hospital in New York City, one of the leading conventional cancer treatment centers in the U.S., and he refused to believe that cancer was incurable. At the time, surgical methods typically involved amputation of the body parts affected by the cancer; understandably, surgeons who had to perform such operations were more than willing to explore alternatives. Bear in mind that radiation therapy and chemotherapy had not yet been conceived.

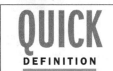

QUICK
DEFINITION

A **vaccine** is a preparation containing a weakened (attenuated) or "killed" solution of a specific bacterium or germ believed to produce a disease. After it is injected into the body, the immune system wages a protective response, developing antibodies to the disease organism's foreign proteins. The theory is that the antibodies "remember" how to respond and neutralize the vaccine antigen in the future, thereby bestowing immunity to this illness. The word vaccine derives from *vacca*, which is Latin for "cow," because the first vaccination in 1796 was for cowpox.

Observing that erysipelas, a dangerous skin infection caused by the bacteria *Streptococcus pyogenes*, was followed by a dramatic tumor regression in a cancer patient with advanced sarcoma, Dr. Coley reasoned that certain infectious diseases might stimulate a therapeutic effect on malignancies. Dr. Coley developed a mixture of sterile bacteria, which became known as "mixed bacterial vaccine," or "Coley's Toxins." Specifically, Dr. Coley used *Streptococcus pyogenes* (the causative agent for erysipelas) and the bacterium *Serratia marcescens*; the product contained the toxins produced by these heat-killed bacteria and the dead bacteria themselves. His idea was that the bacteria would activate the body's anticancer defenses by mobilizing their forces against the bacteria.

Immune Vaccine Predating Chemotherapy

Dr. Coley injected his patients with the bacterial mixture (usually at the site of the tumor or nearby) and claimed success with both partial and complete tumor regression for a number of different types of cancer. If the injection was given in the morning, the patient would typically experience a chill followed by a fever, but would feel normal again by the afternoon. For patients receiving the vaccine for sarcoma (cancer of connective tissue and bone), Dr. Coley reported 41% complete cures. He generally recommended a minimum of five months treatment for effective results; treatments lasting only 4-6 weeks often failed. Dr. Coley's death in 1936 coincided with the explosive growth of chemotherapy; as a consequence, his research was buried in the decade that followed. However, during his lifetime, about 50 physicians in the U.S. (including one at the Mayo Clinic) as well as Europe, treated cancer patients with Coley's Toxins.

For information about **Coley's Toxins,** contact: Innovative Therapeutics, 2020 Franklin Street, P.O. Box 512, Carlyle, IL 62231; tel: 618-594-8244 or 888-688-9922; fax: 618-594-7712. People Against Cancer, 604 East Street, P.O. Box 10, Otho, IA 50569; tel: 515-972-4444; fax: 515-972-4415. For a clinic using Coley's vaccines, contact: GenesisWest Research Institute for Biological Medicine, Del Agua #256 Secc. Jardines, Fracc., Playas de Tijuana, Baja California, Mexico 22700; or P.O. Box 3460, Chula Vista, CA 91909; tel: 619-424-9552; fax: 619-424-7593.

Five-year survival rates after treatment with Coley's vaccine based on data collected in the 1970s showed the following: 65% for patients with inoperable breast cancer; 69% for patients with inoperable ovarian cancer; and 90% for those with bone cancer.[1] Research conducted at Memorial Sloan-Kettering Cancer Center in New York City showed that patients with advanced non-Hodgkin's lymphoma experienced a 93% remission rate versus 29% for those who had only chemotherapy.[2]

Charles Starnes, Ph.D., an immunologist at Amgen, Inc., a biotechnology company in Thousand Oaks, California, declared that Coley's Toxins is among the most promising cancer treatments in existence. According to Dr. Starnes' review, Dr. Coley accomplished an impressive cure rate using his vaccine to treat primarily inoperable sarcoma. For soft tissue sarcomas, 40 out of 84 patients (48%) were free of disease after five years; 17 of these survived for up to 20 years. In another group, 19 out of 33 cases (58%) of lymphoma were cancer-free after five years; eight of these patients survived for up to 20 years.[3]

Success Story: Reversing Uterine Cancer

Roberta, 78, credits her long-term survival to Dr. Lawrence Burton's IAT. In 1968, Roberta was diagnosed with uterine cancer. Her physician recommended a hysterectomy (removal of the uterus), which she underwent; she also received radiation therapy. However, 11 years later, Roberta was diagnosed with breast cancer, which had spread to her lymph nodes. Although the breast tumor was large, she refused to undergo a mastectomy; she received further radiation therapy, with minimal results. Two years later, she began IAT treatments with Dr. Burton and achieved complete remission of her condition; 12 years later, she was still cancer-free.

Coley's mixed bacterial vaccine can cause some disconcerting side effects, beginning with a shaking chill that lasts 10-15 minutes and typically followed by the development of a fever in the range of 102° F to 105° F. The transient fever is simply the body reacting to the bacterial toxins in the vaccine and has therapeutic benefit to the body. In general, Coley's Toxins are not used in conventional cancer treatment, not because they are judged ineffective or experimental, but mostly because they are inexpensive and unpatentable.

Immuno-Augmentative Therapy

Immuno-Augmentative Therapy (IAT) was developed by Lawrence Burton, Ph.D., a biologist and cancer researcher at the California Institute of Technology and St. Vincent's Hospital in New York City. Working first with fruit flies and mice, Dr. Burton isolated a tumor-inhibiting factor capable of producing cancer remissions in humans. More specifically, Dr. Burton identified blood protein components that he suspected were associated with the development of cancer. These consisted of tumor complement, a substance derived from the blood clots of patients with cancer that activates tumor antibodies,[4] and deblocking protein factor (DPF), derived from the blood of healthy donors.

According to Dr. Burton's theory, when the blood protein components are balanced, the body should be able to subdue cancer cells; but if any of the components are out of balance, the body cannot adequately defend itself. Dr. Burton discovered that by injecting certain amounts of these components into his patients, he could bring about remissions in many forms of cancer. He was quick to point out that his treatment was not a cure for cancer: "It is like using insulin for diabetes. It controls the cancer and the patient can live a normal life span." Dr. Burton claimed that IAT achieved tumor reduc-

For information about **Immuno-Augmentative Therapy**, contact: Immuno-Augmentative Therapy Center, P.O. Box F-42689, Freeport, Grand Bahama; tel: 242-352-4755.

tion and even complete remission in 40% to 60% of patients. Particularly impressive were the recoveries of patients with advanced colon cancer and cancer of the abdomen; the five-year survival rate with conventional therapies for both of these diseases is zero.

According to Dr. Burton's records, IAT has shown good results as a treatment for cancers of the bladder, prostate, pancreas, and lymphomas; since IAT builds on the body's anticancer immune function, it is virtually nontoxic. Although the Office of Technology report *Unconventional Cancer Treatments* stated that Dr. Burton's IAT method had not definitively been shown to shrink human tumors, it acknowledged the results of another important study. Here, of 79 advanced cancer patients receiving IAT, 50 patients (63%) were alive an average of 65 months (longer than five years) after diagnosis. The 29 deceased patients survived an average of 59 months, or nearly five years.[5] These findings are remarkable, given that the expected survival for these patients was 36 months or less. Although Dr. Burton died in 1993, IAT is still offered today at the clinic he founded in Freeport on Grand Bahama Island.

T/Tn Antigen Breast Cancer Vaccine

Cancer cells have proteins, or antigens (SEE QUICK DEFINITION), on their surfaces that can be recognized by the immune system. The identification of certain cancer-related antigens forms the basis for the approach embraced by Georg Springer, M.D. Dr. Springer, an immunologist who founded the Heather Bligh Cancer Research Laboratories at the Chicago Medical School, has shown that two antigens, called T and Tn, play a vital role in the immune system's ability to respond to cancer. Since the early 1980s, Dr. Springer has repeatedly shown that the immune system's reaction to T and Tn antigens results in strong cancer cell–killing activity in both animal and human studies.[6]

Using biochemical tests, Dr. Springer has detected the T and Tn antigens in over 90% of all cancers. The less aggressive cancers produce a higher proportion of the T antigen, while the Tn antigen predominates in the more aggressive cancers.[7] The overall concentrations of the T and Tn antigens correlate specifically with the aggressiveness of breast cancer.[8]

In 1974, Dr. Springer had his first opportunity to test his experimental vaccine when his wife, Heather

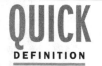

QUICK DEFINITION

An **antigen** is any biological substance (a toxin, virus, fungus, bacterium, amoeba, or other protein) that the body comes to regard as foreign and dangerous to itself. As such, an antigen induces a state of cellular sensitivity or immune reaction that seeks to neutralize, remove, or destroy the antigen by dispatching antibodies against it.

For information about the T/Tn vaccine, contact: The Heather Bligh Clinic, Georg Springer, M.D., 3333 Green Bay Road, North Chicago, IL 60064; tel: 847-578-3435; fax: 847-578-3432.

Bligh, developed breast cancer and was told she had only a year to live. After receiving the T/Tn vaccine, however, she lived a full six years. Encouraged, Dr. Springer began a pilot study with 19 breast cancer patients, all of whom went on to survive at least five years on the T/Tn vaccine; 16 of these women (84%) are still alive, 11 of them after a decade or more of their supposedly terminal diagnosis. In another study, 26 women with advanced breast cancer were given the T/Tn vaccine after undergoing an operation for their primary cancer or after the first recurrence. All survived over five years, and only five out of the 26 patients died within 5-10 years; 14 of 18 patients (78%) who were vaccinated over ten years ago are still alive.[9]

Dr. Springer emphasizes that nutritional support is also important. He advises his patients to take, once daily, a multivitamin, vitamin C (3-4 g), beta carotene (20,000 IU) and vitamin E (1,600 IU). "The nutritional component is extremely important, because nutrients have been shown to influence both cell-mediated and antibody facets of the immune response," says Dr. Springer. "I recommend that my patients consume a wholesome, high-fiber diet that includes fish and liver to obtain the beneficial nutrients from these foods." In theory, says Dr. Springer, his immune-stimulating vaccine could be used for the treatment of all cancers. However, since the T antigen has not been found in brain tumors or in sarcomas (bone and muscle), the vaccine is unlikely to have any therapeutic impact on these cancers.

Bacillus Calmette-Guérin Vaccine

A good example of immunotherapy as applied to cancer treatment is the vaccine called Bacillus Calmette-Guérin (BCG) commonly used against tuberculosis since its introduction in 1921. When used against a highly aggressive form of bladder cancer, the BCG vaccine evokes a strong immune response to the presence of the highly weakened tuberculosis microbes in the vaccine. Introduced into the bladder by catheter, BCG produces an inflammatory response—in effect, a curative fever. The activated immune cells destroy all preexisting cancer cells in the bladder, thus lowering the recurrence of bladder cancer.[10] The BCG vaccine was found to be considerably superior to chemotherapy in dealing with this cancer. Whereas chemotherapy resulted in complete reversal of the disease in 50% of patients, with fewer than 20% still disease-free after five years, BCG had a response rate of 87%, with more than 80% of patients still disease-free after five years.[11] In other words, this immunotherapy approach led to a four-fold improvement in five-year survival. The advantage of BCG and other immunotherapies may be the ability to prevent recurrences.

Autogenous Bacterial Vaccine

Virginia C. Livingston, M.D., who was in her 80s when she died in 1990, was one of the few women physicians of her time. Graduating from New York University in 1936, she became the first woman resident at a New York hospital and went on to develop a germ theory of cancer and vaccines that she successfully used on patients to eliminate cancer. She was an Associate Professor of Biological Sciences at Rutgers University and founder of the Livingston Medical Clinic of San Diego, which specializes in the outpatient treatment of immunodeficiency diseases.

Dr. Livingston's theory arose out of her experience with tuberculosis, leprosy, and scleroderma (a skin disease) among her patients. She discovered certain organisms in scleroderma that were similar to those in tuberculosis and leprosy and set out to discover if they were also found in cancer. She writes, "I reasoned that perhaps scleroderma was a kind of slow cancer. Upon examining all kinds of cancerous tissues, I found that a similar microorganism was present in all of them."[12]

In further research, she proved through recognized scientific principles that a bacterium called *Progenitor cryptocides* fuels the development of cancer. According to Dr. Livingston, *P. cryptocides* is present in everyone from birth, but is held in check by the immune system. When immunity becomes suppressed by poor diet, chemical toxins, emotional distress, and other factors, the dormant microbe can multiply and promote the growth of tumors.[13] Dr. Livingston's research indicated that *P. cryptocides* exists in very high concentrations in cancer patients.

Even more intriguing, Dr. Livingston discovered that *P. cryptocides* is actually a pleomorphic organism, capable of changing its shape and evolving through a series of forms, from simple to complex, from latent to active, depending on the health of the individual, or "host." Dr. Livingston reported that *P. cryptocides* can exist as virus-sized bodies, as larger elementary bodies, but it may also appear less distinctly shaped, as rods or filaments of different lengths without cell walls called mycoplasma. Of these varying forms,

When used for bladder cancer, BCG tends to produce side effects in 50% of cases, including a burning sensation and increased urgency and frequency of urination; occasional blood upon urination; fever and fatigue have also been reported.

For information about **BCG**, contact: Burton A. Waisbren, Sr., M.D., 2315 North Lake Drive, Suite 815, Milwaukee, WI 53211; tel: 414-272-1929. BCG is approved by the FDA for use in the treatment of carcinoma *in situ* of the bladder, but it is not advised for patients with immune deficiencies. BCG is available as TICE® from: Organon, Inc., 375 Mt. Pleasant Ave., West Orange, NJ 07052; tel: 973 325 4500; fax: 973-325-4896.

Dr. Livingston identified the virus stage as the "causative agent in human and animal cancers. When our immune systems are weakened, this microbe gains a foothold and starts cancer cells growing into tumors." In effect, Dr. Livingston suggests that *P. cryptocides* acts similarly to an oncogene, a term oncologists use to denote a gene believed to start the cancer process.

With a microorganism identified as the source of cancer, a vaccine was the likely solution to treatment because, as she explained, "autogenous vaccines are prepared and used all over the world in the treatment of chronic, ongoing infections in the sick." Her theories and clinical results were met with opposition in the conventional medical community. According to Dr. Livingston, pressure exerted by researchers at Memorial Sloan-Kettering Cancer Center in New York forced her to close her laboratory.[14] She continued her research in San Diego, California, and developed vaccines for treatment of cancer after successfully treating a man with malignant lymphoma of the thymus gland with an autogenous vaccine (a vaccine cultured from his own blood or urine).

The concept was to use the bacteria in a person's body to fight that same bacteria; in this way, the vaccine was tailored precisely to match each individual. The vaccines Dr. Livingston developed also included vitamins and minerals to strengthen the immune system.[15] Doses are typically given every 3-5 days, depending on a patient's reaction, which may include soreness or redness at the site of injection, hypersensitivity, mild fever, and muscle or joint pains.

Dr. Livingston designed a complete treatment protocol which included a largely vegetarian raw foods diet, gamma globulin, vitamin and mineral supplements, attention to dental problems, heat therapy, and detoxification. More specifically, the Livingston therapy calls for eliminating from the diet all poultry and egg products, sugars, white flours, and processed foods. Tobacco, and alcohol are also to be avoided. Spleen glandular extracts, the BCG vaccine (to stimulate the patient's immune system), and sometimes hydrochloric acid (to acidify the patient's blood and urine) are administered. However, in her view, the protocol is aimed less at cancer than at reversing a state of immunological dysfunction.

Anti-Mycoplasma Auto-Vaccine

Another approach involves the culturing of a patient's blood for a cell wall–deficient bacterium called mycoplasma, found in the blood of all cancer patients. The process produces a vaccine, called the anti-mycoplasma auto-vaccine, for reintroduction into the patient's system.

Originally developed in Germany, the anti-mycoplasma auto-vaccine technique is now practiced in North America by Filibert Muñoz, M.D., and Fernando C. Ramirez del Rio, M.D., at the Instituto Medico Biologico (IMB) in Tijuana, Mexico. When this mycoplasma vaccine is given to the patient from whom it was made, the cancer often arrests or regresses. IMB physicians are qualified in the handling of different biological medicine modalities for the nontoxic treatment of chronic degenerative conditions, including cancer. Drs. Muñoz and Ramirez use the anti-mycoplasma vaccine as part of a multi-faceted cancer treatment program that involves ultraviolet photophoresis of the patient's blood, detoxification, dietary change, and nutritional supplementation.

Success Rate is High with Livingston Vaccine

According to the Livingston Foundation, for people whose tumors are localized, such as in the prostate or the breast, the remission rate ranges from 70% to 95%. If the cancers have moved into the bone, local lymph nodes, or other areas considered signs of metastasis, the remission rate drops to 40% to 50%. In cases considered terminal, the patient may have three months to live according to conventional standards, but remission rates of 20% are reported with the Livingston approach.[16]

Success Story: Reversing Metastatic Prostate Cancer

Manuel, 73, was diagnosed with Stage IV prostate cancer with metastases to the spine that were dangerously compressing the spinal cord. Manuel refused chemotherapy, radiation, and surgery, and was willing to try the vaccine protocols used by Dr. Muñoz.

First, Dr. Muñoz had to study Manuel's blood. Specifically, he used a darkfield microscope to study a living sample of Manuel's blood for platelet shape. Platelets are disc-shaped cellular elements in blood that are essential for clotting. Blood platelets can be compromised by bacteria, mycoplasmas, viruses, and parasites such that their shape and ability to clot may be impaired, Dr. Muñoz explains. "These changes may be observed during a period of platelet cultivation for several days using darkfield microscopy. The culture allows for the identification of platelet forms typical of many illnesses, particularly of malignant cancers." As a result, very early detection of tendencies to develop cancer can be made. "This test confirmed that there was a prostate cancer with metastasis to the

For more information about **pleomorphic theory**, see Chapter 2: Cancer and Its Causes, pp. 48-93.

For more about **Livingston therapy** and to order her books *The Conquest of Cancer: Vaccines and Diet* (1984), *The Microbiology of Cancer Compendium* (1977), and *Cancer: A New Breakthrough* (1972), contact: The Livingston Foundation Medical Center, 3232 Duke Street, San Diego, CA 92110; tel: 619-224-3515; fax: 619-224-6253.

What is Mycoplasma?

A mycoplasma is a tiny biological life form without a cell wall, normally harmless, but capable of becoming harmful in a cancer process. Mycoplasma is also known as a cell wall–deficient organism. According to Dr. Muñoz, mycoplasma is a bacteria that grows on the surface of the cells such as platelets, lymphocytes, red blood cells, and on malignant cells. "When we take a sample of blood, we separate the serum, then culture the mycoplasma. After 4-6 weeks, the mycoplasma is separated from the culture and broken down into its biochemical components. We use the polysaccharide portion of it to develop the vaccine." It takes about two months to grow the vaccine in the laboratory from the cancer "germs" or mycoplasma, and other blood-borne cancer factors.

bones, and that Manuel had a high amount of toxins in his blood coming from bacterial infections in a root canal tooth and from his dental amalgams," explains Dr. Ramirez.

Next, Dr. Muñoz drew 120 cc of Manuel's blood as the basis for preparing the anti-mycoplasma vaccine. Generally, the results of the platelet test indicate if it is appropriate to prepare an anti-mycoplasma vaccine from the patient's blood, says Dr. Muñoz. Dr. Muñoz explains that a single blood culture from the patient is sufficient to produce enough vaccine to last 4-5 months at the rate of 2-3 injections weekly.

Dr. Ramirez adds that the purpose of the vaccine is to enhance and strengthen the immune system. "It helps the immune system recognize the 'germs' that were formerly blocking its own response, creating a condition in which the body did not act against the mycoplasma, viruses, and other cancer-related factors."

Manuel received the vaccine three times weekly for several months, then as his cancer began to reverse itself and he became healthier, the injections were gradually reduced to once monthly. According to Dr. Ramirez, Manuel will need to receive the anti-mycoplasma injection about once every month for the rest of his life as a precaution against any further cancer activity.

During the two months culturing time for the anti-mycoplasma vaccine, Dr. Muñoz drew a pint of Manuel's blood and ran it through an ultraviolet photophoresis machine. The process of ultraviolet light therapy killed viruses and bacteria and neutralized toxins in the blood; ozone, a form of oxygen, was also introduced into the blood sample to further purify it, then the blood was reinfused into Manuel. "For patients with advanced cancers, we do this once daily for the first 1-2 weeks," says Dr. Ramirez.

There was also chelation therapy (SEE QUICK DEFINITION), sauna, massage, and supplements, including *L. acidophilus*, enzymes, glutathione,

N-acetyl-cysteine, and both herbal and synthetic antiviral substances, says Dr. Muñoz. These included echinacea, goldenseal, interferon, Pranosine, and Zovirax. In addition, Manuel's diet underwent significant changes, based on a modified macrobiotic (SEE QUICK DEFINITION) approach. He was to eat only fresh fruits and vegetables and fish, and to avoid red meats and minimize his poultry consumption. He also started a regular exercise program to induce sweating and the discharging of toxins through the skin, and he received regular intestinal colonics.

A prime source of Manuel's toxins was his teeth, specifically a toxic substance called di-methylsulphite released from several root canals. Di-methylsulphite is a by-product of the interaction of bacteria and heavy metals placed in the mouth by dental procedures such as amalgam fillings, says Dr. Ramirez. "This substance will depress the immune system and can even weaken the heart." As part of his cancer treatment program, Manuel had his root canal teeth extracted.

For more about the anti-mycoplasma vaccine, contact: Filibert Muñoz, M.D. or Fernando C. Ramirez del Rio, M.D., Instituto Binacional de las Californias de Traumatologia Ortopedia, Rehabilitacion y Ciencias Afines A.C., Edificio Allen W. Lloyd, Paseo Tijuana 406, Suite 203, Segundo Piso, Zona del Rio, Tijuana, Baja California, Mexico C.P. 22310; tel: 52-6683-2944 or 52-6683-6225. Or write Dr. Ramirez at: P.O. Box 451, Bonita, CA 91908. Also contact both Drs. Muñoz and Ramirez at: Instituto Medico Biologico, Paseo Tijuana 406-203, Tijuana, Baja California, Mexico: fax: 526-682-4030. U.S. address: P.O. Box 431697, San Ysidro, CA 92143; tel: 619-216-1455; fax: 619-482-4394.

Finally, Manuel required spinal surgery for the nerve compression produced by the bony metastases. "Once his cancer was completely controlled and the cancer markers and antigen factors were down to zero, meaning there was no cancer activity, we still had to deal with Manuel's spinal cord compression at the lumbar nerve roots," says Dr. Ramirez, who is an orthopedic surgeon. This operation was necessary to allow Manuel to regain the use of his lumbar nerves and the ability to walk again without pain or fatigue.

In less than one year of receiving the anti-mycoplasma vaccine, Manuel's cancer markers were down to zero. Two years later, Manuel remained healthy and active, and had taken to traveling all over Mexico, "happy, with no pain," says Dr. Ramirez.

Immuno-Placental Therapy

Cancer immunologists have long proposed that by stimulating the immune system in specific ways they could stop and possibly reverse cancer. The use of vaccines and interleukin-2 has worked well with malignant melanoma and kidney cancer.[17] Dr. Springer's vaccine has shown effectiveness against breast cancer. In treating bladder cancer, the BCG vaccine has proved far superior to even the most aggressive forms of chemotherapy,[18] while monoclonal antibodies appear to be promising for the treatment of melanoma. For other cancers, however, these treatments have yielded inconsistent results.

The main reason for this inconsistency, according to immunologist Valentine I. Govallo, M.D., Ph.D., is that cancer has a unique immunologic character that, in most cases, enables it to evade the immune system. Dr. Govallo is the director of the Moscow Medical Institute's Laboratory of Clinical Immunology. Over the years, Dr. Govallo observed that a large number of the women who came to him indicated miscarriages as part of their health history. His observations led him to conclude that the problem was due to a general deterioration of the fetal-placental immune system as a result of environmental pollution. Dr. Govallo's approach is based on an understanding of the way a fetus relates to its mother on an immunological level.

For more about **ultraviolet light therapy**, see Chapter 10: Energy Support Therapies, pp. 298-316.

Although it is dependent on its mother for everything, the fetus has a primitive immune system with features slightly different from its mother. The fetus and the mother actually have competing immune systems. It sounds strange but it is possible for the mother's immune system to regard the fetus as foreign protein and set out to eliminate it. Under normal, healthy circumstances, the fetus is not rejected because its placenta-based (SEE QUICK DEFINITION) immunity manages to block the mother's immune system.

In the case of miscarriage, the mother's immune system recognizes in the fetus proteins from the father, and since her immune system perceives these as alien to her, the fetus is rejected. Environmental pollution, which is quite fierce in Russia, further adds to the problem, because it gives the mother's immune system even more foreign proteins and materials to react against, and thus further jeopardizes the fetus. Based on this medical insight, Dr. Gavallo was able to prevent miscarriages with a 91% success rate by stimulating the development of the placenta, thus strengthening placental immunity and protecting the fetus against rejection by the mother's immune system.

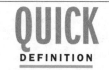

DEFINITION

Chelation therapy refers to a method of binding ("chelating") an organic substance known as a chelating agent to a metallic ion with a positive electric charge (e.g., a heavy metal) and removing it from the body. One type of chelation therapy involves the chelating agent disodium EDTA given as an intravenous infusion over a $3^1/_2$ hour period. Usually 20 to 30 treatments are administered at the rate of 1-3 sessions per week. Chelation therapy is especially beneficial for all forms of atherosclerotic cardiovascular disease including angina pectoris and coronary artery disease.

Macrobiotics is a specialized diet and food philosophy roughly based on Chinese medicine and filtered through contemporary Japanese culture and American representatives such as Georges Ohsawa and Michio Kushi. The diet emphasizes balancing the energy qualities of fresh, whole foods to maximize their delivery of *Qi*, or vital life force, to the body. The diet comprises cooked whole grains, beans and bean products, vegetables, fruits, nuts, seeds, small amounts of saltwater fish (salmon), fermented soybean products (miso), seaweeds, shiitake mushrooms, and special pickles and condiments. Macrobiotics has been used successfully when clinically prescribed as a curative and restorative diet in treating chronic and serious illness, including cancer; as a health maintenance diet, it has produced excellent results for many people.

This discovery gave Dr. Govallo a key insight into the riddle of cancer. He reasoned that just as the placenta synthesizes "blocking factors" to keep it from being rejected by its mother, so might tumors have this ability to hamper the immune system using a kind of immunological "cloaking device" that shields it from the host. In a sense, the tumor uses the same technique as the fetus to avoid being rejected by the host's immune system.

Today, scientists know that tumors produce blocking factors[19] and that some of these blocking factors appear to be proteins that are "shed" from the tumor as it interacts with the host's immune system. For example, one type of tumor protein may shut down the tumor-killing activity of natural killer cells;[20] another is the immune system cytokine called tumor necrosis factor, which in addition to its ability to cause tumor cells to die may also turn off the body's immune response to foreign tissues.[21] The secretion of these blocking factors may be one mechanism by which the tumor cells gain advantage over the antitumor immune responses of the host.

"Cancers have figured out a way of turning off the host's immune system, like a burglar who first turns off the burglar alarm before he goes about stealing things," Dr. Govallo says. "If it is possible to breach the tumor's immunological shield, the organism should be in a position to neutralize the tumor." The healthy human placenta contains factors that appear to suppress the defense mechanism of malignant cells. Dr. Govallo's placenta-derived vaccine basically provides a way to "decloak" the tumor.

The vaccine is produced from human placental tissue after a live human birth. Dr. Govallo called his approach immuno-placental therapy or IPT, but it is now known as VG-1000. The kinds of cancer for which IPT seems particularly effective include malignant melanoma, lung, breast, kidney, and colorectal cancers.[22] "The therapy works best with a small tumor mass, even if this reduction is obtained through surgical intervention." The vaccine is administered only after an evaluation of the status of the patient's immune system. Usually tumor reduction becomes noticeable within a few weeks after beginning the injections; however, most patients experience sensations at tumor sites within minutes of the injection.

VG-1000 has been used effectively in the treatment of advanced cancers. Dr. Govallo's first pilot study focused on 45 patients with advanced cancer; today, 29 of the original 45 remain alive—a 64.4% survival rate after 20 years. A more recent study of advanced-cancer patients compared their survival with VG-1000 to survival following other immunotherapy approaches; the survival in the IPT group was far supe-

Placental Blood Increases Leukemia Survival

Physicians at Duke University observed a 50% survival rate over a period of 7-32 months when 25 leukemia patients received infusions of blood from the placenta (which would otherwise be discarded) of newborn humans, according to the *New England Journal of Medicine* (July 1996). While all 25 patients required marrow to replace stem cells destroyed by the cancer, the use of placental blood produced a better survival rate than standard bone-marrow transplantation and made it easier to match donors with recipients.

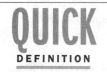

DEFINITION

The **placenta** is the disk-shaped organ responsible for metabolic exchange between a fetus and its mother; it is made partly from the fetal embryo and partly from the mother's uterine mucosa. The placenta receives nutrients and oxygen (and toxins, if present) through the mother's blood, and it can discharge carbon dioxide and nitrogen waste products back into the mother for elimination. The placenta is, on average, ⅙ the weight of the infant at birth; the umbilical cord of the fetus attaches to the middle of the placenta.

rior—77% versus 6% after five years. Dr. Govallo notes that if the tumor is destroyed too suddenly, it can release massive amounts of toxins that can actually kill the patient. For this reason, the body must be well-supplied with nutrients to accelerate its detoxification capacities.

Pleomorphism and SANUM Remedies

The German researcher Guenther Enderlein, M.D., Ph.D. (1872-1968), opened up a new vista in understanding cancer and devising treatments through his use of darkfield microscopy. In the course of studying live blood under the darkfield microscope, Dr. Enderlein observed protein-based microorganisms, which he called protits, that flourish in the blood cells, tissues, body fluids, and plasma. Protits appear to live in a mutually beneficial or symbiotic relationship with the body under healthy conditions, but when the body's internal environment—its cellular terrain—changes in terms of pH (acidity/alkalinity ratio), toxin load, or the availability of oxygen and/or nutrients, the protits develop into a disease-causing form. The ability of organisms to undergo sequential shape changes is a theory of bacteriology called pleomorphism.

The microbe that Dr. Enderlein linked with cancer is primarily *Mucor racemosus Fresen*. Under certain conditions, biochemical factors in the body foster development of the protits into more lethal forms. It has been more specifically identified as the blood parasite *Siphonospora polymorpha*—the most advanced stage of the *Mucor racemosus Fresen*, according to Dr. Enderlein—a major cancer-promoting agent.[23]

Dr. Enderlein noted that a diet rich in animal fats and proteins seemed to promote changes in pH and cause these normally harmless microbes to change into the harmful *Mucor* fungi. Thus, the typical American diet provides the ideal conditions for transforming protits into their harmful forms. This situation is made worse by carcinogenic substances—dietary factors (food additives, pesticides), viruses, alcohol, tobacco, radiation—which can alter the cell's ability to metabolize proteins and fats and to make energy.

Dr. Govallo's immune therapy is contrain-dicated for liver can-cer, because it can destroy the liver tumor so quickly that the liver cannot adequately process and eliminate the dead cancer cells. Consequently, the per-son tends to develop a hepatitis-like condition.

The protit, in its altered form, leads to faulty genetic mechanisms which result in incorrect synthesis of proteins such as those used by the immune system.[24] This situation, combined with the "blocking factors" mentioned earlier, may help explain why the immune system often fails to respond appropriately to cancer cells.

Dr. Enderlein theorized that disease must be treated at the cellular level and he formulated his remedies accordingly. His formulas, known as SANUM remedies, are dilutions of bacteria and fungi that, once injected into the cancer patient, work according to the principles of homeopathy. By injecting harmless forms of bacteria exemplifying the microorganism in its benign state, the disease-causing protits revert to their benign form, which promotes normal immune function.[25]

Erik Enby, M.D. of Gothenberg, Sweden, has carried forth the work of Dr. Enderlein and confirmed all his original findings. During Dr. Enby's initial eight-year experience with the darkfield microscope and Enderlein remedies, he successfully treated more than 100 cases of prostate and uterine cancer and effectively stabilized or reversed many cases of breast cancer and leukemia.[26] Dr. Enby notes that Enderlein remedies are most successful when used with an effective program of detoxification. Dr. Enby also recommends the following measures to max-imize the effectiveness of Enderlein remedies: (1) remove metal fillings or mercury dental amalgams; (2) avoid or minimize the intake of animal pro-teins and fats; (3) eat pesticide-free raw vegetables and fresh fruits; (4) avoid chemotherapy and other anticancer drugs; (5) avoid unnecessary antibiotics and other synthetic infection-reducing drugs; (6) avoid steroid medications; (7) avoid taking medications that reduce fever during an ill-ness, unless health is impaired; and (8) keep X rays to a minimum.

Dr. Govallo's placental vaccine is now available in North America at two alternative cancer clinics: Max Gerson Memorial Center Hospital in Tijuana, Mexico, and Immuno-Augmentative Clinic (IAT) in Freeport, Bahamas. The arrival of VG 1000 in North America was made possible by the efforts of medical historian Harris L. Coulter, Ph.D., director of the Center for Empirical Medicine in Washington, D.C. For preliminary screening information, contact: People Against Cancer, Box 10, Otho, IA 50569; tel: 515-972-4444. To contact Dr. Coulter about licensing VG-1000: Harris L. Coulter, Ph.D., Empirical Therapies, Inc., 4221 45th Street, N.W., Washington, D.C. 20016; tel: 202-362-3185; fax: 202-362-3407. For information about **Enderlein medicine**, contact: Biological Medicine Institute, Avenida de la Paz, No. 16420 Colonia Mineral Sante Fe, Tijuana, B.C. 22360 Mexico; for mailing, Biological Medicine Institute, P.O. Box 433656, San Ysidro, CA 92173; tel: 52-66-240786, 52-66-240939, or 52-66-245110; fax: 52-66-240786. For more about **SANUM remedies**, contact: Enderlein Sales Group, P.O. Box 2352, Santa Rosa, CA 95405; tel: 800-203-3775 or 707-537-9505; fax: 707-538-9179.

8 Enhancing Metabolism

METABOLISM IS THE SUM TOTAL of all the biochemical processes going on inside the body, and metabolic therapies focus on ways to balance these chemical processes—enabling normal cells to thrive and cancer cells to become depleted and die, or revert back to normal. The therapeutic goal of metabolic therapies is to rebuild and revitalize all of the body's life-sustaining functions, thereby helping to stop and reverse cancer, or to prevent a recurrence. In this chapter, we examine different therapies, such as the use of hydrogen peroxide, ozone, enzymes, and glandular extracts, vital to the functioning of all systems of the body. Along with diet and nutritional factors, these make up what we call metabolic therapies.

Making and Using Energy at the Cellular Level

First, we need to briefly review the metabolism of healthy and cancerous cells as a background to understanding metabolic therapies.

The primary goal of metabolic therapy is to alter the cancer cells' chemical processes and thereby promote their vulnerability or reversion to normal cells. Some of these processes—the metabolism of oxygen and glucose, for example—are directly aimed at the cancer cells. Others exert an indirect influence by boosting the patient's immune system, influencing cancer tissue damage by free radicals, and detoxifying the body. Most standard

Metabolism: How We Get Energy From Foods

Metabolism is the biological process by which we extract energy from the foods we eat, producing carbon dioxide and water as by-products for elimination from the body. More generally, metabolism refers to any of the chemical reactions that take place in our cells. These chemical reactions are controlled by enzymes, which are specialized proteins produced by the cells. Enzymes initiate and regulate the speed of all chemical reactions; hence they are known as catalysts.

There are two kinds of metabolism: anabolic and catabolic. The anabolic function produces substances for cell growth and repair, while the catabolic function controls digestion, disassembling food into forms the body can use for energy. For example, proteins are broken down into amino acids, fats into glycerol and fatty acids, and carbohydrates into monosaccharides or simple sugars. Anabolic and catabolic metabolism are constantly under way in the cells. Under healthy, normal conditions, both phases operate in balance with each other so that energy needs do not outstrip energy supply.

Biochemically, metabolism involves hundreds of chemical reactions, necessitating the involvement of hundreds of different enzymes, each of which handles a specific reaction. Some chemical reactions have a number of stages that must occur in a certain order. A different enzyme will be responsible for each stage and they must work together to ensure the proper sequence. This sequence of enzyme-controlled reactions is known as a metabolic pathway.

The carbohydrate pathway is one example of a metabolic pathway. When carbohydrates enter the body as food, amylase breaks them down into monosaccharides (the main one is glucose); these can be converted into energy via the catabolic pathway or converted via the anabolic pathway into glycogen or fat for storage.

Another metabolic process is called cellular respiration. This involves the breakdown of glucose and other substances and the release of energy from them. Through chemical reactions occurring in cells, glucose is converted to citric acid and energy is transferred to ATP (adenosine triphosphate), an energy-carrying molecule. At this point, the Kreb's cycle begins. In this, during another series of chemical conversions, molecules of carbon dioxide and hydrogen atoms are released. The carbon dioxide is transported into the blood and the hydrogen atoms are joined with oxygen. Again, the chemical reactions release energy, some of which is transfered to ATP for use by the cell and the remainder is expended as heat. The entire process represents the "breathing" of the cell.

chemotherapy drugs, hydrogen peroxide, and ozone work by producing free-radical damage to cancer cells at greater rates than to non-cancerous cells.

When it comes to understanding how healthy and cancerous cells make and use energy, the key is oxygen. The metabolism of cancer cells is similar to that of normal cells in many respects, but there are crucial differences. In normal cell metabolism, oxygen is used in the cell along with glucose (blood sugar) to produce energy for the cell to function. This aerobic (oxygen/air-dependent) form of energy production is about 18 times more efficient than its opposite, anaerobic metabolism, in which the cell burns glucose in the absence of oxygen. For this reason, anaerobic cells must work harder than aerobic cells to derive energy, burning far more glucose to generate the same amount of energy as aerobic cells.

Cancer cells exhibit the anaerobic mode of metabolism, which means they are not dependent on oxygen, a characteristic that seems related to the fact that the mitochondria, or primary energy-producing components of cells, are defective in cancer.[1] Mitochondria are often called the cell's "powerhouses" because they generate energy. Mitochondria contain enzymes that help them break down fats and carbohydrates in the presence of oxygen.

Under normal conditions of aerobic metabolism with healthy mitochondria, the cell takes in glucose and oxygen and releases carbon dioxide; with its defective mitochondria, the tumor cell is incapable of carrying out this elementary cell respiration. Cancer cells only partially metabolize glucose, producing lactic acid rather than carbon dioxide in the process. Cancer cells thrive under the conditions of high-sugar low-oxygen associated with fermentation, but fare poorly under low-sugar high-oxygen conditions.

As cancer cells begin to multiply, forming a tumor, the liver must expend a considerable amount of energy converting the toxic lactic acid back to glucose. Also, most cancer cells can function only at a low pH—a very acidic state—because of the lactic acid they constantly produce. The combined effect of the tumor's metabolism is to tax the liver and acidify the body. This leads to frequent bouts of fatigue, an early warning sign of cancer.

Over time, the cancer cell's highly inefficient use of energy places a huge burden on the host. As the cancer grows, ever more lactic acid is produced, creating an even larger energy drain. This has the effect of drawing amino acids such as glutamine and alanine (which can be used for energy) out of the muscles, thereby causing physical wasting or loss of lean tissue mass.

Success Story: Taking Charge of Her Healing

Jane, 65, a highly successful realtor, investor, and developer, was diagnosed with Stage IV breast cancer which had metastasized from her left breast to her bones. She underwent a lumpectomy. At the same time, she refused radiation, but accepted chemotherapy and had two cycles of Cytoxan, methotrexate, and 5-FU. Based on research she conducted herself, Jane decided that she did not want any more chemotherapy; she believed it was doing her body more harm than good.

Jane went to James W. Forsythe, M.D., H.M.D., director of the Cancer Screening and Treatment Center of Nevada in Reno. "She was feeling awful, very tired and weak, having some hair loss and nausea, and decided she wanted to go on her own," says Dr. Forsythe, who helped her design a program that included the following vitamins, minerals, herbs, and other substances:

■ Germanium (an antioxidant trace mineral): 150 mg every 12 hours

■ DHEA (an immune stimulant and hormone vital to the production of other hormones): 25 mg daily

■ Bovine (or shark) cartilage (for antitumor activity): 4-12 g daily in powder or 500 mg capsules

■ Thymus glandular extract (to enhance the immune system, specifically T cells): 200 mg, three times daily

■ Evening primrose oil (a botanical high in essential fatty acids, for antioxidant support): one capsule every 12 hours

■ Red clover (for herbal anticancer support): 300 mg every eight hours

■ Vitamin C (an antioxidant): 2.5 g every six hours

■ Garlic (for immune support and anticancer activity): three capsules every eight hours

■ Glucosamine (for bone pain relief and bone repair): 500 mg every eight hours

■ Calcium citrate (for bone growth and prevention of osteoporosis): 500 mg every eight hours

■ Armour natural thyroid glandular extract (to enhance metabolism and speed healing): two grains daily

■ Chlorella (a blue-green algae, to aid in detoxification): three capsules daily

■ Pau d'arco (for herbal antitumor support): 200 mg daily

■ Essiac tea (a combination of herbs used to treat cancer, for herbal antitumor support): three cups daily

■ Glutathione (an amino acid complex, for immune support): 500 mg daily

For **Dr. Forsythe's cancer protocols**, see *Alternative Medicine Definitive Guide to Cancer* (Future Medicine Publishing, 1997; ISBN 1-887299-01-7); to order, call 800-333-HEAL.

James W. Forsythe, M.D., H.M.D.: Cancer Screening and Treatment Center of Nevada, Hematology Oncology Ltd., 75 Pringle Way, Suite 909, Reno, NV 89502; tel: 702-329-5000; fax: 702-329-6219.

Jane began this program immediately after discontinuing chemotherapy and remained on it faithfully for 3½ years, says Dr. Forsythe. Her cancer markers, which had been elevated before, became normal. "Here is a woman with a Stage IV cancer who didn't take the prescribed radiation and chemotherapy. She did not have what we call a complete cancer surgery, yet she is doing beautifully, extremely well," reports Dr. Forsythe. "Jane is a very assertive person who runs her own business. She really took charge of her disease and did the healing her own way. She's been very successful."

Oxygen (Hydrogen Peroxide and Ozone)

Cancer only grows in the absence of oxygen, which means if you introduce sufficient oxygen into the body's cells, this will help reverse the cancer process by suffocating the tumor with too much oxygen. Physicians working with oxygen therapy find that hydrogen peroxide and ozone can produce excellent results.

Most health-minded people are aware of the harmful effects of free radicals caused by oxidation. What is not well-known is that when produced under controlled circumstances, as in oxygen therapy, free radicals are deadly to bacteria, viruses, and fungi. Oxygen therapy stimulates the immune system and various enzyme systems, probably through increasing the production of cytokines, immunologically active proteins that destroy or inhibit the growth of microorganisms and tumor cells.

Recent research has begun to show the precise immune changes that occur in oxygen therapy. German scientist Otto Warburg, M.D., was the first to propose that a lack of oxygen at the cellular level may be the prime cause of cancer and that oxygen therapy could be an effective treatment for it. He showed that normal embryonic cells, when subjected to reduced oxygen concentrations, quickly adopt the fermentative metabolism typical of cancer cells. The lack of oxygen apparently alters the normal cell's respiration during growth, triggering the development of cancer. When oxygen levels surrounding the cells are raised, cancer cells do not form.

Dr. Warburg proposed that normalizing the metabolism of cancer cells was the key to effective treatment and that the prime means to accomplish this was through oxygen. Specifically, Dr. Warburg suggested as the first priority of treatment "that all growing body cells be saturated with oxygen."[2] The second priority was to avoid further exposure to toxins, as a way to help shift the enzyme balance of the cancer cell and restore normal cellular metabolism.

Oxygen's Role in the Growth of Cancer Cells

According to Dr. Warburg, almost anything can cause cancer, but even for cancer there is only one prime cause—the replacement of the respiration of oxygen in normal cells by a fermentation of sugar. "All normal body cells meet their energy needs by respiration of oxygen, whereas cancer cells meet their energy needs in great part by fermentation.[3]

The metabolic approach originally proposed by Dr. Warburg entails exposing the cancer cell to high levels of oxygen. Since the cancer cell can participate only in fermentative metabolism, oxygen at high levels is toxic. The cancer cell has a very low production of superoxide dismutase (SOD), an antioxidant enzyme that protects normal cells from high oxygen concentrations.[4] This lack of SOD may make cancer cells particularly vulnerable to high oxygen concentrations. Oxygen can be used in various forms to promote healing and to destroy pathogens in the body. These therapies have been used to treat a wide variety of conditions, including cancer, infections, circulatory problems, chronic fatigue syndrome, arthritis, allergies, and multiple sclerosis. There are two principal types of oxygen therapy, classified according to the chemical process involved: oxygenation and oxidation.

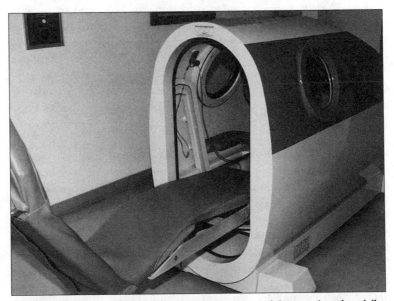

A hyperbaric oxygen chamber, somewhat resembling a miniature submarine, delivers pure oxygen under pressure to all the cells of the body, including the brain.

Oxygenation—This is the process of enriching the oxygen content of the blood or tissues. Using oxygen as a safe, selective "chemotherapy" for cancer patients has been found to be effective when used in combination with regular aerobic exercise, hyperthermia (heat therapy) induced by infrared light, intermittently induced high blood sugar (by giving glucose intravenously), and daily administration of 30 mg of vitamin B1, 100 mg of magnesium orotate, and 75 mg of dipyridamol (a drug that prevents blood clotting).[5]

Hyperbaric oxygen therapy introduces oxygen to the body in a pressurized chamber. A clinical process called hyperoxygenation saturates the body with oxygen through the use of gas, sometimes at high pressure. The application is based on the principle that insufficient oxygenation promotes the growth of pathogens whereas excessive oxygenation damages normal tissues. Oxygenation employed under strictly controlled conditions can have positive therapeutic effects.

Oxidation—Oxidation is a chemical reaction occurring when electrons (electrically charged particles) are transferred from one molecule to another. Oxygen molecules are frequently, but not always, involved in these reactions. The molecules that give up their electrons are referred to as oxidized; the molecules that accept electrons are referred to as oxidants. Although uncontrolled oxidation can be destructive—as is the case when free radicals are produced in excess—it can also be therapeutic when carefully used on weak and devitalized cells as the targets. These weak cells are metabolically broken down, permitting the formation of new, healthy cells that are better able to resist disease.[6] Oxidation therapy may help by "jumpstarting" the body's oxidative processes and returning them to normal, according to Charles Farr, M.D., Ph.D., a leading researcher in oxygen therapy.

Hydrogen Peroxide as a Metabolic Cancer Therapy

Hydrogen peroxide (H_2O_2) is a natural substance made by healthy cells in the body to regulate metabolism and to destroy invaders. In 1920, the prestigious British journal *The Lancet* reported the use of intravenous hydrogen peroxide by British Army doctors in India treating troops suffering from influenza. It reduced their death rate from 90% to 50%. In the 1950s, hydrogen peroxide was approved by the FDA as a food additive and was used by farmers to retard spoilage in animal feed. Following this, farmers noted an unexpected health benefit in the livestock and started using hydrogen peroxide themselves as a folk remedy. Since that time, physicians have experimented with intravenous hydrogen peroxide treatment

Glyoxylide—A New Way to Deliver Oxygen to the Cells

During the 1940s, William F. Koch, M.D., Ph.D., a physiology professor at Detroit Medical College (later part of Wayne State University) reasoned that cells become cancerous because the blood's oxygen levels get depleted. If sufficient oxygen were continually delivered to the body's tissues, cancer pathology would be virtually impossible.

Dr. Koch proposed to supply oxygen by means of carbonyl and ethylene, a compound he called glyoxylide.[10] Rather than intravenous delivery, Dr. Koch preferred to give glyoxylide once or twice in the form of intramuscular injection of a solution diluted to 6X, a mild homeopathic level.[11]

Harold R. Stark, M.D., a physician who studied with Dr. Koch, explains that glyoxylide promotes vigorous oxygenation and oxidation activity in spite of its great dilution. The cell is literally forced to take on oxygen through aerobic metabolism and give up waste products. With the Koch remedies, the cancer cell gradually dies and is eliminated.[12]

Dr. Koch monitored the patient's diet and drug intake, attempting to minimize the latter. Because of his desire to keep cancer patients off anti-cancer drugs that might interfere with metabolism, Dr. Koch was harassed and eventually sued by the FDA. He was exonerated, but he decided to continue his studies of glyoxylide in Brazil. Due to FDA obstruction, the substance is not available in the U.S.; however, physicians may import it from Germany for single patient use.

in a number of conditions, including heart disease, emphysema, bronchitis, asthma, influenza, Lyme disease, chronic fatigue, *Candida*, parasitic infections, and arthritis, with excellent results. Research indicates that H_2O_2 stimulates natural killer cells, which attack cancer cells throughout the body.[7]

Hydrogen peroxide is a simple compound made up of a molecule of water (H_2O) with an extra atom of oxygen (O) attached. It is produced in cells during normal metabolism. Hydrogen peroxide, when given at the correct dosage, can have an oxidizing or cleansing effect, although excessive amounts can be harmful.

Oxygen or oxidative therapies today are based on *dilute* H_2O_2, which is relatively harmless, particularly when the individual is taking antioxidant supplements that help protect the body's normal cells. Macrophages and other immune cells generate H_2O_2 to help kill bacteria, parasites, viruses, and other pathogens. Research indicates H_2O_2 helps enzymes remove toxins and can directly destroy invading microbes;[8] the H_2O_2 produced by these immune cells has also been shown to have antitumor properties.[9]

According to Dr. Farr, oxidation achieved through H_2O_2 therapy regulates tissue repair, cellular respiration, growth, immune and energy functions, most hormone systems, and the production of cytokines (chemical messengers involved in the regulation of almost every system in the body). Some cytokines, such as interferon and interleukin-2, play key roles in helping the immune system destroy cancer cells, and the anticancer effect of interferon seems to depend on the H_2O_2 generated by immune cells.[13]

Hydrogen peroxide provides an additional boost to the anticancer defenses by stimulating natural killer cells, which are needed to stop the spread of cancer.[14] Intravenous H_2O_2 also stimulates the oxidative enzymes in the body, helping them remove toxins and exert a direct cancer-killing effect on tumor cells.[15] Dr. Farr discovered that these intravenous H_2O_2 infusions almost doubled the metabolic activity of detoxifying enzymes.[16] Taken together, these effects could account for the positive clinical results observed when oxygen therapies are used to treat cancer.

Most of the studies that have examined the ability of H_2O_2 to improve the survival rates in cancer are based on animal research. A study of rats implanted with tumors found that when their drinking water was replaced by a dilute H_2O_2 solution, the tumors completely disappeared within two to eight weeks.[17] When oral H_2O_2 was given to mice preinjected with cancer cells, death rates declined and onset of palpable tumors was delayed.[18] Researchers at Rockefeller University in New York concluded that H_2O_2 could exert a "direct antitumor effect and thereby prolong survival."[19]

Many studies have documented the value of combining H_2O_2 with conventional cancer treatments. In one, H_2O_2 improved the outcome of chemotherapy;[20] in another, H_2O_2 injected into the arteries for ten days, followed by mitomycin C (an antibiotic showing antitumor activity), enhanced the effectiveness of the anticancer drug.[21] H_2O_2 has also been shown to make cancer cells more sensitive to the effects of radiation therapy.[22]

There are cautions to observe regarding hydrogen peroxide. Ross Pelton, Ph.D., reports that the medical staff at the Hospital Santa Monica in Mexico administered over 30,000 infusions of dilute hydrogen peroxide without a serious reaction.[23] On some occasions, however, a stinging or burning sensation occurred at the infusion site; patients with smaller veins tended to experience more of this transitory discomfort. In rare cases, inflammation of the veins at the site of injection will occur. Hydrogen peroxide should not be taken orally as it causes nausea and vomiting, and rectal administration can lead to inflammation of the lower intestinal tract. Other effects can include temporary faintness, fatigue, headaches, and chest pain.

Ozone Can Stimulate Energy-Producing Activity

Another oxygen therapy uses ozone and relies on both oxidation and oxygenation pathways. Approximately 20% of the air we breathe is comprised of oxygen, which has two atoms (O_2). Ozone (O_3) contains three oxygen atoms and is a less stable form of oxygen. Due to this added molecule, ozone is more reactive than oxygen and readily oxidizes other chemicals. During oxidation in the body, the extra oxygen molecule in ozone can break away, leaving a normal O_2 molecule. Often it does this by combining with water to form hydrogen peroxide and oxygen. The net result is to increase the oxygen content of the blood or tissues.

The Ozone Story

Around 1900, interest began to focus on the uses of ozone in medical therapy. It is estimated that more than ten million ozone treatments have been given over the last 40 years worldwide and more than 1,000 articles on the subject have been published in scientific journals.

Used primarily to kill viruses, bacteria, and fungi, ozone produces important benefits in the human body, including the oxygenation of blood, improved circulation, and stimulation of the immune system. The range of human health problems that respond favorably to ozone therapy includes AIDS, arthritis, asthma, cancer, fungal diseases, hepatitis, sinusitis, atherosclerosis, and more.

Many Americans think of ozone as an air pollutant. Although it is true that high concentrations of ozone may be irritating to the lungs and cause free-radical damage, controlled use of ozone may be beneficial for many purposes, such as the purification of air and water. The City of Los Angeles uses ozone to purify its water system and many swimming pools are now kept clean with an ozone water purification system rather than with chlorine. What is generally not known is that ozone has many medical uses as well.

Ozone can be administered intravenously, intramuscularly, into the joint, and subcutaneously (just beneath the skin). In the case of intravenous use of ozone, this is usually done by removing up to one quart of the patient's blood, mixing it with ozone, then reinjecting it into the body. Ozone may be applied topically as a gas or dissolved in water or olive oil, then applied to the skin. As a gas, it may be applied vaginally or rectally; it may also be taken orally, rectally, or vaginally in the form of ozonated water. One of the most effective methods is to inject humidified ozone into the rectum; this is ozone dissolved in water vapor.[24]

Evidence shows that ozone has strong therapeutic value. It can selectively inhibit cancer cell growth in tissue culture for cancers of the lung, breast, and uterus when given in doses of as little as 0.3-0.8 parts per million (ppm) over a period of eight days.[25] Exposure to the 0.8-ppm dose inhibited cancer cell growth more than 90%. The growth of normal cells was not inhibited, which suggested that "cancer cells are less able to compensate for the oxidative burden of ozone than normal cells."[26] Ozone therapy can also enhance the tumor-fighting ability of standard cancer drugs.[27] Test doses of ozone were found to selectively block the division of cancer cells; this positive effect increased as the ozone doses got stronger until all cancer cell activity was virtually halted at high doses.[28] Ozone seems to stimulate the activity of cytokines, natural cancer-killing proteins.[29]

German surgeon Joachim Varro, M.D., has worked with hundreds of cancer patients, most of whom had received chemotherapy and radiation. Dr. Varro found that ozone therapy greatly reduces pain while increasing energy levels and appetite. Dr. Varro noted the following: (1) patients were free of metastases and recurrences for long periods of time; (2) the survival time could be prolonged, far exceeding the prognoses of conventional treatment; and (3) most patients who had undergone ozone therapy shortly after surgery and radiation could return to full-time work.[30]

According to Jonathan Wright, M.D., medical director of the Tahoma Clinic in Kent, Washington, any time oxygen therapies are used, the possibility of generating excess free radicals must be guarded against by taking antioxidants. "You can't use ozone alone," says Dr. Wright. "You need to combine it with a proper diet, supplements, herbs, botanicals, acupuncture, and chiropractic." Antioxidants (substances that can neutralize free radicals) such as vitamin C should be given to all patients who are receiving any form of oxygen therapy.

Adverse effects associated with intravenously administered ozone can include phlebitis (inflammation of a vein), circulatory depression, chest pain, shortness of breath, fainting, coughing, flushing, and cardiac arrhythmias. Although it is easily tolerated in other tissues, ozone in high concentrations can cause severe inflammation of the lung tissues and even coughing up of blood.

Enzymes

One of the factors that can impede the body's ability to ward off cancer is a lack of enzymes. These are molecules that speed up biochemical reactions and keep metabolism running efficiently. Diseases result when enzymes are inadequately produced or when essential elements are lacking in the diet; when minerals or trace elements are missing, the enzymatic action can be upset.

For example, the trace element selenium is needed for the enzyme glutathione peroxidase, one of the body's essential antioxidant enzymes; manganese, copper, and zinc are required by another important antioxidant system, called superoxide dismutase (SOD). When these trace elements are inadequately supplied, the resulting enzyme dysfunction can increase the body's vulnerability to toxins and harmful free radicals, which can promote the growth of tumors.

Enzyme dysfunction can affect digestion, and the body's inability to effectively metabolize protein may promote cancer. This inability may be linked to improper amounts of protein-digesting enzymes such as pepsin from the stomach and proteases from the pancreas which, along with hydrochloric acid (HCl) in the stomach, are the body's first defense against cancer development.

The Nature and Work of Enzymes

An Enzyme Primer

The following are some of the health conditions commonly associated with shortages of each of the four basic enzymes:

- **Protease (digests proteins)—** Anxiety; low blood sugar; kidney problems; water retention; depressed immunity; bacterial and viral infections; cancer; appendicitis; bone problems, such as osteoporosis, arthritis, and bone spurs.

- **Amylase (digests non-fiber carbohydrates)—**Skin problems such as rashes, hives, fungal infections, herpes, and canker sores; lung problems such as asthma, bronchitis, and emphysema; liver or gallbladder disease.

- **Lipase (digests fats)—**High cholesterol; obesity; diabetes; "hardening" of the arteries and other cardiovascular problems; chronic fatigue; spastic colon; dizziness.

- **Cellulase (digests fiber)—**Gas and bloating; acute food allergies; facial pain or paralysis; candidiasis (bowel and vaginal yeast infections).

As people age, they tend to lose their capacity to produce sufficient amounts of digestive enzymes, as well as HCl. Protein is normally broken down into smaller nutritive units, called amino acids, which are then absorbed in the small intestine; these eventually become neurotransmitters (chemical messengers in the brain), hormones, antibodies, metabolic and digestive enzymes, cell membrane receptors, and other components the body needs for healthy functioning. Approximately 50% of the daily utilization of protein goes into producing enzymes, mostly digestive enzymes.[31]

When protein is inadequately broken down, it putrefies in the intestinal tract and tends to form nitrosamines and ammonia, highly toxic compounds and known carcinogens. Although the extent to

For information about **enzymes** developed by Howard Loomis, D.C., contact: 21st Century Nutrition, 6421 Enterprise Lane, Madison, WI 53719; tel: 800-662-2630 or 608-273-8100; fax: 608-273-8111. For **Gastroprotective Enzymes** (a plant enzyme combination), contact: Health Restoration Systems, P.O. Box 832267, Richardson, TX 75083; tel: 972-480-8909;

which ammonia may contribute to the development of cancer is unknown, some researchers speculate that it may significantly increase one's susceptibility to colon cancer.

The effective action of digestive juices is critical not only for protein digestion, but also for processing of essential micronutrients—both vitamins and minerals. To make these micronutrients available to the body, digestive enzymes and HCl must be secreted in adequate amounts. A lack of such secretions in later life is one of the reasons older people are more prone to mineral deficiencies and vitamin B12 deficiency, for example, regardless of the presence of these in their food. The absorption of many other vitamins and essential nutrients can be similarly impeded by a lack of hydrochloric acid and digestive enzyme activity.

The human body makes approximately 22 different types of digestive enzymes, capable of digesting protein, carbohydrates, sugars, and fats. Most of the digestive enzymes are produced by the pancreas and include proteases, amylases, and lipases. Pancreatic enzymes function in both the intestine and in the blood. Supplemental pancreatic enzymes can aid digestion, sharing the workload of the body's own enzymes.

The Therapeutic Role of Enzymes

Enzyme therapy can be an important first step in restoring health and well-being by helping to remedy digestive problems. Plant enzymes and pancreatic enzymes are used in complementary ways to improve digestion and absorption of essential nutrients and to enhance the immune system's ability to recognize and destroy cancer cells. Both plant-derived enzymes and animal-derived pancreatic enzymes are used in enzyme therapy, independently or in combination.

Plant enzymes are prescribed primarily to enhance the digestive system, while pancreatic enzymes have historically been used to benefit both the digestive system and immune system. As proper digestive functioning is restored, many acute and chronic conditions are usually improved. For strict vegetarians and those persons allergic to beef and pork, plant enzymes can be used efficiently to aid the immune system as well as to support digestion.

Pancreatic enzymes can help in the treatment of cancer in several ways. Enzymes help expose foreign antigens on the surface of cancer cells so they can be recognized and destroyed by the immune system. They also help destroy CICs (circulating immune complexes) produced when cancerous cells shed antigens into the blood to avoid

Metabolic Therapies at American Biologics Hospital

One of the largest metabolic treatment centers in operation today is the American Biologics Hospital in Tijuana, Mexico, headed by Robert Bradford, D.Sc., and Rodrigo Rodriguez, M.D. The elimination of dietary sugar, excess animal protein, refined carbohydrates, and stimulants such as caffeine, and the use of amygdalin (laetrile) as well as nutritional supplements, such as vitamin C and other antioxidants, are emphasized.

In addition, the clinic uses embryonic live-cell therapy to bolster the patient's endocrine system; for example, embryonic brain and adrenal tissue are used to replenish DHEA, a hormone necessary for the proper function of the immune system. Detoxification therapy in the form of enemas and colonic irrigation is also important.

In 1987, American Biologics Hospital (ABH) presented an overview of its first 5,000 cancer cases to the Office of Technology Assessment of the U.S. Congress. Among these cases, of which more than 90% were supposedly terminal, ABH achieved a five-year survival rate of about 20% with few or no symptoms reported by patients.

For example, a male engineer had bone cancer of the thigh, with a tumor the size of a bowling ball. According to Michael Culbert, D.Sc., information director for ABH, "His doctors told him he would have to have his leg and part of his groin removed and undergo radiation. We placed him on a metabolic program and infused ozone gas directly into the tumor on alternate days; we also applied herbal poultices. Over a couple of months, the tumor became soft, then it popped open and oozed out. That was ten years ago. At last report, the patient is still doing well."

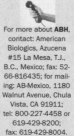

For more about **ABH**, contact: American Biologics, Azucena #15 La Mesa, T.J., B.C., Mexico; fax: 52-66-816435; for mailing: AB-Mexico, 1180 Walnut Avenue, Chula Vista, CA 91911; tel: 800-227-4458 or 619-429-8200; fax: 619-429-8004.

detection by the immune system. Pancreatic enzymes can stimulate natural killer cells, T cells, and tumor necrosis factor, all toxic to cancer cells.

The metastatic potential of a tumor depends, in part, on the adhesiveness of the cancer cells, their capacity to adhere to cell walls. Adhesiveness, in turn, seems to depend on the blood's "stickiness" or ability to coagulate. The greater this adhesive quality, the greater the capacity of the tumor to develop metastases.[32] The use of anticoagulants and proteolytic enzymes can effectively reduce the invasive or metastatic potential of cancer cells.[33] In addition, it is now thought that the cancer cell uses a protein called fibrin (or sometimes fats and lipids) to mask its identity, effectively hiding from the immune system. A logical therapeutic strategy would involve degrading the cancer cell's coating, allowing it to be identified by the immune system and halting metastasis.[34]

See *The Enzyme Cure*
by Lita Lee, Ph.D., and
Lisa Turner, with
Burton Goldberg
(Future Medicine
Publishing, 1998;
ISBN 1-887299-22-X);
to order,
call 800-333-HEAL.

Enzymes also play a vital role in the relationship between digestion and immune overload. Protein molecules that are only partially digested in the small intestine can be absorbed into the bloodstream. The immune system treats these substances as invaders, causing antibodies to form, couple with these antigens, and create circulating immune complexes (CICs). In a healthy person, CICs may be neutralized in the lymphatic system, but in a person with cancer, CICs tend to accumulate in the blood where they burden the detoxification pathways or initiate an allergic reaction.

If too many CICs accumulate, the kidneys cannot excrete enough of them. The CICs then accumulate in soft tissues, causing inflammation and bringing unnecessary stress to the immune system. Enzyme expert Howard Loomis, D.C., comments: "I always wonder why the diets for cancer and AIDS include such high amounts of protein when an excess of undigested protein can so obviously lead to demands on the immune system." It is here that pancreatic enzymes come into play. Pancreatic enzymes break down CICs enabling them to pass through the kidneys for excretion. High concentrations of CICs are associated with poorer prognoses in cancer patients.[35]

When too much of the enzyme production is allotted for digestion of food, less may be available for systemic protection against cancer (such as reducing CIC levels). "Ideally, you want to make it unnecessary for the digestive system to have to produce so many enzymes," says Jack Taylor, D.C., who uses enzymes in his anticancer program. "If you assist in the process of digestion by providing food enzymes, you can divert the body's overall enzyme production so that it can channel more enzymes to the site of malignancy."

Also, if a patient eats a lot of dairy products, meats, and cooked foods (whose own enzymes are destroyed in the cooking), then most of their pancreatic enzymes will be used up digesting foods, but if mostly raw fruits and vegetables are eaten, the active enzymes in these foods can assist in their own digestion, leaving more of the patient's pancreatic enzymes available to digest CICs.

Some European physicians addressing cancer and other illnesses use special enzyme formulations called Wobenzyme® and Wobe-Mugos®, first developed in Germany. These formulas contain pancreatin, papain, bromelain, trypsin, chymotrypsin, lipase, amylase, and rutin (a bioflavonoid), and are administered by injection, tablets, or suppositories. The German physician Max Wolf, M.D., started using Wobe-Mugos and other multi-enzyme formulas in 1949. He treated over

1,000 patients using oral doses of 200 mg daily, then raising it to 2-4 g daily. For 107 women who had undergone mastectomies, their five-year survival rate was 84% under Wobenzyme therapy compared to 43% to 48% with conventional therapy, reported Dr. Wolf. Localized application produced better results than systemic uses, and long-term use produced the best results in stopping the spread of cancer.

Research reported by the product's manufacturer indicated that pancreatic cancer responded well to this treatment, with 30 patients still alive two years after receiving the enzymes; some of these patients survived 5-9 years. All of this must be seen in contrast to the "standard" survival expectation of seven months for pancreatic cancer. For postsurgical breast cancer patients with Stage I and III cancers, the use of Wobe-Mugos produced five-year survival rates of 91% and 58%, respectively, compared to 78% and 42% under conventional treatment.[36]

Glandular and Organ Extracts

Glandular and organ extracts, usually taken from animals, can be an important component of a complete nutritional program. These include extracts from the pituitary, thyroid, adrenals, pancreas, heart, liver, kidney, and thymus; they are called for when a patient's endocrine system is underproducing a specific hormone or when an organ is weakened or diseased. The efficacy of these extracts is generally recognized, yet they are often overlooked in conventional medicine.

Prior to the 1940s, glandular extracts were in wide use and a considerable amount of research was in progress to support their use. World War II sparked a shift in priority to the development of antibiotics. Government funding by the United States and other nations soon resulted in the discovery of penicillin and other antibiotics. As drug companies launched their lucrative ventures into the drug business, research in glandular therapy came to a halt. However, the fact that the glandular approach was set aside does nothing to diminish the validity of its therapeutic value.

Glandulars are used nutritionally for three reasons:

■ Active components—These are the biochemical substances particular to the glandular tissue being administered. The effect of the biochemical compound often is one of "substituting" an external source to make up for the internal deficiency.

■ Associated nutritional factors—Numerous nutrients are naturally present in glandular tissue, including vitamins, minerals, amino acids,

Metabolic Therapies at Advanced Medical Group

The Advanced Medical Group in Juarez, Mexico, a major metabolic treatment center, was the brainchild of H. Ray Evers, M.D., a pioneering alternative physician who died in 1990.

According to former medical director Francisco R. Soto, M.D., "Treatments rest on a foundation of nutrition, oxidative therapy (hyperbaric oxygen and ozone), Koch vaccination, and antioxidant chelation therapy. The Koch vaccine derives from work originally done by German bacteriologist Robert Koch, who developed it in 1883 as a medical response to tuberculosis. AMG uses the Koch vaccine as a preventive inoculation to enhance the immune system. It acts as an antibody, targeting cancerous cells."

AMG also employs cell therapy administered in the form of frozen live-cell and whole-cell injections; in addition, magnetic field therapy, amygdalin, shark cartilage, and detoxification are also important.

In one case, William, a retired banker, was diagnosed with Stage IV bladder cancer. A biopsy showed that the tumor was growing directly on the lining of his bladder and there was indication that it had invaded the muscle wall as well. William's urologist advised him to have his bladder removed within the next two weeks; instead, he went to AMG. There he received chelation therapy, megadoses of vitamin C, and hyperbaric oxygen to increase the oxygen content of his blood and enhance the effectiveness of the chelation. William's bladder cancer went into a complete remission within 20 days and, six years later, he was still cancer free.

For more about the **Koch vaccine**, contact: Advanced Medical Group, 5862 Cromo Drive, Suite 100, El Paso, TX 79912; tel: 800-621-8924 or 915-581-2273.

For information about **glandular extracts**, contact: Innovative Therapeutics, 2020 Franklin Street, Carlyle, IL 62231-0512; tel: 888-688-9922 or 618-594-7711; fax: 618-594-7712. Professional Health Products, P.O. Box 80085, Portland, OR 97280; tel: 503-245-2720 or 800-952-2219; fax: 503-452-1239.

fatty acids, polypeptides, enzymes, and many other substances. These can supply essential nutritional needs in a highly efficient manner.

■ Adaptogenic effect—For a tissue cell to repair or replace itself, it must have the raw materials necessary. "Like supports like" is the concept here: failing organs, glands, and tissues should be treated biologically with material corresponding in its entirety to these organs, glands, and tissues.

Biochemist Jeffrey Bland, Ph.D., proposes a rational explanation for how these products work. "Glandular-based food supplements may contain small polypeptides, protein-like substances that have specific messenger activity and which act on target tissues."[37] Many of the hormones found in the glandular tissues, even at low concentrations, still have potent tissue-specific activities, according to Dr. Bland.

The raw materials for the glandular products come preferentially from lambs raised in New Zealand. "Lamb is preferred over other animals because of their resistance to disease," says Dr. Taylor, who uses them as part of his cancer treatment protocols. Dr. Taylor cautions that glandular extracts are not intended as a "cure" for any specific disease or condition: "The [extracts] provide nutritional support to assist normal cellular function and repair. Specific supplementation advice for glandular extracts should be made only after a determination of need. If you experience difficulty with a glandular, consult your physician."

A Glossary of Useful Hormones and Glandular Extracts

DHEA (Dehydroepiandrosterone)—DHEA is a naturally occurring hormone produced in the adrenal glands. In fact, it is the most abundant hormone found in the human bloodstream, until the normal course of aging depletes it dramatically. If you live to be 80, your body will probably have only 10%-20% of the DHEA it had when you were 20 years old. The healthiest older humans usually have the highest DHEA levels, while the sickest individuals have the lowest levels. Low DHEA levels can leave you vulnerable to breast, prostate, and bladder cancer, atherosclerotic plaque, nerve degeneration, and other age-related conditions.

DHEA is called the "mother of all hormones" because not only does it have many functions in the body pertaining to health and longevity, but it is the substance from which other

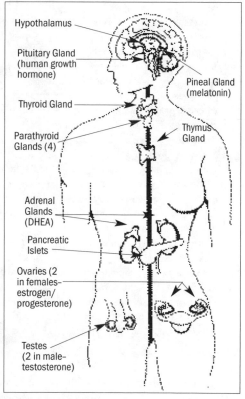

Hypothalamus

Pituitary Gland (human growth hormone)

Pineal Gland (melatonin)

Thyroid Gland

Thymus Gland

Parathyroid Glands (4)

Adrenal Glands (DHEA)

Pancreatic Islets

Ovaries (2 in females- estrogen/ progesterone)

Testes (2 in male- testosterone)

The glandular system.

Metabolic Therapies at BioPulse

A new therapy uses insulin-induced hypoglycemia to create an internal biological environment that cancer simply can't survive in. Insulin-induced Hypoglycemic Therapy (IHT), available at the BioPulse Rejuvenation Center, in Tijuana, Mexico, involves intravenously introducing insulin to produce a state of profoundly lowered blood sugar. This state lasts for a period of about an hour, with the patient under careful clinical supervision. This hypoglycemic condition changes the environment in the body to one in which cancer cells cannot survive.

Oxygen and glucose are normally metabolized together. When glucose levels are lowered by the hormone insulin, metabolism slows, oxygen accumulates in the blood, and the production of carbon dioxide decreases. This increases the pH of the blood and tissues, from an acidic to an alkaline condition. Cancer cells cannot survive in an oxygenated, alkaline environment. It has been theorized that the extreme pH of the blood inactivates enzymes responsible for cancer cells' energy and their ability to replicate. Repeated exposure to these conditions does not harm healthy cells, but it kills cancer cells.

It takes five days of preparation once a patient arrives at BioPulse before IHT is formally commenced. Initial small insulin injections are given on a daily basis, with the patient's blood glucose constantly monitored to determine the proper dosage. The blood is also analyzed to detect any nutritional deficiencies or abnormalities. Based on this, an IV (containing vitamins and minerals tailored to the patient's needs, including high amounts of vitamin A and melatonin to protect brains cells from a lack of glucose) is prepared and given an hour prior to the insulin.

Then the insulin itself is administered with a physician continually monitoring to maintain the desired glucose level. Oxygen is also administered during the entire session. Glucose is then gradually reintroduced into the patient's system so that they emerge from the session, without side effects. They are generally soaked with sweat and almost always hungry, both positive therapeutic signs for a cancer patient. About 75% of the patients report a reduction in pain from the first session. Virtually all feel substantially better after the third session, and some are completely pain-free. The present course of treatment consists of 30-35 sessions over eight weeks.

Patients at BioPulse are never treated by IHT alone. This kills the cancer cells, but cancer is a systemic disease, and the entire environment of the body must be changed. The body must be detoxified, the immune system rebuilt, nutritional deficiencies rectified, and biological functions normalized as much as possible.

The **BioPulse Rejuvenation Center** is located in Tijuana, Mexico. For more information, call 888-552-2855 (from U.S.), 801-233-9094 (outside U.S.), or 011-526-686-1880 (international direct); fax: 801-233-9089; website: www.alternativemedicine.com (click the BioPulse link in the Clinics section).

important hormones, such as estrogen, progesterone, and testosterone, are made. Evidence strongly suggests that DHEA hormone replacement therapy can work wonders for your health as you age.

"This common, powerful hormone is clearly important in cancer prevention," states naturopathic physician Eileen Stretch, N.D., of the Institute of Complementary Medicine in Seattle, Washington. Dr. Stretch notes that premenopausal women with low circulating levels of DHEA tend to have a higher incidence of breast cancer, while postmenopausal women with breast cancer have higher than normal DHEA levels.[38] DHEA can inhibit the proliferation of cancer cells by blocking an enzyme required for cell division.[39] Many physicians state that DHEA is effective in treating premenopausal breast cancer, but the only controlled studies in support of this claim have been done with animals.[40]

Many uncertainties remain concerning the use of DHEA in cancer therapy; hormone-sensitive cancers such as prostate cancer may actually be promoted by the compound. Those people diagnosed with hormone-sensitive cancers should generally avoid taking DHEA. Most physicians who use DHEA recommend frequent measurements and careful monitoring of circulating levels of DHEA.

Melatonin—Melatonin is a potent immune-enhancing hormone produced by the human pineal gland, a tiny gland inside the brain. Although known mainly as a sleep promoter—brain melatonin levels rise dramatically at night—melatonin also appears to have substantial cancer-repelling power. In addition to boosting the activity of key immune cells called T helper cells,[41] melatonin stimulates natural killer cells by increasing the production of the cytokine interleukin-2 (IL-2).[42]

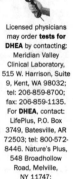

Licensed physicians may order tests for DHEA by contacting: Meridian Valley Clinical Laboratory, 515 W. Harrison, Suite 9, Kent, WA 98032; tel: 206-859-8700; fax: 206-859-1135. For DHEA, contact: LifePlus, P.O. Box 3749, Batesville, AR 72503; tel: 800-572-8446. Nature's Plus, 548 Broadhollow Road, Melville, NY 11747; tel: 800-645-9500.

A recent study of 60 cancer patients found that melatonin combined with synthetic interleukin-2 may be more effective than chemotherapy in treating patients diagnosed with aggressive lung cancer. Whereas only 19% of those receiving chemotherapy were still alive after one year, 45% of those receiving the melatonin/IL-2 therapy survived the year.[43]

Melatonin treatment also appears to give certain cancer patients a survival advantage—those with inoperable brain tumors,[44] metastatic gastric cancer,[45] and metastatic colon cancer.[46] Other cancers that may benefit from melatonin treatment include metastatic breast cancer[47] and advanced endocrine tumors.[48] Aside from the improved survival among patients taking melatonin, these patients also report consistent improvement in quality-of-life issues and a reduced frequency of cancer-related complications. Melatonin has sedative qualities and helps reduce anxiety, panic disorders, and migraines as well as inducing sleep. It is also a powerful antioxidant and is a primary regulator of the immune system.[49]

Factors that are known to lower the brain's melatonin production include high-protein diets, overeating, chronic stress, alcohol, medications, tobacco, caffeine, lack of natural light exposure during the daytime, sleep deprivation, electromagnetic fields, geopathic stress, and sleeping in a room that is not pitch black.

Thymosin—Moderate success has been reported with this active ingredient from the thymus. In animal research focusing on lung cancer, a combination of thymosin and interferon caused a "dramatic and rapid disappearance of tumor burden."[50] Animals treated with thymosin had more vigorous natural killer (NK) cell activity—a measure of the body's ability to repel cancer—and significantly longer survival compared to those that received chemotherapy. Similarly, in trials involving people with lung cancer, patients receiving thymosin had "significantly prolonged survival times relative to the other treatment groups."[51] Trials with thymus hormones have found reduced immunosuppression in patients with breast cancer and other cancers.[52]

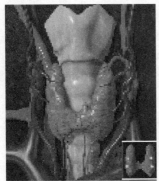

The thyroid gland, one of the body's seven endocrine glands, is located just below the larynx in the throat, with interconnecting lobes on either side of the trachea. The thyroid is the body's metabolic thermostat, controlling body temperature, energy use, and, in children, the body's growth rate. The thyroid controls the rate at which organs function and the speed with which the body uses food; it affects the operation of all body processes and organs. Of the hormones the thyroid synthesizes and releases, T3 (tri-iodothyronine) represents 7% and T4 (thyroxine) accounts for almost 93%. Additional T3 is made available to the body by the conversion of T4 outside the thyroid. Iodine is essential to forming thyroxine.

T3 Thyroid Hormone—In the 1990s, E. Dennis Wilson, M.D., described a medical concept he called Wilson's Syndrome. Dr. Wilson had treated hundreds of patients with low body temperatures (and a multitude of other symptoms) using a sustained-release form of active thyroid (T3) hormone. Dr. Wilson documented significant improvement in symptoms and normalization of temperatures in the majority of patients treated in this fashion. Dr. Wilson is not an oncologist and did not pursue the relationship between the treatment with active T3 hormone and cancer. However, if Dr. Barnes and fellow researchers were correct in their observations about the relationships among depressed thyroid, goiter, and cancer, this type of thyroid condition should be looked for in cancer patients.

It is important to note that standard T3 and T4 thyroid blood tests will not detect this condition. The only way to uncover the condition is by measuring underarm

The Thyroid's Role in Cancer Resistance

From 1930 to 1980, Broda Barnes, M.D., Ph.D., a researcher at the University of Chicago, sought to uncover the thyroid's role in cancer. According to his estimates, approximately 40% of the U.S. population suffers from chronically low thyroid function, or hypothyroidism. Most doctors would consider this figure absurd until they understand that the manifestation of this problem is quite different from that of an acute thyroid problem.

Dr. Barnes' pioneering research indicated that low thyroid function may manifest simply as a relatively constant (basal) body temperature of less than 97.8° F. Among the many symptoms of low thyroid function are coldness, constipation, weight gain, heavy periods, regular miscarriages, elevated blood fats,

For more on the **thyroid and cancer**, see Chapter 2: Cancer and Its Causes, pp. 48-93.

mental confusion, depression, and hypoglycemia, as well as an increased risk for both diabetes and cancer.[53]

To test for suboptimal thyroid function, take your body temperature first thing in the morning on several consecutive days before getting out of bed. If your temperature is below 97.8° F, you may benefit by taking an iodine or kelp supplement. Other alternatives for reviving normal thyroid function include ginseng, chromium, and L-carnitine.[54] If the patient is deficient in various nutrients that support the thyroid (iodine, chromium, copper, L-carnitine, and selenium, for example), this gland's function becomes depressed, and the functioning of the immune system declines accordingly. If one's temperature is consistently less than 98.2° F, the immune system is suboptimal and thyroid medication may be indicated.

temperature for ten minutes every morning with a thermometer, before getting out of bed; if the temperature is consistently below 97.8° F, the physician should assume that the person may need thyroid treatment. The second-best thyroid medication to use after active T3 is a glandular thyroid hormone derived from beef, pork, or sheep thyroid glands. Giving T4 either has no effect on this condition or makes it worse.

Physical Support Therapies

THE SUCCESSFUL APPROACH to reversing cancer and preventing its future recurrence is always multimodal. No single therapy, technique, or substance can prevail against the complexity of this disease. The exact combination of therapies and substances depends entirely on the individuality of the patient and the skill and knowledge of the physician. In this chapter, we present detailed information regarding several highly useful therapies that provide physical support to the body as it struggles to overcome cancer.

Specifically, we will discuss detoxification, or ways of getting the cancer toxins out of the body; biological dentistry, the crucial role your teeth play in both contributing to and reversing cancer; hydrotherapy and hyperthermia, how water and heat can fortify the body; therapeutic massage and exercise, which can relax the tension and stress associated with serious illness; and *qigong*, a form of relaxed, meditative movement that weaves together body and mind for therapeutic benefit.

Success Story: Naturopathic Support During Conventional Leukemia Treatment

Tommy, 11, suffered from an early form of leukemia. His parents had been advised to enroll him in a bone marrow transplant program and that his chances for survival were slim without it. They decided to consult naturopathic physician Dan Labriola, N.D., of Seattle, Washington.

Tommy's immune system was highly dysfunctional, providing little "raw material" capable of responding to natural support, says Dr. Labriola. In addition, Tommy had multiple risk factors. He had a high degree of toxicity as he had been around motors, automotive chemicals, and solvents for years, and had lived close to a garbage dump where he inadvertently inhaled the toxic fumes when the garbage was burned. Industrial toxins from these sources had compromised his immune system, says Dr. Labriola.

A bone marrow transplant was decided upon and Dr. Labriola agreed to provide naturopathic support. In this medical procedure, bone marrow is harvested from the patient and set aside; then high-dose chemotherapy and, in Tommy's case, total body irradiation, are administered; the bone marrow is then returned to the patient. Tommy's bone marrow was not good enough for the procedure, so his doctors used bone marrow from his sister.

In the time before the combined chemotherapy and radiation, Dr. Labriola built up Tommy's immune system and general health, using nutritional and botanical supplements. Dr. Labriola worked in collaboration with Tommy's attending physician; the hospital eventually gave Dr. Labriola attending status and was highly cooperative with his program, he says. "I was there every day for months," says Dr. Labriola. Using a classical naturopathic technique, he gave Tommy hot and cold packs (hydrotherapy) and mild electrical stimulation to get the immune system "up and kicking." During the recovery stage, Dr. Labriola repeated the hydrotherapy to reduce the side effects of the treatment.

Tommy not only survived the treatment and the cancer but, ten years later, was "an adult and doing wonderfully." There had been some fear that the toxic treatments might stunt his growth (at the time he was 5'5"), but the naturopathic immune support avoided this and Tommy eventually grew to be 6' tall.

For **Dr. Labriola's cancer protocols**, see *Alternative Medicine Definitive Guide to Cancer* (Future Medicine Publishing, 1997; ISBN 1-887299-01-7); to order, call 800-333-HEAL.

"The bone marrow graft went well and he had an absolutely spectacular recovery," comments Dr. Labriola. "He had some mouth sores and hair loss, but he fared not nearly as badly as other patients receiving similar treatments without the naturopathic support. This is in part because Tommy received considerable nutritional care and because

Dan Labriola, N.D.: P.O. Box 99157, Seattle, WA 98199; tel: 206-285-4993; fax: 206-285-0085.

the hospital was skilled in providing their care. Choosing your hospital and oncologist carefully has a great deal to do with your survival." As a health maintenance plan, Dr. Labriola advised Tommy to stay away from petrochemicals whenever possible and to wear a respiratory mask and gloves when he worked around gasoline engines. Eventually he abandoned this work in favor of his health.

Detoxification

One of the most essential practices in any cancer-reversal program, and for prevention, too, is to detoxify the body, down to the level of its cells, of a myriad of toxins, chemicals, parasites, and foreign substances, and to open up clogged elimination channels to move them out of the body.

Each year, people are exposed to thousands of toxic chemicals and pollutants in air, water, food, and soil. People carry within their bodies a "chemical cocktail" made up of industrial chemicals, pesticides, food additives, heavy metals, and the residues of pharmaceuticals, as well as of legal (alcohol, tobacco, caffeine), and illegal drugs (heroin, cocaine, marijuana). Today, people are exposed to chemicals in far greater concentrations than were previous generations. For example, over 70 million Americans live in areas that exceed smog standards; most municipal drinking water contains over 700 chemicals, including excessive levels of lead. Some 3,000 chemicals are added to the food supply; and as many as 10,000 chemicals in the form of solvents, emulsifiers, and preservatives are used in food processing and storage.[1] To make matters worse, food and product labels do not always list every ingredient. When people consume these foods—especially seafood, meat, and poultry—they ingest all the chemicals and pesticides that have accumulated in the food chain.

CAUTION

People with cancer should almost always assume that a detoxification program is necessary; however, any effort at detoxifying should be planned and executed under direct supervision of a physician. Those recovering from substance abuse, alcoholics, diabetics, people with eating disorders, and those who are underweight or physically weak or who have a hypothyroid or hypoglycemic condition should not detoxify without strict medical supervision.

These pollutants lodge in the body and manifest in a variety of symptoms, including decreased immune function, nerve cell toxicity, psychological disturbances, environmental illness and chronic fatigue, degenerative diseases, and cancer. "The current level of chemicals in the food and water supply and the indoor and outdoor environment has lowered our threshold of resistance to disease and has altered our body's metabolism, causing enzyme dysfunction, nutritional deficiencies, and hormonal imbalances," says Marshall Mandell, M.D., a pioneer of environmental medicine.

"A body with a healthy immune system, efficient organs of elimination and detoxification, and a sound circulatory and nervous system can handle a great deal of toxicity," states Leon Chaitow, N.D., D.O., of London, England. "But if a person's immune system has been damaged from chronic exposure to pollutants, restoring these functions can be accomplished only through detoxification therapies, including fasting, chelation, and nutritional, herbal, and homeopathic methods, which accelerate the body's own natural cleansing processes."

Most alternative physicians agree that detoxification is essential and that it brings many benefits to the person undertaking it. "Detoxification is the missing link to rejuvenating the body and preventing such chronic diseases as cancer, cardiovascular problems, arthritis, diabetes, and obesity," says Elson Haas, M.D., director of the Marin Clinic of Preventive Medicine and Health Education in San Rafael, California. "The cleansing of toxins and waste products will restore optimum function and vitality." One of the most important and longest lasting effects of detoxification therapy is the reduction of stress on the immune system, says Dr. Haas. Other benefits can include increased vitality, reduced blood pressure and blood fats (cholesterol and triglycerides), improved assimilation of vitamins and minerals, and mental clarity.

Everyone has a natural, specific level of tolerance for toxins that cannot be exceeded if good health is to be maintained. When the body gets overwhelmed with toxins, the immune system mechanisms malfunction, and fatigue, confusion, aggression, or mental disorder may occur. Symptoms indicating that you may need detoxification are headaches, joint pain, recurrent respiratory problems, back pain, nasal or sinus inhalant allergy symptoms, insomnia, mood changes, and food allergies. Conditions such as arthritis, constipation, hemorrhoids, ulcers, psoriasis, and acne can also indicate the need for detoxification.

Seven General Steps to Improve Detoxification
There are seven steps anyone can adopt starting today to improve their detoxification capabilities as a way of preventing illness.

First, make some dietary changes. Start eating a diet that is high in fiber, fresh raw vegetables and fruits, and very low in mucus-producing foods. It would be wise to completely stop eating all milk products from cows and all refined white flour products, such as pastas, breads, and baked goods. It is also advisable to reduce your intake of sugar, eggs, meats, fowl, most fish, nuts, seeds, and unsprouted beans and grains.

Second, reduce your stress load. Practice stress-reduction techniques before each meal. These might include muscle relaxation, deep breathing, or the visualization of a favorite natural setting. It is also advisable to eat in a calm, pleasant environment, either by yourself or with a companion whose presence does not produce stress.

Third, practice lymphatic drainage. It is important to take steps to clean out your lymphatic system, especially the lymph vessels that attach to the intestines. You can do this by gently bouncing on a mini-trampoline or rebounder for 5-15 minutes daily. This will stimulate the lymph nodes in your neck, chest, and groin to start draining toxins into the bloodstream for removal from the body.

Fourth, brush your skin. In the early morning, soon after you get up, take a wooden brush with stiff natural bristles and lightly brush your skin. Move the brush across the skin towards the middle end of the collarbones on each side of the body, as important lymph drainage sites are located here. Spend 8-10 minutes dry brushing your entire body. This procedure will mechanically aid your lymph system in its detoxification efforts. Do the dry brushing before taking a bath, but be aware that skin brushing just before bedtime can make it difficult to fall asleep.

Fifth, try ozonated bathing. Many of the toxins that build up in the body are fat soluble and gather in the fatty tissues. If you immerse yourself in a tub of warm ozonated water for 30 minutes once daily for 2-3 weeks, this will aid in removal of the toxins from your body. Ozone (SEE QUICK DEFINITION) is used to purify the bath water by killing viruses, bacteria, fungi, and parasites. It will also oxidize the water-insoluble toxins on the skin, turning them into water-soluble toxins. Once water soluble, they may be flushed from the system.

Purify the tap water by running it through a KDF solid charcoal showerhead filter as you fill the tub. A solid charcoal filter can remove up to 99% of the toxic substances found in tap water. Next, bubble ozone into the water using an ultraviolet ozone generator and an ozone-diffusing bath bubbler. While you remain in the bath, scrub your entire skin surface with a loofah sponge or natural fiber brush three times. Bubble the ozone for 15 minutes before you get into the tub and also during your 30-minute soak.

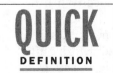

QUICK

DEFINITION

Ozone (O_3) is a less stable, more reactive form of oxygen, containing three oxygen atoms. This extra atom enables ozone to more readily oxidize other chemicals. In oxidation, the extra oxygen atom breaks off, leaving ordinary oxygen (O_2), thereby favorably increasing the oxygen content of body tissues or blood. Ozone is a commonly occuring natural substance. Medical-grade ozone is used as part of oxygen therapy to increase local oxygen supply to lesions, speed wound healing, reduce infections, and stimulate metabolic processes. Ozone may be administered by physicians intravenously, by injection, or applied topically as a gas or dissolved in water or in olive oil; it may also be taken orally or rectally as ozonated water.

Adding to your bath water ½ cup of Body Soak Gold, increasing this amount to one cup over 2-3 weeks, will usually produce a faster removal of toxins from the body than ozonated water alone. After you have used one full bottle of Body Soak Gold, you may gain additional detoxification benefit by switching to ¼ cup of Liquid Needles Foot Soak added to the bath water; over a period of several days, increase this amount to one cup for each bath.

Sixth, fortify yourself with nutrients. Take at least 400 IU of vitamin E, 25,000 IU of beta carotene and/or mixed carotenoids, 2,000 mg of vitamin C, and 100 mg of grape seed extract (pycnogenol), 30-40 minutes before your ozonated bath or 10-15 minutes after it.

Seventh, take one lozenge of superoxide dismutase (SOD) and 100 mg of L-glutathione powder. Dissolve both substances under your tongue before each bath; this enables it to be absorbed faster and more completely. These nutrients will facilitate toxin removal from your system. SOD is an antioxidant (SEE QUICK DEFINITION) enzyme that protects against free-radical damage. L-glutathione is a sulfur-containing peptide made of amino acids (protein building blocks) and antioxidants essential to the body's toxic waste disposal system.

For **Body Soak Gold,** (containing water, sea minerals, and glycerin) and **Liquid Needles Foot Soak** (containing electrolytes from mineral particles), contact: Health Restoration Systems, P.O. Box 832257, Richardson, TX 75083; tel: 972-480-8909. For a source of **SOD,** contact: Optimal Nutrients, 1163 Chess Drive, Suite F, Foster City, CA 94404; tel: 650-525-0112 or 800-966-8874; fax: 650-349-1686.

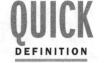

QUICK
DEFINITION

An **antioxidant** (meaning "against oxidation") is a natural biochemical substance that protects living cells against damage from harmful free radicals. Antioxidants work against the process of oxidation—the robbing of electrons from substances. If unblocked or left uncontrolled, oxidation can lead to cellular aging, degeneration, arthritis, heart disease, cancer, and other illnesses. Antioxidants in the body react readily with oxygen breakdown products and free radicals, and neutralize them before they can damage the body.

Seven-Day Rapid Colon Cleanse

This approach works rapidly and involves semi-fasting in conjunction with taking fiber, nutritional supplements, and ozonated water delivered directly to the intestines. This program is helpful for people with cancer that is rapidly spreading.

Preliminaries—The night before beginning this program, take two tablets of *Cascara sagrada* herbal laxative to stimulate the colon to begin detoxifying. If you have a history of chronic constipation, use four tablets. During the seven days you will be on this program, it is necessary that you eat nothing except 2-5 servings of vegetable broth daily; be sure the broth contains no beans or grains.

In addition, melt 10 mg of superoxide dismutase (SOD) powder under the tongue, along with 100 mg of L-glutathione powder each morning and again each evening just before the ozonated

Mayr Intestinal Detoxification

Various methods are used to purge the small intestine of a pasty layer of mucus under which most parasites originate and propagate. Parasites and pathogenic yeasts that produce toxins live between this lining and the true lining of the intestine, producing ill health for their human host. This "false lining" also inhibits nutrient absorption.

Helpful in eliminating this false lining is the detoxification program of Franz Xavier Mayr (1875-1965), an Austrian physician who lived to be 90 and attributed this, in part, to his intestinal health. Dr. Mayr explained that if the digestive system and particularly the intestines are not unobstructed and free of toxins, they cannot operate efficiently and become a breeding ground for disease.

Dr. Mayr's program does not involve colonics, but cleans the intestines through dietary changes. The program calls for a diet based on avoiding whole grains, margarine, decaffeinated coffee, and alcohol. Other aspects of his diet include eating only cooked food, chewing thoroughly, eating only when hungry, not drinking beverages with meals, drinking pure water, and not eating again after dinner. The Mayr program calls for taking natural products such as the Bittersalz drink (magnesium sulfate or Epsom salts) that acts as a natural laxative, plus homeopathic remedies and botanicals. Dr. Mayr's program (in use today by hundreds of physicians worldwide) includes a 15-minute abdominal treatment technique, manually performed on patients to increase intestinal activity and improve circulation throughout the abdomen.

The Mayr diet is designed to help move accumulations of mucus out of the intestinal tract. The goal is to slough off the small intestine's false lining. When this happens, three benefits accrue: (1) nutrient absorption is increased; (2) the buildup of toxins is reduced; and (3) antiparasite medicines work more effectively.

A "tea fast" requires the patient to consume only herbal tea (typically chamomile, mint, sage, or peppermint), honey, and mineral water, and a small amount of vegetable broth for 1-2 weeks. This is usually followed by a diet consisting of a teaspoon of yogurt or milk and a single hard wheat roll taken in the morning; the purpose of the old, crusty rolls is to force the patient to thoroughly chew the food (70-80 times) so that it becomes liquified. Other than the wheat rolls and ½ cup daily of uncooked rice, most cereal grains are avoided because grains are directly converted into sugar (glucose), which can be used by tumor cells to stimulate growth, Dr. Mayr explained. The sugar also stimulates the release of the hormone insulin, which in turn activates a set of hormone-like substances (prostaglandins) that trigger tumor growth and inflammatory processes.

In the absence of a blood sugar surge, the body produces another kind of hormone, glucagon, which stimulates prostaglandins that inhibit tumor and clot formation and increases oxygenation of the tissues.

For information about **Mayr therapy**, contact: Occidental Institute Research Foundation, P.O. Box 100, Penticton, B.C., V2A 6J9 Canada; tel: 800-663-8342 or 250-497-6020.

colemics. Immediately following this, mix and consume the following two drinks. Drink No. 1 contains cool purified water (10 oz), pure organic apple juice (4 oz), psyllium seed husk powder (1 tbsp), and 1-3 tablets of NatureSpring's small bowel and tissue cleanser. Drink No. 2 contains 10 oz hot pure water (but not heated by a microwave), organic apple cider vinegar or fresh lemon or lime juice (1 tbsp), and raw unfiltered honey (1 tbsp). Consume this drink immediately after Drink No. 1. The pair of drinks is mixed and consumed in rapid sequence five times daily during the seven-day program.

For **NatureSpring** products and colonic equipment, contact: Health Restoration Systems, Inc., P.O. Box 832267, Richardson, TX 75083-2267; tel: 972-480-8909; fax: 972-480-8807.

Ozonated Colemics—Twice daily, shortly after the first and fourth pairs of drinks are consumed, the next step is to combine ozonated water with the use of a colema board. This is a device that enables one to use an enema and empty one's bowels while lying on a sanitary plastic board stretched between a chair and the toilet bowl.

First, run five gallons of body-temperature water through a KDF solid charcoal showerhead filter into the five-gallon bucket that has a special top to prevent ozone from escaping into the room. Next, bubble ozone for 15 minutes into the water in the bucket with the top closed securely. The bucket stands on a high stool or platform so that its contents flow by gravity into the colon. Place the colema board over the toilet and the other end on a chair or stool so that it is two inches higher than the end over the bowl. The person lies down on the colema board with the buttocks centered over the toilet bowl. Lubricate the tip of the plastic tube from the water drain on the bucket with coconut, grape seed, or olive oil and gently insert into the rectum.

Next, push one finger deep into the abdomen for three minutes at a point that is one inch above and one inch to the left of the belly button. This will help relax the small intestine before running water into it; this point is usually tender if the small intestine is stressed. Open the valve on the tube from the five-gallon bucket so that the ozonated water can run slowly into the colon for 30-45 minutes. While the ozonated water is running into your colon, it is important to manually keep the ileocecal valve closed. This valve controls the passage of material from the small into the large intestine. Use one or both hands to press firmly on your right lower abdomen.

For more on the **use of ozone for cancer**, see Chapter 8: Enhancing Metabolism, pp. 232-253.

Periodically, the water inflow hose may be clamped off. Then push the water out of the intestines into the toilet by contracting the abdominal muscles; only after this should you release the hand that is blocking the ileocecal valve. Then massage your abdomen, especially around the belly button, to stimulate movement of the false lining in the small intestine through the ileocecal valve into the large intestine. When you restart the flow of water, the false lining may be flushed into the toilet. Be sure to hold the ileocecal valve closed as the hose clamp is opened and water runs into the colon again.

After each ozonated colemic, take a 30-minute bath in ozonated water. Prepare the bath by running very warm water through the KDF filter to a depth of 8-10 inches. Next, bubble ozone into this water for 15 minutes before and continually during immersing yourself. Scrub your skin with a loofah three times during the bath.

Nutrient Fortification—About 15 minutes before the morning colema, take niacin (100 mg) and flaxseed oil (three capsules). Before the first colema, consume Drinks No. 1 and 2 and dissolve under your tongue 100 mg of L-glutathione powder and 10 mg of SOD powder.

After the morning ozonated bath, take the following nutritional supplements:

- Vitamin C (2,000 mg)
- Protease (an enzyme; two capsules)
- NatureSpring Gastro-Protective enzyme
- NatureSpring Essential Nutrients (one capsule)
- Cracked chlorella (six capsules; 335 mg per capsule)
- Nature's Sunshine CA-ATC (a mixture of herbs high in calcium; two capsules)
- Dulse (two tablets or one dropperful)
- Colloidal minerals (1 tbsp)
- Magnesium malate or magnesium citrate (two capsules)
- Potassium (200 mg)
- EPA fish oil (one capsule)
- Beet crystals (five tablets; 400 mg per tablet)

Take this group of supplements again, either late in the morning or early afternoon, then again just before receiving the second colema in the late afternoon. You may complement the nutrients with warm vegetable broth.

When you have completed the seven-day program, it's advisable to restock your intestines with friendly bacteria, or probiotics, such as Nature's Sunshine Bifidophilus Flora Force (three capsules, three times daily) and NatureSpring Lactobacillus Plantarum (three capsules, three times daily). Take both for the next ten days.

Additional Detoxification Programs

If there is one thing that most alternative medicine doctors agree on, it is that too many toxins in the body produce illness. Increasingly, toxicity is being identified as the predisposing factor in a long list of acute and chronic degenerative illnesses. Signs and symptoms of the toxic body can include being overweight, bloating and intestinal gas, insomnia, nausea, bad breath, asthma, constipation, tension, headaches, depression, stress, allergies, menstrual problems, and many others. In addition to the commercial products mentioned above, there are several others available over-the-counter, enabling anyone to start a self-care detoxification program.

A.M./P.M. Ultimate Cleanse™–"When was the last time you cleaned your liver, your heart, your lungs, or your body's sewage system?" asks nutritionist Lindsey Duncan, C.N., chief nutritionist for Home Nutrition Clinic in Santa Monica, California. Duncan offers a practical way to accomplish this with the A.M./P.M. Ultimate Cleanse.

This program is set up as a two-part vegetarian detoxification formula. It involves 29 cleansing herbs, amino acids, antioxidants, digestive enzymes, vitamins, minerals, and five kinds of fiber. Both Multi-Herb™ and Multi-Fiber™ formulas are taken in the morning and evening in gradually increasing dosages, for several weeks. Positive signs that the detox program is working include flu-like sensations, runny nose, transient pimples, headaches, "brainfog," or fatigue, all of which will pass in one to two days. "The goal is to stimulate, feed, and detoxify the complete internal body, not just the bowel," states Duncan. At the end of the program, a person should be having two to three bowel movements every day. Once the internal system is cleaned out, nutrient absorption can proceed much more efficiently. The key to the effectiveness of the program, Duncan explains, is that of timing: the morning formula stimulates, the evening formula relaxes. Following your body's natural digestive and cleansing cycles is the key to proper detoxification, says Duncan.

For information about **A.M./P.M. Ultimate Cleanse™**, contact: Nature's Secret, 4 Health, Inc., 5485 Conestoga Court, Boulder, CO 80301; tel: 303-546-6306; fax: 303-546-6416. For **Nature's Pure Body Program™**, contact: Pure Body Institute of Beverly Hills, 423 East Ojai Avenue, #107, Ojai, CA 93023; tel: 800-952-7873; (orders); 805-653-5448 (customer service).

Nature's Pure Body Program™–Another cleansing herbal formula is called Nature's Pure Body Program made by Pure Body Institute of Beverly Hills, California. The program is a blend of 27 herbs specifically chosen for their ability to flush toxins out of the organs and old fecal matter from the intestines. For example, buckthorn bark stimulates bile secretion; chickweed and black cohosh root combat blood toxicity; *Cascara sagrada* bark promotes intestinal peristalsis (natural contraction rhythms); yarrow flower regulates liver function; peach leaves are a natural laxative; and licorice root stimulates the adrenal glands.

The program consists of two sets of pills: colon and whole-body blends. Users start with one colon and three whole-body pills taken twice daily with water, 30 minutes before breakfast and 30 minutes before dinner. The colon pills can be increased to three pills twice daily, or more, until the bowels move twice daily; the whole-body pills are increased to 4-7, taken two times daily. Users need to double their intake of pure water (to at least 64 ounces daily), take one day off from the pills every week, and take a daily multivitamin. The program is designed to last about 30 days, although first-time users may find that three courses are required for complete detoxification.

Restoring the Intestine's Friendly Bacteria—Under the best of conditions, the estimated 100 trillion bacteria that live in the human intestines do so in a delicate balance. Certain bacteria such as *Lactobacilli* and *Bifidobacteria* are beneficial "friendly" bacteria that support numerous vital physiological processes. Other bacteria, such as *E. coli*, *Staphylococcus*, and *Clostridrium* may be present in smaller numbers, but they are considered "unfriendly," even dangerous bacteria. A healthy intestine maintains a balance of the various intestinal flora, but with current lifestyles and the use of antibiotics, drugs, and processed foods, this balance is often upset. Practitioners of alternative medicine often recommend using probiotics, introducing live bacteria into the system through food products (yogurt, *acidophilus* milk) or through special supplements.

A new approach, developed in Japan in the mid-1980s, is called prebiotics. Here you introduce nutrients that directly feed the beneficial bacteria already in place, most typically *Bifidobacteria* and *Lactobacilli*. Researchers determined that a naturally occurring form of carbohydrate called fructo-oligosaccharides (FOS), found in certain foods in minute amounts, could act like an intestinal "fertilizer," selectively feeding the friendly microflora so their numbers can usefully increase. *Bifidobacteria* work to lower the pH (acidity/alkalinity balance) in the large intestine to a slightly more acidic condition; this discourages the growth of unfriendly bacteria. Benefits from

For **FOS and NutraFlora®**, contact: GTC Nutrition Company, 1400 W. 122nd Avenue, Suite 110, Westminster, CO 80234; tel: 303-254-8012; fax: 303-254-8201. For a source of **friendly bacteria, or probiotics**, contact: Nature's Way Products, 10 Mountain Springs Parkway, Springville, UT 84663; tel: 800-962-8873 or 801-489-1500. Futurebiotics, 145 Ricefield Lane, Hauppauge, NY 11788; tel: 800-FOR-LIFE or 516-273-6300.

For more information about **toxic chemicals**, see Chapter 2: Cancer and Its Causes, pp. 48-93.

increasing *Bifidobacterium* levels include relief of constipation or diarrhea, promotion of regularity, serum cholesterol reduction, control of blood sugar levels, immune function enhancement, improved calcium absorption and B vitamin synthesis, and a reduction of the detoxification load on the liver.

See "Colon Therapy,"
pp. 143-148;
"Detoxification
Therapy," pp. 156-166.

Coffee Enema—Many alternative cancer physicians use the coffee enema as part of their detoxification program. One of the first to do so was Max Gerson, M.D., founder of the Gerson Diet Therapy for cancer. The following is a review of the procedure, according to Howard Straus, vice president of the Gerson Institute in Bonita, California.[2]

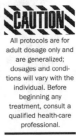

All protocols are for adult dosage only and are generalized; dosages and conditions will vary with the individual. Before beginning any treatment, consult a qualified health-care professional.

First, it is essential to start with organically raised coffee beans to avoid introducing pesticides, fungicides, and other toxic chemicals into the intestines. Second, the water used for the enema must be free of chlorine and fluoride; Straus recommends using distilled water. Straus suggests mixing three rounded tablespoonsful of drip-grind coffee to one quart of water. The coffee is boiled for three minutes, simmered for 15-20 minutes, then strained and cooled to body temperature. This produces enough coffee for a single enema.

As a shortcut, Straus suggests preparing a "concentrate or instant enema" mix. He suggests boiling two quarts of water to which three cups of organic drip-grind coffee is added; this boils for another three minutes, then is simmered for 12-15 minutes, then strained. If the resulting product is less than two quarts, add enough distilled water to bring the volume to two quarts. Straus then advises using four ounces of this concentrate mixed with 3½ cups of water for each enema. Refrigerate the unused amounts of prepared coffee. Do not prepare the enema coffee as though you were brewing coffee for consumption, Straus says, because the potassium normally present in coffee, which is of considerable benefit to the body, is lost.

The Link Between Lymph Circulation and Cancer

The lymphatic system comprises a network of lymph ducts or channels and transports lymph fluid. Lymph is a clear fluid that accumulates in the tissue spaces between cells and in the tiniest blood vessels to eventually enter the lymphatic network. Interspersed throughout the lymph channels are tight clusters of cells called lymph nodes, which act as primary filters protecting the bloodstream from foreign and toxic substances. Each lymph node contains vari-

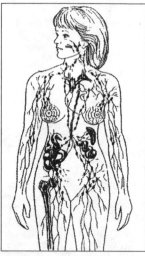

Lymph nodes are clusters of immune tissue that work as filters or "inspection stations" for detecting foreign and potentially harmful substances in the lymph fluid. Lymph nodes are part of the lymphatic system, which is the body's master drain.

ous scavenger cells that help break down toxins and microbes.

Since the lymph also carries essential nutrients and various immune components, any interference with its flow can adversely affect the body as a whole. Unlike the blood, which is moved primarily by the action of the heart, the lymphatic system lacks a pump. Its movement depends entirely on the body's own movements, including contractions of the diaphragm in the act of breathing and muscular contractions during physical activity. The lymphatic system has to be capable of flowing freely and filtering out the toxins. Otherwise, the liver, kidneys, and lungs have to work much harder to keep the system clean. Eventually, these other organs become weakened by the flow of toxins from the polluted lymph nodes and channels.

Few people actually die of cancer. Rather, they die of toxemia, produced by an excessive buildup of toxins. This is where the lymph system comes into play. As people age or become less physically active, the flow of lymph is impaired; muscle tension from chronic stress can further promote accumulations of toxins. The lymph vessels and nodes become stagnated and inflamed; the result is a kind of "traffic jam" in the lymph channels.

The function of the lymphatic system is linked with two factors that have generally eluded modern medicine: a person's psychological state and the electromagnetic energy surrounding and permeating the body. First, stressful emotional experiences can constrict the lymphatic system and lead to increased accumulations of toxins. Second, the body's electromagnetic energies can be affected by the state of one's psyche. Problems in metabolism appear to be influenced by a toxic chemical environment, but these problems become amplified when the person is experiencing some form of extreme distress. In addition, many important lymphocytes, including natural killer (NK) cells, are formed in the lymph nodes. Taken together, these points highlight important links between the lymphatic system, stress, toxemia, and cancer.

When the lymph fails to function properly, the clear lymph fluid becomes cloudy and thick, progressively changing from its watery condition to the consistency of milk, then yogurt, then cottage cheese. Thickened, stagnant lymph overloaded with toxic wastes is the ideal condition for the development of cancer. Lymph starts backing up in the system creating a toxic, oxygen-deprived environment conducive to degeneration. This is when cancer and other degenerative ailments can accelerate.

There are many interlinked conditions that contribute to sluggish lymph circulation and that improve during lymphatic treatment. These include hormonal imbalances; chronic constipation and intestinal blockages; muscle tension, including structural misalignment in the neck and shoulders; and emotional disorder. The lymph system is the beginning and end of all disease. Once you get the lymph circulating freely again, this enhances recovery from any illness by reversing the slow, possibly lifetime, poisoning your body has endured.

How Lymphatic Therapy Works

Lymphatic therapy may benefit cancer patients by enhancing the immune system's capacity for destroying the metastatic cancer cell or it may make establishment of the cancer cell at a new site much more difficult. In this way, the use of lymphatic therapy should actually lower the risk of early metastatic disease.

Manual lymph drainage, developed in the 1930s by Danish scientist Emil Vodder, Ph.D., consists of specific massage movements performed by a trained practitioner that enable the lymph to begin draining. Dr. Vodder described these as "circular pumping and draining movements" of sufficiently light pressure so as to prevent blood congestion. "We employed gentle stationary circles on the lymph nodes, an area that no one had previously dared to massage, palpating with the tips or the entire length of the fingers," Dr. Vodder explained. "Massaging was always in the direction of the collarbone, the terminus of all lymph pathways in the body." Dr. Vodder noted that the method

The Negative Health Impact of Bras

The lymph channels and nodes of the armpit tend to become congested from wearing bras and from lack of exercise. This observation has recently been confirmed by Sidney Singer and Soma Grismaijer, who present compelling evidence for a connection between bras and breast cancer in *Dressed to Kill* (Avery, 1995). The authors conducted a three-year study of 4,700 women living in cities throughout the U.S.

Women who wore their bras over 12 hours daily but not to bed—the majority—were 21 times more likely to develop breast cancer compared with women who wore their bras less than 12 hours a day. On extreme ends of the bra-wearing spectrum, women who also wore bras to bed had a 125-fold greater chance of getting breast cancer than did women who refrained from wearing bras altogether.[3]

Limit Your Exposure to Toxins in the Home

Be wary of cancer-causing chemicals and contaminants found in common consumer items, including household products, cosmetics, processed foods, beverages, paints, paint thinners, furniture polishes, and the like. They all contain carcinogens ranging from formaldehyde to crystalline silica. Although none of these products alone may present a critical carcinogenic exposure, they present a cumulative toxic load that stresses the body's immune system and damages cells until, over time, cancer can set in.[4]

Generally, it is wise to be cautious about nearly all products. Many chemicals used in cosmetics, pesticides, and other products do not require full safety testing before they are allowed to be marketed and used by millions of consumers. Therefore, one must become a prudent, wary, and skeptical shopper. "This sort of conscientious buying will enable people to vote with their dollars for an environmental clean-up of all carcinogenic substances used in manufacturing, including those found in pesticides," according to Samuel Epstein, M.D. Dr. Epstein recommends boycotting all consumer products containing known carcinogens, then finding healthy, natural substitutes. "For example, a combination of plain water mixed with distilled white vinegar and a small amount of baking soda, Borax, and lemon juice can clean the home and bathroom as effectively as many higher-priced cleaners."

Avoiding electromagnetic exposure (especially while you are asleep) by measuring your environment with a gauss meter and unplugging all electric appliances that have high gauss readings (a basic unit of electromagnetic energy) reduces your cancer risk. Avoiding geopathic exposure by measuring your immediate environment with a geomagnetometer also significantly reduces cancer risk. Radiation exposure from televisions, computer monitors, microwave ovens, and fluorescent lights should also be minimized or avoided.

---

had benefits not only for cosmetic and preventive measures, but also "to cure illnesses." Providing slow and rhythmic movements, Dr. Vodder obtained positive results for conditions such as skin rejuvenation, hematomas produced by accidents, eczema, varicose veins, and ulcerous legs. He noted that an average of 35 billion lymphocytes enter the blood every day through the lymph nodes, but during stress this number can climb to 562 billion. "One thing, however, is certain, said Dr. Vodder. "The lymph system not only serves to clean tissues through the drainage, but is also a protection, a defense mechanism, and carries out vital functions."[5]

Light Beam Generator (LBG)—To free up a clogged lymphatic system as part of a detoxification program, the Light Beam Generator™ and

Lymph-Pho Laser™ are highly effective. The devices radiate photons (light) to help restore the cells' normal energy state, allowing the body to heal itself more readily. The equipment used resembles a flashlight with a long, extensible housing. Noble gases such as argon and neon are stimulated by an electric current to emit a diffuse purple light through its "flashlight" head. The practitioner projects the light onto the skin, often focusing on lymph nodes and channels. "The Light Beam Generator can be used anywhere on the body where there is a problem," says Robert Jacobs, N.M.D., D.Hom. (Med), of London, England, "and because of its deep penetration, it can help heal organs and structures deep within the body, as well as skin problems." Dr. Jacobs also points out that since healthy cells are in a stable energetic state, there are no adverse effects when the LBG is used in 30-45 minute sessions.

For information about **lymph detoxification**, contact: Marika von Viczay, Ph.D., N.M.D., 16 Arlington Street, Asheville, NC 28801; tel: 704-253-8371; fax: 704-258-1350. For the **Light Beam Generator**, contact: ELF Teslar, Star Route 1, Box 21, St. Francisville, IL 62460; tel: 618-948-2393; fax: 618-948-2650.

Dry Skin Brushing—Dry skin brushing is based on concepts from acupuncture, which states that there are an estimated three million nerve points spread over the surface of the skin, 700 of which are nodal, meaning they can serve as treatment nodes in acupuncture. Dry skin brushing, by applying friction to these acupuncture nodal points, can take advantage of these energy connections, stimulating and invigorating the entire nervous system, such that every organ, gland, muscle, and ligament benefits. Dry skin brushing helps to physically move fluid through the lymph vessels so that toxins can be cleared from the body by the kidneys, liver, intestines, and lungs. This dumping of toxins significantly improves the function of the immune system and most other organ systems.

You will need a moderately soft, natural vegetable fiber bristle brush, preferably with a removable wooden handle. (Nylon or synthetic fibers build up undesirable static electromagnetic energy, in addition to being too sharp and possibly hurting the skin.) Brush gently at first, as some parts of the body are more sensitive than others; within a few days, your skin will become conditioned. As you become accustomed to dry brushing, the process should take no more than ten minutes daily. It would be a good idea to brush your skin daily for three months, then twice weekly as a lifetime practice. Your brush will rapidly fill with impurities and should be washed regularly. Every two weeks or so, wash your brush with soap and water and dry it in the sun. For hygienic reasons, each member of the family should have a separate brush.

Detoxify Your Fruits and Vegetables

Here's how to get the pesticides and poisons off your foods, according to the late naturopathic physician Hazel Parcells, N.D., of the Parcells Center in Santa Fe, New Mexico. This technique will rid food of harmful toxins, chemicals, and poisons, and it will noticeably improve their flavor and shelf life.

Before cooking, soak all your fruits, eggs, meats, and vegetables in a bath of Clorox and water, at the rate of ½ teaspoon Clorox to one gallon water. Make sure it is the old-fashioned, pure Clorox; this is hydrochloric acid, not chlorine. Divide your foods into the following categories and soak no longer than the time listed: leafy vegetables (10-15 minutes); root vegetables (15-30 minutes), thin-skinned berries (10-15 minutes), heavy-skinned fruits (15-30 minutes), eggs (20-30 minutes), and thawed meats (5-10 minutes per pound). Prepare a fresh batch of Clorox water for each category of foods; dispose after use. Soak all Clorox-treated foods in fresh water for 5-10 minutes before using.

Parasite Removal is Essential in Detoxification

Most conventional doctors are unaware of the connection between parasites and health and thus fail to recognize the clinical symptoms. These include joint and muscle aches, anemia, allergy, skin conditions, nervousness, diarrhea, bloating, constipation, chronic fatigue, and immune dysfunction, among others. In fact, members of the same family can have the same species of parasites yet show completely different symptoms—emotional upsets, food allergies, fatigue, bowel discomfort—or no symptoms. That is why nutrition educator Ann Louise Gittleman, M.S., states, "If these symptoms sound familiar, then you may be an unsuspecting victim of the parasite epidemic that is affecting millions of Americans." With this information in mind, here are practical steps often employed to start detoxifying one's system of parasites.

1. Cleanse the Intestines: Parasites tend to embed themselves in the intestinal wall, but over the course of several weeks, you can flush them out by using some of these natural substances (preferably in combination): psyllium husks, agar-agar, citrus pectin, papaya extract, pumpkin seeds, flaxseeds, comfrey root, beet root, and bentonite clay (take bentonite only in combination with another substance, such as psyllium). You might also take extra amounts of vitamin C (minimum 2 g daily, but higher amounts up to individual bowel tolerance are more useful) to help flush out your intestine.

2. Do a Colon Irrigation: Irrigate the colon with 2-16 quarts of water. To the water you may add black walnut tincture or extract, garlic juice, vinegar (two tablespoons per quart of water), blackstrap molasses (one tablespoon per quart of water), or organically raised coffee. Use filtered or distilled water for the enema; further sterilize it by boiling or ozonating it for 10-15 minutes before use, including before using it to prepare the coffee.

3. Prepare Your System: It is prudent to give your gallbladder and liver a week to prepare for a parasite program. To flush the gallbladder of its toxins, take lime juice in warm water or Swedish Bitters before each meal. Eliminate all refined and natural sugars, meats, and dairy products during the parasite program; even better, start cutting back on them during this preparatory week. Take barberry bark capsules, dandelion, or a similar herbal extract to help cleanse the liver.

4. Herbs for Parasites: Herbs are a safe and effective alternative to drug therapies for ridding yourself of parasites. They are free of side effects and often work better than their synthetic counterparts. Purgative herbs such as pumpkin seeds act as mild intestinal cleansers. Decoctions and powders of pumpkin seeds have shown effects against tapeworm and other intestinal parasites in humans and in animals. A typical dose consists of 10-12 seeds in the morning on an empty stomach for two weeks. If the parasites are systemic and have entered the bloodstream, antibiotic herbs such as Coptis (a Chinese herb high in berberine) may also be used.

For information about **Dr. Hulda Clark's program**, contact: Self-Health Resource Center, 757 Emory Street, No. 508, Imperial Beach, CA 91932; tel: 619-429-4408. Another option is Parasite Out®, a blend of wormwood, black walnut seeds, and grapefruit seed extract, available from: Carotec, Inc., P.O. Box 9919, Naples, FL 34101; tel: 800-522-4279. For Wormwood Combination capsules, contact: Hanna's Herb Shop, 5684 Valmont Road, Boulder, CO 80301; tel: 800-206-6722.

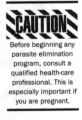

Before beginning any parasite elimination program, consult a qualified health-care professional. This is especially important if you are pregnant.

■ Garlic—One of the least expensive yet most effective ways to deal with parasites is to use an extract of garlic (*Allium sativum*). Raw garlic and garlic extract have been shown to destroy common intestinal parasites, including roundworms and hookworms. As an oral supplement, typically take two cloves of fresh garlic daily; in capsule form, 500 mg, twice daily.

■ Goldenseal—The alkaloid berberine is found in many plants and in particularly high concentrations in goldenseal (*Hydrastis canadensis*). Berberine inhibits the growth of several common parasites that invade the intestine and vagina. Typical dosage: 500 mg, three times daily.

■ Thyme (*Thymus vulgaris*)—The principle chemical components of thyme are the volatile oils, namely, phenol, thymol, and carvacrol. Thymol is one of the most potent anti-microbial substances known, and even surpasses many of the strongest antibiotics. Typical recom-

Important Reminders During Any Parasite Treatment

Whatever treatment you employ to rid your body of parasites, the following recommendations can help ensure that the program is a success:

■ If you have children and/or pets, they must be treated at the same time as the adults in the household to prevent re-infection.

■ Drink more pure water (not from the tap) than usual to help the body flush out the dead parasites from your system; at least 64 ounces of water per day for a 150-pound adult.

■ Sanitize your environment. When you have almost finished treatment, wash all pajamas, bed clothes, and sheets before using them again.

■ Eat antiparasitic foods. According to Ann Louise Gittleman, a nutrition educator in Bozeman, Montana, these include pineapple and papaya, either as fresh juice or in organic supplement form, in combination with pepsin and hydrochloric acid. Avoid all meats and dairy products for at least one week. You can also use pomegranate juice (four 4-ounce glasses daily), papaya seeds, finely ground pumpkin seeds (¼ to ½ cup daily), and two cloves of raw garlic daily. Do not drink the pomegranate juice for more than four to five days.

■ Modify your diet. For people with heavy parasitic infection, nutritionist Gittleman recommends a diet comprised of 25% fat, 25% protein, and 50% complex carbohydrates. You also need a regular intake of unprocessed flaxseed, safflower, sesame, or canola oils (two tablespoons daily) and extra vitamin A. Flaxseed oil is preferable because it has much higher levels of alpha-linolenic acid (an omega-3 essential fatty acid that is commonly deficient in many people) than the other oils.

■ Recolonize your intestines. You need to reintroduce beneficial, friendly bacteria (probiotics) into your intestinal system once you have flushed out the parasites, Gittleman advises. The bacterial strains most helpful here are *Lactobacillus plantarum*, L. salvarius, L. acidophilus, L. bulgaris, and B. bifidum, and *Streptococcus faeceum*, which are available as nutritional supplements. L. plantarum is the most effective of these in resolving parasite problems.

mended dosage is five drops of thyme essential oil diluted in a quart of pure water as an enema solution. You may also take thyme orally at the rate of two or three drops of oil extract diluted in one cup of water, three times a day for two weeks.

For **grapefruit seed extract**, contact: Imhotep, Inc., P.O. Box 183, Ruby, NY 12475; tel: 800-677-8577.

■ Grapefruit Seed Extract—Grapefruit Seed Extract (GSE) offers some of the benefits of antibiotics (in a natural format) without the side effects. Clinical tests by the U.S. Food and Drug Administration, Pasteur Institute in Paris, and University of Georgia at Athens, have successfully treated bacterial, fungal, and viral infections. Very little is known about the active components of GSE, but it contains bioflavonoids (vitamin C enhancers) and hesperidin, a natural immune booster. Typically, a few drops are taken with each meal or diluted in vegetable or fruit juice if the taste is too bitter.

■ Worm Seed (Mexican Tea)—Epazote (*Chenopodium ambrosoides*), also called worm seed or Mexican tea, is often used in the Caribbean and Central America for worms. Worm seed should never be given to children under the age of six; for those ages six and older, a typical dose is 3-5 drops per day. Make a tea by steeping 3-4 teaspoons of the dried or fresh herb in one cup of water for 20 minutes; drink one cup per day. Dosage: 50 mg, three times daily.

■ Chinese Wormwood (*Artemesia absinthium*)—*Artemesia absinthium* has a long history of use as a vermifuge or "worm expeller," hence its common name, wormwood. However, some caution is advised: it may initially worsen symptoms and cause some intestinal irritation. It is often combined with citrus seed extract and other anti-parasitic herbs. Although it may be toxic if used alone in large quantities, it is usually mixed in formulas with other herbs that offset its possible toxic effects. Typical recommended dosage: 150 mg, three times daily.

Wormwood is also part of the anti-parasite protocol of naturopathic physician Hulda Regehr Clark, N.D., Ph.D. She recommends using a blend of three herbs to flush the parasites out of your system: black walnut hull tincture, wormwood capsules, and fresh ground cloves (to kill the parasites' eggs). This program should only be undertaken with professional guidance from a licensed health-care practitioner.

5. Dietary Changes: If an intestinal parasite infection is diagnosed or suspected, we advise you to eliminate all uncooked food (which may contain parasites) from your diet and to cook all meats until well done. Soak all vegetables, including those organically grown, in salted water (one tablespoon salt for five cups of water) for at least 30 minutes before cooking to kill parasites and their eggs. Avoid coffee, sugars (including fruit and honey) and all milk and dairy products, since these substances lower immunity and make it more difficult for the body to fight off parasites. Raw goat milk is excepted because it contains IgA and IgG immunoglobulins, which help protect the intestinal lining from infectious agents.

Certain foods inhibit worm growth, such as garlic, onions, papaya, pineapple, pumpkin seeds, figs, pomegranate seeds, and the seeds of the rangoon creeper fruit (*Quisqualis indicae*). Since much of commercial fruit is irradi-

For more information about **Dr. Hulda Clark's anti-parasite program**, see *Alternative Medicine Definitive Guide to Cancer* (Future Medicine Publishing, 1997; ISBN 1-887299-01-7); to order, call 800-333-HEAL.

ated, the amount of enzymes found in fresh pineapple and papaya, unless organic, is minimal. The enzymes are needed to break down parasites inside the body. Digestive pancreatic enzymes as well as bromelain and papain should be taken as supplements both with and between meals. When taken with meals, they aid with digestion; when taken between meals, they help to destroy parasites and other cellular debris. Pomegranate juice (four 4-ounce glasses daily) can aid in the expulsion of worms. Wheat germ can be used to inhibit various amoeba from binding to target cells in the intestines.

Biological Dentistry

Biological dentistry stresses the use of nontoxic materials for dental work and focuses on the unrecognized impact that dental toxins and hidden dental infections can have on overall health. Typically, a biological dentist will emphasize the safe removal of mercury dental amalgams; in many cases, the avoidance or removal of root canals; the investigation of possible jawbone infections as a "dental focus" or source of bodywide illness centered in the teeth; and the health-injuring role of misaligned teeth and jaw structures. There is a slowly building recognition among dentists and physicians practicing alternative medicine that dental health has a tremendous impact on the health of the body. European researchers estimate that perhaps as much as 50% of all chronic degenerative illness can be linked either directly or indirectly to dental problems and the techniques of modern dentistry.

One of the first Western practitioners to address the hidden dental connection to cancer was the German physician Josef Issels, M.D., who understood that in a person who has cancer, the entire body is involved. Therapeutic attention must be directed at healing the whole organism and changing the biochemical milieu that enables cancer cells to thrive. To reverse the cancer, the body needs to be detoxified, nourished, and biochemically rebalanced, said Dr. Issels.

In the late 1940s, Dr. Issels proposed that a healthy body would not develop cancer and that the best way to attack cancer was not to attack the tumor alone but to strengthen the individual's metabolism. In his words, "The tumor is merely a late-stage symptom, accidentally triggered off, but able to exist and grow only in a bed already prepared for it."[6] Like other chronic illnesses, cancer can lie dormant and be activated only when the defense mechanisms are no longer capable of destroying the malignant cells.

Dr. Josef Issels is the senior consulting physician at the Max Gerson Memorial Cancer Center of CHIP-SA, located at 670 Nubes, Playas de Tijuana, Mexico; U.S. address: Gerson Research Organization, 7807 Artesian Road, San Diego, CA 92127-2117; tel: 800-759-2966; fax, 619-759-2967.

From this realization Dr. Issels developed his whole-body therapy (WBT), which integrates many modalities into a single protocol aimed at improving the body's natural defense systems. Wolfgang Wöppel, M.D., an associate of Dr. Issels, states that WBT focuses much attention on the contributions of "genetic traits, microbes, dental amalgams and infections, abnormal intestinal flora, faulty diet, neural interferences, chemical toxins, and radiation." One of the first steps in WBT is the removal of infected teeth and mercury fillings, a tremendous source of toxic stress on the body.

Regarding the cancer-promoting potential of an infected tooth and root canal, Dr. Issels states, "Even after the most precise preparation of the main root canal, protein will always remain in the tiny interconnecting canals...If this protein becomes infected, toxic products will be produced, and conveyed into the organism." A root canal procedure can "literally convert a tooth into a toxin-producing 'factory.'"[7] The primary toxin generated by infected teeth is dimethyl sulfide, a major carcinogen. According to Dr. Issels, 98% of his adult cancer patients have teeth whose root canal fillings have

Chelation Removes Heavy Metals

Chelation therapy refers to a method of binding ("chelating") an organic substance known as a chelating agent to a heavy metal and removing it from the body. One type of chelation therapy involves the chelating agent disodium EDTA given as an intravenous infusion over a $3\frac{1}{2}$ hour period. Usually 20 to 30 treatments are administered at the rate of one to three sessions per week.

Infusions of EDTA are extremely beneficial for all forms of atherosclerotic cardiovascular disease including angina pectoris and coronary artery disease, intermittent claudication and gangrene, atherosclerotic disease of the legs and feet, and strokes.

Chelation reduces abnormal tissue calcification, enhances and stimulates a variety of enzymes, improves circulation throughout the body, and reduces free-radical damage—one of the major common denominators of cancer and other degenerative diseases. By reducing the body's free-radical burden (which would otherwise promote tumor growth), chelation probably enhances one's ability to fight cancer.[9]

become sources of toxins. Unless these teeth are removed, the dental toxins are released continuously into the blood and adversely affect the liver, heart, nervous system, endocrine glands, and the lymph system.[8] Removal of the tooth—including its roots—means drilling thoroughly through the tooth socket and up to the healthy bone.

Dr. Issels also notes that toxins from degenerated tonsils probably exist for years prior to the onset of cancer. Patients with this condition often have never been ill with tonsillitis nor can they recall any pain or swelling in their tonsils. Yet, these clinically unremarkable tonsils prove to be foci of the most dangerous kind whose toxins are drained into the bloodstream, thereby lowering immune function. Dr. Issels and his colleagues conclude that there is a correlation between tumor growth and the extent of tonsil infection. Upon removing this obvious source of toxins, tumor growth is halted or markedly depressed.

Dr. Issels' program uses botanical and homeopathic remedies to encourage cell regeneration and to stimulate the body's anticancer defenses. The body's detoxification system—which includes the liver, kidneys, intestines, and skin—is thus stimulated to start eliminating the toxins associated with the tumor. Patients are encouraged to drink plenty of water and herb tea to irrigate the kidneys and to take mild herbal purgatives to cleanse their colon. The approach also uses hyperthermal techniques to re-energize the immune system. By provoking a fever with mixed bacterial vaccines, Dr. Issels can increase the number of white blood cells.

He employs vaccines for specific types of cancer, using ultrafine filtrates of cancer tissues in much the same way as modern vaccines use infectious agents. Dr. Issels also uses oxygen therapy: blood is drawn from the patient, oxygen is bubbled through it, it is exposed to ultraviolet rays, then returned to the patient.

Dr. Issels realized that this approach gave cancer patients a valuable survival advantage over those treated conventionally alone.[10] In one long-term study, Dr. Issels' treatment protocol was applied to 252 patients who had previously undergone conventional surgery and radiation therapy. These patients were considered "terminal" when they came to him for help; i.e., they were not expected to live more than one year. After five years, 16.6% were still alive and functioning, compared to a worldwide average rate of 2%; after 15 years on the program, over 92% of the original survivors were still alive and showed no signs of cancer.[11]

The Advantages and Methods of Mercury Amalgam Removal

Charles Gableman, M.D., of Encinitas, California, who is a leader in the field of environmental medicine, always advises the removal of his patients' amalgam fillings. According to Dr. Gableman, patients with chronic fatigue syndrome, or with a lack of resistance to infections, allergies, and thyroid damage, all improve after their fillings are properly removed. He believes it is possible that these patients have suffered from basic allergies all their life and that the mercury toxicity from the fillings adds to the body's toxic load and "pushes them over the edge," resulting in chronic medical problems.

Once mercury toxicity has been demonstrated, by tests such as high electrogalvanism (electrical conductivity in the metals of the teeth), high mercury vapor emissions, and/or high mercury tissue deposits, mercury amalgam removal and replacement with alternate, nontoxic materials is the recommended step, advises Dr. Daniel Royal, D.O., of Las Vegas, Nevada.

For more on **the health hazards of mercury toxicity and other dental factors,** see Chapter 2: Cancer and Its Causes pp. 48-93.

Colorado biological dentist Hal Huggins, D.D.S., recommends that people who choose to have their amalgams removed ask their dentists to use a rubber dam, a thin sheet of rubber that slips over the teeth. "Dams prevent over 95% of the mixture of mercury and water produced by the drilling out

Daniel F. Royal, D.O.: The Nevada Clinic, 3663 South Pecos McLeod Road, Las Vegas, NV 89121; tel: 702-732-1400; fax: 702-732-9661.

of old fillings from going down your throat. They also reduce the amount of mercury that you might absorb from your cheeks and under your tongue." Dr. Huggins suggests that people consider early morning appointments for amalgam removal, rather than later in the day, because the mercury vapor from other patients' sessions can linger in the air for hours and be absorbed by breathing. Some dentists use mercury vapor filter systems, he points out, but they are rare.

While removal of amalgam fillings stops any further poisoning from mercury, you still need to detoxify the body to eliminate the residual effect from mercury that remains behind. The following guidelines for detoxifying mercury come from the clinical practice of Dr. Royal.[12] Ideally, for those who are about to have amalgams removed, this detoxifying program should be initiated at least two weeks before removal and continued for at least three months after the last amalgams are removed, Dr. Royal says. The usual length of time required for body elimination of mercury is 3-6 months.

Chlorella—This medicinal green algae helps move mercury out of connective tissue so that substances such as DMPS can then remove it from the body. Begin with only one chlorella capsule daily for the first few weeks after amalgam removal, then gradually increase to three daily.

L-glutathione—This natural detoxifying substance (made from the amino acid cysteine) improves liver function, thereby helping the body detoxify. Typically take 150 mg once daily.

Garlic Extract—Garlic's high sulfur and cysteine content enable it to bind up (chelate) toxic metals and to work against harmful microbes. Take one capsule with meals three times daily.

Silymarin–Also known as milk thistle, silymarin has long been used as a liver-purifying agent. Take one capsule twice daily.

On the day of amalgam removal, vitamin C should not be taken until after the procedure; otherwise, it may interfere with the anesthesia.

Vitamin C–Ascorbic acid has a protective effect against free-radical damage, which can occur as heavy metals are being removed and excreted through the kidneys. On the day before amalgam removal, take your bowel tolerance of vitamin C (the amount your system can tolerate before producing diarrhea, usually 8,000-16,000 mg, divided into hourly doses of about 2,000 mg for a 150-pound person). Typical recommended daily dosage is 2,000-8,000 mg.

Vitamin B complex–Take 25-100 mg daily to help replenish nutrients lost when heavy metals are bound up and excreted.

DHEA–This is an adrenal hormone precursor. The adrenal glands of patients with mercury toxicity are often weak, contributing to an inability to handle stress. Recommended dosage is 5 mg for men and 2.5 mg for women, to be taken daily with pregnenolone.

Pregnenolone–This substance (a steroid building block made from cholesterol, usually extracted from soybeans or wild yam) aids in the formation of key brain chemicals associated with memory and thinking. The recommended daily dosage is 10 mg for men and 30 mg for women. This dosage should initially be taken daily and may be decreased as symptoms improve.

DMSA–DMSA (2,3-dimercaptosuccinic acid) is an effective agent for binding up heavy metals because it crosses the blood-brain barrier and thus helps remove toxic residues from the central nervous system. Take three 100-mg capsules in the morning on the day of amalgam removal and the same dosage in the morning on the day after removal. Take 30 minutes before or after eating. Once the amalgams have been removed and after you have been on this supplement program for three months, on one occasion only, take two capsules (100 mg each) three times daily for three days.

DMPS–DMPS (2,3-dimercaptopropane-1-sulfonate) is the chelating agent of choice for the removal of mercury from the human body.

DMPS can be given orally, intravenously, or intramuscularly with a maximum dose of 3 mg/2.2 pounds of body weight, with 250 mg being the typical dose, taken once a month. On the day of the last amalgam removal, the first DMPS treatment may be given. People who have had exposure to amalgam through their fillings will usually require 3-5 injections. Those who have never had amalgam fillings, but show evidence of heavy metal toxicity, may require only 1-2 injections. An injection every 4-6 months thereafter is recommended for maintenance.

Heavy metal–related symptoms, such as joint pains, depression, burning sensations, digestive problems, and fatigue can be temporarily aggravated as DMPS removes toxins from the cells. The routine use of intravenous DMPS is not advisable for patients who still have mercury amalgam fillings. This is because DMPS may dissolve the surface of the existing amalgam fillings. The potential outcome is acute toxicity from heavy metal injury to the lining of the gut.

Essential minerals–As DMPS and DMSA remove vital nutrients from the body, zinc, copper, magnesium, selenium, and manganese should be taken in addition to the other vitamin supplements.

Homeopathic amalgam drops–This is a combination of homeopathically prepared elements found in amalgam fillings given for the purpose of enhancing the removal of heavy metals from the body. Beginning one week prior to amalgam removal, take ten drops, three times daily; continue this dosage for one week after amalgam removal. Once all the amalgams have been removed, begin taking homeopathic mercury (*Mercurius Solubilis* 30C) at the rate of 30 drops, 2-3 times weekly, for the duration of the oral detoxification program.

Acidophilus–Removing mercury-based fillings without intestinal cleansing can accomplish only partial detoxification. A toxic bowel can repollute the mouth through the acupuncture meridians that connect the intestines and the teeth. Therefore, a complete bowel cleansing program must be undertaken at the same time as any removal of mercury fillings. *Acidophilus* helps to restore the microflora of the intestine, which can be adversely affected by the presence of mercury. Take one teaspoon daily, or more if diarrhea or constipation are present.

Psyllium husk–This acts as a bulk fiber laxative to absorb toxins and facilitate the removal of fecal debris from the intestines. Drink at least 6-8 glasses of water daily and slowly build up the amount of psyllium consumed. Begin with one teaspoon in liquid once daily and gradually increase to three teaspoons once daily (three times daily if constipation is present). Take psyllium separately from vitamin and mineral supplements as the fiber will reduce their effectiveness.

Dietary changes—A high-fiber diet, consisting primarily of fruits, vegetables, and legumes, will tend to decrease fecal transit time, reducing the amount of time that liquids containing heavy metals remain in the colon and thus reduce the quantity. Decrease consumption of refined carbohydrates including simple sugars, white flour, and saturated fats, because they may reduce the availability of essential enzymes and nutrients.

Avoid fish, which is the largest dietary source of mercury. While some fish have comparatively lower mercury content (sardines, herring, pollack, mackerel, cod, redfish, and Greenland halibut), most tuna and shellfish have a fairly high level of mercury. Individuals who are sensitive to mercury usually have some type of adverse reaction to shellfish. Also reduce chicken/egg consumption. Fish meal has become a major source of feed for chickens. Depending on the mercury content of the fish meal, chickens and eggs have the potential of containing a significant amount of mercury.

Water Therapy

Water therapy, also called hydrotherapy, is the use of water, ice, and steam to maintain and restore health. Treatments include full-body immersion, steam baths, saunas, sitz baths (in which the pelvis is immersed in hot and/or cold water), colonic irrigation, and the application of hot and cold compresses. Hydrotherapy is effective for treating a wide range of conditions and can easily be used as part of a self-care program. Today, many alternative practitioners prescribe baths, Jacuzzi, steam saunas, mineral and mud baths, wraps, rubs, sitz baths, and wet compresses to remedy a great variety of health conditions, ranging from stress and pain to the many toxins, parasites, bacteria, and viruses that can cause disease.

Hydrotherapy Method #1: Hot Blanket Packs

A hot blanket pack involves the use of a hot water bottle or nonelectric heating pad. The purpose is to produce a mild increase in body temperature (the pack serving as a form of hyperthermia, or heat therapy) for immune stimulation or detoxification.

See "Hydrotherapy," pp. 281-298.

The following guidelines are for the health practitioner: In a typical application, assemble a dry cotton sheet, two wool blankets, two hot water bottles (or a nonelectric heating pad), and a cold compress. Spread out the two blankets and cover them with a dry sheet. Have the patient undress and wrap them in the sheet. Place one hot water bottle on the abdomen and one at the feet, or place the heating pad on the abdomen; wipe the face with the cold compress as needed. Leave the patient in the pack for 20-60 minutes, depending on the amount of heating desired. The goal is to heat the body and induce sweating.

Where it is desirable to heat only the lower half of the body, a hot half-pack may be used. In this case, wrap the body only from the waist to the feet with a hot water bottle or heating pad between the legs. This treatment may be used with people who have peripheral vascular diseases or loss of peripheral sensations. Take care not to overheat the patient with the hot water bottles or heating pad and always follow the hot blanket pack with a cool rinse.

Hydrotherapy Method #2: Self-Applied Hyperthermia

This local or whole-body treatment can be used in home treatment to raise the temperature of the tissues, a process called artificial fever. The purpose is to destroy heat-sensitive organisms (viruses and bacteria), to enhance immune function, and to encourage elimination of toxic material. The technique may also be useful as an adjunctive treatment of the upper respiratory infections that are a common complication of many types of cancer, including advanced cases of lung cancer.

Materials required include a hot tub or deep bath with water at 103°-104° F; a basin of ice water and towel; and pure drinking water. A typical treatment may be performed by immersing the body in hot water for up to 60 minutes at a time; maintain bath temperature for the entire time. To prevent a headache, apply a cold compress to the head early in the treatment and maintain it throughout. Check oral temperature every 10-15 minutes; if it exceeds 104° F, cool the bath and apply more cold compress. Following the treatment, rinse in a cool shower, then wrap up and stay warm. If a bath or hot tub are not available, heat the body in a steam bath or sauna.

Take the following precautions when using hyperthermia treatment:

1) Consult your physician before doing this treatment if you have any of the following: high or low blood pressure, serious illness, diabetes, or multiple sclerosis. Do not use this treatment if you are or may be pregnant.

2) Watch for signs of hyperventilation. These include numbness and tingling in the lips, hands, or feet. If hyperventilation occurs, reduce the bath temperature; breathe from the abdomen, not the chest; or breathe into a paper bag until the tingling passes.

3) Stand slowly after finishing the treatment and be especially careful during the cool rinse in the shower so as not to faint. It is advisable

Aromatherapy Aids Cancer Treatment

Researchers at Memorial Sloan-Kettering Cancer Center in New York City used aromatherapy to ease the anxiety attacks of patients who received magnetic resonance imaging (MRI), a high-tech diagnostic procedure that involves being fully enclosed inside a large machine. Before their MRIs, some patients were exposed to the fumes of heliotropin essential oil, a scent often prescribed by aromatherapists for relaxation. Compared with those who received no aromatherapy, the heliotropin group experienced significantly less anxiety during the MRI.[13]

to have an attendant at hand for the first few treatments.

Hydrotherapy Method #3: Wet Sheet Packs

This procedure begins with a full-body wrap in a cold wet sheet. Typically, the treatment progresses in three phases; cold or cooling, neutral, and heating. The purposes are to stimulate, relax, and detoxify, respectively. The cold phase is stimulating and tonifying if it is stopped after the sheet loses its cool temperature. The cold application is useful to control a fever that is rising too rapidly or is too high. The neutral temperature phase is useful to relax and sedate. Heating is used to promote sweating and detoxifying from environmental or chemical exposure or from drug, alcohol, or tobacco use.

Materials for this treatment include a bed or treatment table, wool blankets (1-3 may be needed), two pillows (one for the head and one for under the knees), a polyester or cotton sheet soaked in ice water, a bath towel, and a hand towel. The procedure (for the health-care practitioner) is typically done this way: Spread one blanket, placing a pillow at the head and another to support the knees. The blanket should be large enough to fold over the shoulders of the patient. Thoroughly wring out the ice water sheet and lay it out over the blanket. Have patient undress and lie down on the center of the wet sheet and pull the far half of the wet sheet toward you. Have patient place their arms in a comfortable position across the abdomen. Wrap the near half of the sheet over the shoulders, arms, and around the near leg. Add extra layers of blanket over the patient to hold in the heat produced by the patient to warm the sheet.

If the treatment is used to reduce fever, extra blankets are not needed. If general detoxification is desired, leave the patient in the wet sheet until profuse sweating occurs and for as long as can be tolerated. This may take 2-4 hours. The heating/detoxifying stage will be reached sooner if the patient has undergone some sort of heating activity before getting into the wet sheet pack, such as exercise or a hot shower. If relaxation is the primary goal, remove the patient from the pack before perspiration begins; then follow with a warm (not hot) wet sheet wrap. If tonifying, fever-reducing effects are sought, remove the patient as soon as the sheet begins to heat up. It may be necessary to use the cold wet sheet several times to reach the desired effect.

Take the following precautions when using wet sheet packs:

1) Hot drinks such as ginger tea will promote sweating. Don't give too much fluid because the need to urinate could end the treatment too soon. Have the patient drink ample purified or spring water during elimination/perspiration phase.

2) The bath towel may be used to cover the patient's head and eyes to enhance the heating phase and shade the eyes. The hand towel may be used as a cold compress and to mop the patient's face once perspiration begins in the elimination phase.

Heat Therapy

The body uses its own internally generated heat to protect itself from viruses, bacteria, and other harmful substances. A fever is the body's attempt to destroy invading organisms and to sweat impurities out through the skin. Fever is an effective natural process of curing disease and restoring health; heat therapy, or hyperthermia, represents a way to create fever to call out this natural healing process. A state of natural hyperthermia exists when body temperature rises above its normal level of 98.6° F. An increase in body temperature causes many physiological responses to occur. For one, by increasing the production of antibodies and interferon, it stimulates the immune system. Practitioners of alternative medicine have long recognized hyperthermia as a useful technique in detoxification therapy because it releases toxins stored in fat cells, such as pesticides, PCBs, and drug residues from the body.

The principle behind hyperthermia is simple: heat cancer cells and they can be killed easily. Direct killing of cancer cells begins to occur when the cancerous tissue reaches about 104° F to 105.8° F.[14] "Only a relatively small rise in body temperature can make a huge difference," says Robert Atkins, M.D., who includes it in his cancer protocols. Though the principle sounds simple, the technique is far more complicated, thanks to the body's ability to regulate its internal temperature. As any sauna enthusiast will attest, the human body likes heat only to a point. When the body temperature rises, blood flow increases to dissipate the

See "Hyperthermia," pp. 299-305.

Detoxify and Enhance Immunity with an Aromatherapy Spa

Physicians have long known of the many therapeutic benefits of steam heat, also known as hyperthermia or heat stress detoxification. Similarly, the benefits of aromatherapy—the inhalation of the vapors of essential plant oils—are widely recognized among alternative practitioners. Now Variel Health International has combined both modalities in the form of the aromaSpa™ for home use. In the self-contained aromatherapy and steam heat diffuser, soothing aromatic mists envelop the entire body surface for maximum absorption and benefit.

The unit stands 5'6", weighs about 68 pounds, and plugs into any standard outlet. Any of at least 250 aromatherapy oils may be used, singly or in combination, to support muscle relaxation, detoxification, immune system stimulation, eliminate fatigue, lift mood, or revitalize skin. Other self-care benefits include general mind and body relaxation, energization, emotional cleansing, and general rejuvenation, says Variel's Cathy Dammann.

The aromaSpa was tested by Jerry Schindler, Ph.D., director of the Sports Health Science Human Performance Lab at Life College School of Chiropractic in Marietta, Georgia. Dr. Schindler reported that the unit was effective in decreasing the risk of everyday and athletic injuries, primarily by increasing muscle flexibility, blood flow, and oxygen delivery to the muscles. Steam heat therapy may heighten immune response by stimulating white blood cell production, Dammann says. Heat therapy is also one of the most effective ways to remove fat-stored toxins from the body. The aromaSpa can produce detoxifying effects in only ten minutes compared to standard hot body wraps which require 60 minutes, says Dammann.

See "Aromatherapy," pp. 53-62.

For information about **aromaSpa™**, contact: Variel Health International, 9618 Variel Avenue, Chatsworth, CA 91311; tel: 818-407-4717; fax: 818-407-0738.

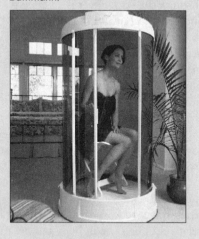

excess heat. One way to circumvent the body's ability to regulate its temperature is to apply the heat locally, targeting a specific tumor. This can be done with the use of microwaves and ultrasound, which can be directed at parts of the body with great precision. Unlike normal tissue, tumors have poor blood flow relative to their metabolic needs and cannot dissipate the heat, so they tend to get hotter than the surrounding area and are more vulnerable to the effects of heat.

At the Duke Hyperthermia Program of the Duke University Medical Center in Durham, North Carolina, considerable success has been reported in using hyperthermia to treat soft-tissue sarcomas and recurrences of breast cancer. One recent study found that radiation combined with hyperthermia was 30% more effective against breast cancer than radiation treatment alone.[15] Tumors located near the surface of the body appear to be more amenable to treatment than deep-tissue tumors.

"I try never to use radiation treatment—which is even more dangerous than most forms of chemotherapy—without also using hyperthermia," says Dr. Atkins. "Thanks to hyperthermia, we can shrink tumors with far less radiation to get the same therapeutic outcome, and our patients' immune systems and overall health are faring much better as a result."

Body temperature can be swiftly increased by the external application of heat. This approach causes blood vessels to dilate and the body to perspire in an attempt to prevent an increase in temperature. An increase in body temperature may also be accomplished by immersing the body in hot water, sitting in a sauna or steam bath, or wrapping oneself in blankets with a hot water bottle. Other approaches, more commonly found in hospital and medical centers, include the use of shortwave or microwave diathermy, ultrasound, radiant heating, and extracorporeal heating. Diathermy raises body temperature by applying radio-frequency electromagnetic energy. Ultrasound generates heat as a result of friction produced at the molecular level as the high-energy sound waves strike body tissues. Radiant heating devices produce infrared heat that is applied to the body. Extracorporeal heating involves removing blood from the body, heating it, and returning it to the body.

Patients with temperature regulation problems, especially the old and the very young, should not use hyperthermia. Microwave diathermy can burn tissue around the eyes; it should never be used by people with pacemakers. People with peripheral vascular disease (poor blood flow to the legs and feet) or loss of sensation should not use hyperthermia because of the risk of burns. Caution is advised with patients who have cardiovascular disease, in particular arrhythmia (irregular heartbeat) and tachycardia (abnormally rapid heart rate), or severe hypertension or hypotension.

Hyperthermia in the Treatment of Cancer

Studies have shown that hyperthermia treatment modifies cell membranes in such a way as to protect healthy cells and make tumor cells more susceptible to chemotherapy and radiation.[16] For this reason, hyperthermia is a useful adjunct in cancer therapy, largely because it enables the use of lower doses of chemotherapy and radiation. Hyperthermia treatments play a role in stimulating the immune system, as evidenced by the drop in white blood cell counts immediately following treatment and the rise that occurs within a few hours. Not only do the number of white blood cells increase, but their ability to destroy target cells appears to increase as well.[17]

A recent study showed an increase in the production of interleukin-1 (an immune-stimulating compound) with whole-body hyperthermia.[18] Studies indicate that increased body temperature plays a positive role in the healing process of the body. According to Arthur C. Guyton, M.D., an authority on medical physiology, the metabolic rate is increased 100% for every 10° C rise in temperature.[19] An increase in temperature from 98.6° F to 104° F should increase metabolism by about 30%. This increased metabolic rate accounts for some of the increased immune activity and thus hyperthermia's contribution to cancer reversal.

When used knowledgeably and with care, hyperthermia is a safe and effective treatment. However, certain individuals are sensitive to the effects of heat, such as those with anemia, heart disease, diabetes, seizure disorders, or tuberculosis, and women who are or may be pregnant;[20] individuals with these conditions should always consult with a doctor before embarking on self-administered treatments. Other reported risks associated with the use of hyperthermia include herpes outbreaks[21], liver toxicity,[22] and nervous system injury. Hyperthermia used for detoxification should be performed only under medical supervision.

Bodywork and Exercise

The term *bodywork* refers to hands-on therapies such as massage, deep tissue manipulation, movement awareness, and energy balancing, among others, which are employed to soothe injured muscles, stimulate blood and lymphatic circulation, reduce pain, and promote deep relaxation as well as to improve the structure and physical functioning of the body.

Movement therapies help realign the body by correcting postural imbalances and thereby promoting more efficient functioning of the nervous and musculoskeletal systems. A form of movement therapy known as Authentic Movement (AM) has been used therapeutically for breast cancer. In a study of 33 breast cancer patients, women attending regular support group sessions were encouraged to share their feelings and concerns. The women were also invited to move spontaneously with their feelings, all the while being observed impartially by a trained AM therapist, called the "witness."

The therapist attends respectfully and sensitively to the other's experience. "A good witness is insightful, impartially attentive, and has the maturity to claim her own projections. Over time, she develops a deep respect and empathy for the mover," says Tina Stromstead of the San Francisco–based Authentic Movement Institute. After a movement session, witness and mover share their feelings, thoughts, and impressions regarding the session. The study's coordinator, psychologist Sandy Dibell-Hope, Ph.D., reports that the AM sessions improve mood, body image, and self-esteem, as well as decrease depression, anxiety, and a sense of social isolation.[23] Such changes translate into an improved quality of life for breast cancer patients, and this shift can help promote long-range survival.

Since the mid-1980s, considerable scientific evidence has supported the claim that massage therapy is beneficial.[24] According to John Yates, Ph.D., author of *A Physician's Guide to Therapeutic Massage*, massage can benefit such conditions as muscle spasm and pain, spinal curvatures, soreness related to injury and stress, headaches, temporomandibular joint (TMJ) syndrome, and respiratory disorders such as bronchial asthma or emphysema. Massage can also help reduce swelling, correct posture, improve

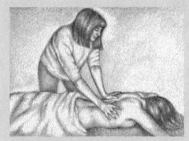

The Therapeutic Effects of Massage

Gertrude Beard, R.N., R.P.T., former Associate Professor of Physical Therapy at Northwestern University Medical School, summarizes the findings of numerous research studies on the therapeutic effects of massage. Studies indicate that massage helps to:

- sedate the nervous system and promote voluntary muscle relaxation
- promote recovery from fatigue produced by excessive exercise
- break up scar tissue and lessen fibrosis and adhesions that develop as a result of injury
- relieve certain types of pain
- provide effective treatment of inflammatory conditions by increasing lymphatic circulation
- reduce swelling from fractures
- improve circulation and increase blood flow through the muscles
- loosen mucus, promote drainage of sinus fluids, and increase drainage of mucus from the lungs
- increase peristaltic action (muscular contractions that move waste through the intestines)
- trigger reflex actions in the body to stimulate organs.

body motion, and facilitate the elimination of toxins.[25]

According to the Quebec Task Force on Spinal Disorders, massage is particularly useful in controlling pain.[26] Massage is also useful for simply relaxing muscle tension and reducing stress. People who face a diagnosis of cancer, particularly for the first time, are often overwhelmed by a sense of anxiety and impending doom. This anxiety triggers the "fight-or-flight" response in the body (notably the release of adrenaline) and leads to heightened muscular tension and elevated blood pressure.

Muscle tension, whether from normal activity or awkward movement or stress, contributes to muscle fatigue and pain by compressing nerve fibers in the muscle. Prolonged contraction interferes with the elimination of chemical wastes in the muscles and surrounding tissues, and can cause nerve and muscle pain. If not properly addressed, these body tensions have a tendency to build into chronic patterns of stress.

For these tension-related conditions, Robert D. Milne, M.D., of Las Vegas, Nevada, coauthor of *Alternative Medicine Definitive Guide to Headaches*,[27] finds that massage can break up muscular waste deposits and stimulate circulation. Accumulated metabolic wastes often form "trigger points" within muscles; these are specific areas that are painful to the touch. By applying deep pressure to these points, the tension or spasm can often be eliminated. Sometimes this deep pressure will even release the assorted toxins from the tissues.

The Therapeutic Benefits of Exercise

The benefits of exercise extend far beyond cardiovascular fitness and the prevention of obesity and heart disease. Exercise aids in detoxification, digestion, and immune processes and can do wonders for mood and attitude. Advanced-cancer patients treated conventionally often end up spending many hours in a hospital bed, in contrast to those who undergo alternative cancer therapies who typically engage in regular exercise or physical activity. A brisk walk several times a week is a good start for any exercise program; low-impact aerobics, calisthenics, *qigong*, yoga, stretching and flexing exercises, and gardening, among others, are all ways of strengthening the body's self-healing system.

Among the anticancer benefits of physical exercise, well-documented by clinical research, are the following:

■ Aerobic activities increase oxygen supply to tissues; because cancer tends to flourish in an oxygen-poor environment, the well-exercised body is more likely to repel cancer cells.

■ Any form of physical activity, because it involves muscle contractions, stimulates the lymphatic system, which filters toxins from the blood and supports the body's immune system.

■ Exercise stimulates the activity of natural killer cells and other components of the body's anticancer defenses.[28]

■ Exercise causes an elevation of body temperature and increases the production of pyrogen, a lymphokine that enhances the function of white blood cells.[29]

People who maintain regular activity are less likely to develop colon cancer, the second leading cause of cancer-related death in the U.S.[30] Female college athletes, when compared to their nonathletic counterparts, have a lower incidence of cancers of the breast, ovary, cervix, vagina, and uterus.[31] In the same study, the risk of developing cancers of the reproductive system was 2.5 times lower for the athletes than it was for the sedentary women.

Keith I. Block, M.D., notes that exercise also helps cancer patients maintain normal muscle mass, which can increase significantly their chances of recovery. "Patients who are overweight or who lose lean tissue or muscle during therapy tend to have poorer prognoses," Dr. Block says. He recommends finding a form of exercise that can be carried out consistently, without causing strain.

In one study, men who burned as few as 500 calories a week in exercise—the equivalent to about an hour's worth of brisk walking—had death rates about 20% lower than men who rarely exercised.[32] Men who walked about four hours each week (about 2,000 calories burned) died of all cancers about 35% less frequently than their less active counterparts. A recent report from the Cooper Clinic in Dallas indicates that even moderate exercise—five hours of walking per week—significantly reduces the risk of developing prostate cancer.[33]

Qigong

Among the more systematized programs of movement therapy that can be applied to treating serious illness is *qigong*. In China, it is estimated

Qigong Proven to Improve Cancer Outcomes

At the Kuangan Men's Hospital in Beijing, China, 93 cases of advanced malignant cancer were treated with a combination of drugs and qigong exercises, while a control group of 30 patients was treated by drugs alone. Of the qigong group, 81% gained strength, 63% experienced improved appetite, and 33% were free from diarrhea compared to comparable control group improvements of 10%, 10%, and 6%, respectively.[35]

See "Qigong," pp. 422-433; "Traditional Chinese Medicine," pp. 450-459.

that nearly 100 million people, from the healthy to the severely ill, practice qigong every day. Qigong plays a central role in the Chinese doctor's anti-cancer arsenal and is used in almost all hospitals in China today.

Qigong movements are gentle and unhurried; the slow rate tends to synchronize with the rate of breathing. People engaged in these activities experience a sense of deep relaxation and heightened alertness. In fact, many derive an immediate positive sensation from the practice, giving them an incentive to continue practicing, even long after recovering from cancer. Qigong literally means to work with or cultivate the qi, the vital life force energy that flows through the body. In one laboratory demonstration performed by a qigong master upon a group of patients, researchers measured the following results: a 30% reduction in cervical cancer cells; a 50% reduction in flu viruses; and a 60%-80% reduction in bacteria.[34]

Qi is a naturally occurring, internally produced, self-healing resource, says Roger Jahnke, O.M.D., an acupuncturist practicing in Santa Barbara, California, who uses qigong as part of his support treatment for patients with serious illness, including cancer. "Qigong can facilitate the free flow of energy throughout the body, which supports and promotes blood and lymph flow and even the flow of neurological impulses necessary for good health," says Dr. Jahnke. "The primary benefit is to activate the bioelectrical currents that flow along the energy channels through breathing regulation, deep relaxation, and gentle movement." One advantage of this kind of exercise is the lack of strain on the body's joints and organ systems, a problem associated with high-impact aerobic activities. "Qigong is simple and easy to learn," says Dr. Jahnke. "My goal is to teach and inspire my patients to learn these techniques, so they can play an active role in their recovery."

How Qigong Helps You Resist Cancer

Medical applications of qigong have been studied in major cancer treatment facilities in China. Immunologists have observed that *qigong* stimulates the activity of lymphocytes, neutrophils, and other immune cells that play a role in fighting cancer.[36] Research conducted at the Beijing Lung Cancer Research Institute has shown that *qigong* increases the immune function of lung cancer patients, as indicated by the activity of their white blood cells.

A study of 122 cancer patients found that *qigong* resulted in better control of tumor growth and that those patients who practiced longer had better results.[37] Most of these patients reported an enhanced quality of life as well as reductions in pain. In another study, 2,873 "terminal" cancer patients practiced *qigong* for six months. The outcome: 12% of the patients were cured while 47% showed significant improvement.[38] These are considerably better outcomes than are achieved through chemotherapy.

In Chinese medicine, cancer exists in two ways: either as "accumulations" (tumorous form in which the cancer is localized) or as a whole-body toxicity problem (metastatic, blood, or lymph forms, in which cancer has spread). As Dr. Jahnke explains: "Tumors and toxicity that contribute to cancer are caused by a severe derangement of the function of the *qi* in its ability to support the body's overall functioning. The *qi* has become disordered, which shows up in numerous ways, such as pain, accumulations of toxins, and immune system deficiency."

From Dr. Jahnke's perspective, the practice of *qigong* has the three following beneficial effects on the individual with cancer:[39]

1. Improved Oxygen Supply—Under healthy conditions, body cells and tissues receive oxygen as needed and this helps repel cancer, since cancer cells cannot thrive in a high-oxygen environment. During *qigong*, the

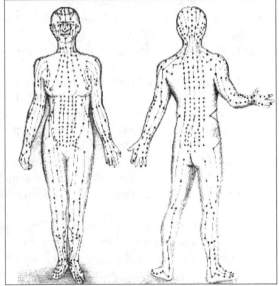

Front and back view of acupuncture meridians.

body becomes deeply relaxed and oxygen is absorbed from the blood by the tissues. "*Qigong* accelerates oxygen distribution in the body at a time when your muscles are not rapidly using it as in high-stress forms of exercise," says Dr. Jahnke. "The higher the oxygen supply, the more readily your body can reverse a cancerous condition." At the same time, there is an increased efficiency of cell metabolism and tissue regeneration through increased circulation of oxygen and nutrient-rich blood to the brain, organs, and tissues.

2. Improved Balance of Autonomic Nervous System—The second major effect of *qigong* involves the person's psyche and its effect on the autonomic nervous system (ANS). The ANS, which controls most of our basic body functions, contains two branches: the sympathetic and parasympathetic systems. The sympathetic nervous system is associated with arousal and stress; this system prepares us physically when we perceive a threat or challenge, by increasing our heart rate, blood pressure, and muscle tension. The hormones released in this process tend to suppress the immune system, which is why a calm way of responding to difficult situations is desirable. The parasympathetic nervous system conserves body energy, slows heart rate, and increases intestinal and gland activity. During *qigong* practice, the individual can achieve a state of deep relaxation, enabling the parasympathetic nervous system to neutralize the stress response, says Dr. Jahnke. This decreases heart rate and blood pressure, dilates the blood vessels (enhancing oxygen supply), and supports optimal immune function. A related benefit, Dr. Jahnke adds, is a reduction in depression and anxiety.

3. Improved Lymphatic Function—*Qigong* exerts a powerful influence on the lymphatic system, the "garbage disposal system" of the body. "People who are not well are generally not mobilizing their lymphatic systems. This system is moved by a kind of composite heart, including all the body's muscles, the breath, the cells' production of water, gravity, and an automatic contraction of the lymph vessels. *Qigong* practice stimulates circulation of the lymph fluid, carrying the immune cells to key areas and eliminating toxins from the tissue spaces."

The cancer patients who come to Dr. Jahnke for medical care are typically receiving some form of conventional treatment. Traditional Chinese doctors regard *qigong* not as an exclusive form of therapy; rather, they emphasize using it in combination with conventional treatment, Chinese herbal remedies, a healing diet, psychotherapy, and regular group activity.[40]

One study compared cancer patients treated with this integrated approach for half a year to those receiving only conventional therapy. Compared to the conventional group, the group treated with the integrated approach experienced clear benefits: the antitumor activity of immune cells increased, their DNA repair ability improved, and the rate of cancer recurrence was reduced. At the same time, patients in the *qigong* group showed improved confidence and optimism, and in a few cases, tumors went into complete remission.[41] Studies of patients with advanced cancer have found that *qigong* helped improve the condition of the immune system, stimulated appetite, and reduced adverse side effects of chemotherapy, such as nausea and vomiting.[42] The response rate to chemotherapy in the *qigong*-treated group was nearly five times better than that of the group that received chemotherapy without *qigong*.

Dr. Jahnke notes that patients practicing *qigong* appear not to suffer from the side effects of radiation treatments and, in addition, maintain their lean tissue mass—a significant factor, since a loss of lean tissue mass can greatly worsen the cancer patient's prognosis. *Qigong* appears to raise energy levels and improve muscle tone and coordination.[43]

An Introduction to *Qigong* Practice
This section contains detailed instructions from Dr. Jahnke on a specific set of therapeutic *qigong* practices.

Tracing Acupuncture Meridians to Circulate Vital Life Energy—The goal of this practice is to move the *qi* along the meridians. Rub your hands together to build up heat and increase *qi*. They will become warmer if you are relaxed and your environment is comfortable. As if washing your face, stroke your palms upward across the cheeks, eyes, and forehead; continue over the top and side of your head, down the back of the neck, and along the shoulders to the shoulder joint. Continue under the arm and down the sides to the rib cage. At the lower edge of the rib cage, move the palms around to the back, across the buttocks, down the back and sides of the legs, and out the sides of the feet. Trace up inside the feet and the inner surface of the legs, up the front side of the torso and onto the face again, beginning the second round.

Directing Vital Life Energy to Internal Organs—Again, rub your hands together to build up heat. Apply the right hand to the area over the liver at the lower right edge of your rib cage. Visualize the liver receiving the *qi* and its benefits. Apply the left hand to the area over the

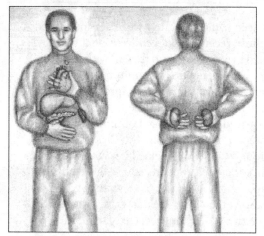
Directing vital life energy to internal organs.

spleen and pancreas at the lower left side of the ribs. The spleen is the producer of white blood cells and the pancreas produces digestive enzymes as well as insulin and glucagon. Move your hands in a circular way, continuing to create heat, breathing restful breaths, and relax. Feel the heat, or *qi*, moving through the surface of the skin and penetrating the organs as the entire metabolic process becomes more efficient. Still holding the hands over the organs, continue to feel the heat penetrate. On exhalation, visualize the *qi* circulating from the center of the body out along the arms, and into the hands, to finally penetrate into the organs.

Now, move your left palm to cover the navel and your right palm to cover the breastbone. The navel is the original connection to life and nourishment, and the Chinese feel that in adulthood it still connects energetically to the whole body. The breastbone protects several vital organs—the heart and the thymus. The heart pumps the blood, of course, but the Chinese believe it is the resting place of one's emotional and spiritual self. The thymus is the original source of T cells, some of the most powerful immune agents. Visualize them benefiting from the *qi* pouring into the navel, heart, and thymus. Move the palms around to cover the lower back. In traditional Chinese medicine, this area is thought to be directly connected to the kidneys, which not only remove toxins from the blood, but also are the storehouse of vital life energies. The adrenal glands rest on top of the kidneys and control the regulation of our energy. Rub these areas, penetrating the *qi* deep into the body to improve the function of the kidneys and adrenals.

Massaging the Acupuncture Microsystems—In modern Chinese medical terminology, the hands, feet, abdomen, and ears are called reflex microsystems. Pressure properly applied to these areas can stimulate *qi* throughout the body. With your thumbs, vigorously press all areas of the palms and the soles of the feet. Find sore points and concentrate pressure on them several times. Press out along each segment of the fingers and toes. At the tips of the fingers and toes press on the lateral sides of the base of the finger or toenails. Continuing to press, roll the receiving finger or toe under the pressure of the thumb and forefinger of the working hand. Give additional pressure to those points that were particularly tender. Now using the thumbs and forefingers, massage both ears simultaneously. Begin with moderate pressure and work over the entire ear on both sides, until the ears begin to feel hot. Rub any areas of discomfort vigorously a second or third time.

Building Up Vital Life Energy with Breathing—Sit or stand, keeping your eyes closed or just slightly open, with your attention focused inward. Be aware of your physical body and emotional state. Relax your shoulders and allow your head to rest directly on top of the shoulders and spine. Hold your hands with palms facing upward, fingertips pointing toward each other two inches below the navel. Slowly inhaling, bring the hands upward to the lower edge of the breastbone. Then, take in three additional short puffs of breath to fill the lungs, raising the hands a bit with each puff to the level of the center of the heart; hold for a movement. Turn the palms face down and exhale slowly, gradually lowering the hands to the navel. Exhale three additional puffs of breath, to empty the lungs completely. Lower the hands a bit to the beginning level; hold for a moment. Turn the palms upward and repeat. On the exhalations, you may feel a warm sensation spreading outward from the center of your body toward your hands. On inhaling, visualize the *qi* accumulating deep inside the abdominal cavity.

Contracting and Relaxing While Breathing—While sitting or standing, bring the hands in front of the heart/breastbone, inhale, and relax. Begin to exhale, pressing the hands forward as if pushing something heavy. Contract as many of the body's muscles as possible. Grip the floor or ground with the toes and, while the hands

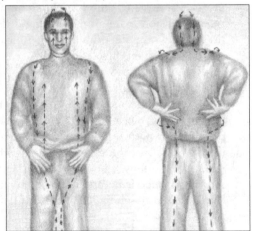

Tracing acupuncture meridians to circulate vital life energy.

Success Story: *Qigong* to Reverse Breast Cancer

When Janice, 50, was diagnosed with breast cancer, she decided to explore the options of alternative medicine. She sought the guidance of Roger Jahnke, O.M.D. Dr. Jahnke encouraged Janice to pursue a therapeutic program that included a mainly vegetarian diet, herbal medicine, acupuncture, and *qigong*.

Janice learned an exercise focused on storing the *qi* in the bone marrow. "According to the Chinese tradition, the practice of *qigong* is believed to support the bone marrow's ability to produce immune cells," says Dr. Jahnke. "Anyone with a cancer diagnosis can benefit from the practice of *qigong*." These benefits include enhancing immune function and increasing blood and lymph circulation, as well as cultivating inner strength, calming the mind, and restoring the body to its natural state of health.

When Janice began *qigong* practice, she noticed that the tumor in her breast would actually feel hot, then would cool off when she stopped practicing. In the following weeks, her energy level increased noticeably. She felt that the practice, as an addition to other natural healing methods and conventional medicine, was helping to restore her health. Janice's health continued to improve and, eight years after her diagnosis, Janice was doing well, living symptom free with cancer in apparent remission.

slowly push forward, contract the perineal muscles (located on the pelvic floor between the genital and anal area, the muscles used to curtail the flow of urine). When the hands are extended and all muscles contracted, the breath is completely exhaled. Now relax, release tension from all muscles, and float the hands back toward the heart with a deep inhalation. Release the toes, the perineum, and the abdomen.

Repeat the same cycle, pressing the hands upward as high as possible, as if lifting a great weight off yourself, exhaling and contracting. Then relax completely, inhale slowly, and return the hands to the position before the heart. Next, repeat pushing out to the sides, then pressing downward. Continue for several rounds, pressing forward, then up, then to the sides, and finally downward. Contraction and release of the muscles pumps lymphatic fluid away from the tissues, carrying metabolic by-products and pollutants to the bloodstream, for elimination through the liver and kidneys.

Qigong Concentration—This practice can be done standing, sitting, or lying down. In the severely ill, it can mobilize important healing resources; in a healthy person, it can help maintain health and coordinate body, mind, and spirit. On inhalation, visualize a concentration of *qi* in the abdominal area. On exhalation, visualize these resources circulating out from the center to all the parts of the body. Continue, through thought and visualization, to circulate healing energy with deep breathing and deep relaxation.

Maintaining the Therapeutic Practice of *Qigong*

If able, one should practice *qigong* for 30-60 minutes daily, says Dr. Jahnke. For those with cancer, if they feel they have the resources and energy to carry out *qigong* practice more aggressively, then they should practice it several times a day. Cancer patients using *qigong* to treat advanced cancer need to apply themselves on a vigilant yet gentle basis, until they begin to experience some benefits. "There is great value in a continuing practice to ensure long-term healing and the increase of vitality," says Jahnke. Practicing *qigong* with other people, as is commonly done in China, provides positive reinforcement and makes the practice easier to maintain.

For more information about *qigong*, contact: Roger Jahnke, O.M.D., Health Action, 243 Pebble Beach Drive, Santa Barbara, CA 93117; tel: 805-685-4670; fax: 805-685-4710.

Some physicians recommend *qigong* to their patients as a "last resort," when other therapies fail. Dr. Jahnke considers this a mistake, since *qigong* aids in the recovery process by enhancing the immune system. "*Qigong* should be incorporated into every cancer treatment approach from day one. It is better as a first resort," he says. "It is an excellent way to improve the cancer patient's appetite and sleep as well as increase their overall immune resistance, energy level, and emotional well-being. Why would anyone want to experience these benefits as a last resort?"

10 Energy Support Therapies

THE REALM OF ENERGY is at the forefront of new alternative approaches to cancer diagnosis and treatment. By energy, we mean a somewhat subtler level of bodily functioning than what is reflected in biochemistry and immunology. Traditional Chinese medicine and acupuncture, for example, talk of *qi*, a basic flow of energy or life force through the body; homeopathy speaks of the *dynamis*, the fundamental self-healing vitality of the human organism. In this chapter, we explore the diagnostic and therapeutic role of energy in addressing cancer, as exemplified in electrodermal screening and the applied energies of magnets and light.

The Growing Importance of Energy Medicine in Cancer Treatment

It may surprise you to note that many of the most sophisticated diagnostic systems used today in conventional medicine—EKG (electrocardiogram, to measure heart activity), EEG (electroencephalogram, to measure brain waves), MRI (magnetic resonance imaging, to "picture" internal organs)— employ the principles of energy medicine. Energy medicine, or bioenergetic medicine as it is sometimes called, refers to diagnostic procedures and therapies that use an energy field—electrical, magnetic, sonic, acoustic, microwave, infrared—to screen for health conditions by detecting imbalances in the body's energy fields, and then correct them.

The detection of energy imbalances in the body provides an early warning system for potential disruptions in biochemical balance and function that may lead to disease. Balance can be restored using a variety of alternative therapies, or with treatment devices that rebalance the energy levels before the actual biochemical or structural disturbances can occur. Through energy medicine, and particularly with electrodermal screening (EDS), you can see disease coming before it manifests and thereby stop it early.

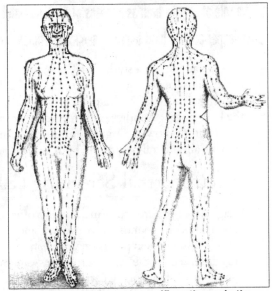

Acupuncture meridians are specific pathways in the human body for the flow of life force or subtle energy, known as *qi* (pronounced CHEE). In most cases, these energy pathways run up and down both sides of the body and correspond to individual organs or organ systems, designated as Lung, Small Intestine, Heart, and others. There are 12 principal meridians and eight secondary channels. Numerous points of heightened energy exist on the body's surface along the meridians and are called acupoints. There are more than 1,000 acupoints, each of which is potentially a place for acupuncture treatment.

Most energy medicine devices are based on the acupuncture meridian system. Acupuncture works on the principle that there is a network of energy channels or pathways, called meridians, running throughout the body. According to acupuncture theory, different organs are associated with different energy meridians, and health problems in organs show up as disturbances of energy in the associated meridians. Acupuncture points, or acupoints, are the points along these meridians where energy flow can be measured and manipulated.

See "Energy Medicine," pp. 192-204.

Although orthodox oncologists have trouble accepting the existence of energy meridians, the effectiveness of acupuncture treatment itself is now beyond dispute, particularly in the realm of pain relief for

At the forefront of new alternative clinical approaches to cancer is recognition of the role of energy, both as a means of diagnosis and treatment. Acting at an even deeper cellular level than biochemicals, energy can make or break health.

cancer patients. In a study of 183 cancer patients attending a London clinic and receiving acupuncture, 82% of the patients reported experiencing pain relief in the early stages and 52% reported benefits in the later stages.[1] Another study found that cancer patients treated with acupuncture showed a significant elevation in their natural killer cell activity, an integral part of the body's anticancer defenses.[2]

Electrodermal Screening (EDS)

Imagine that you are sitting in a doctor's office. The doctor takes a small, handheld probe connected to a meter and, with no further questions, gently presses certain points on your hands or feet while noting the figures displayed on the meter. From this, she can tell you which parts of your body are functioning correctly and which organs are causing problems. Next, she places small glass vials containing colorless liquids into a container, which is also connected to the device. The doctor then remeasures some of the points on your hands. On this basis, the doctor can tell you, in lucid terms, why you are not feeling well or whether you are likely to have a problem in the near future. By way of remedy, the physician gives you a few drops of a tasteless medicine (usually a homeopathic remedy) and, before long, you begin to feel better. This description is not a futuristic fantasy. It is a factual narrative of what practitioners of energy medicine using electrodermal screening are presently doing in medical clinics in the U.S., Europe, and Asia.

Since the 1940s, research has established that acupuncture points possess electrical conductivity. Earlier, German doctors, led by Reinhold Voll, M.D., measured changes in electrical conductivity at the body's acupuncture points and discovered that the electrical resistance of the skin decreases at the acupoints compared to the surrounding skin, meaning the electrical current is conducted more efficiently at these points. They also found that each point appeared to have a standard measurement for anyone who is in good health, but this measurement changes when health deteriorates. For this reason, EDS researcher William A. Tiller, Ph.D., of Stanford University in Palo Alto, California, calls the conductance points "information-access windows." Comparing values before and after treatment provides useful information about a patient's condition.

In the original research, Dr. Voll measured the body's energy using skin resistance: he measured changes in electrical conductivity at each of the body's acupoints. Skin conductance can indicate or register physiological changes in the body. According to James Hoyt Clark of Orem, Utah, an EDS inventor and educator, "Research has shown that skin generally has a resistance of about 2-4 million ohms, but at the conductance points, the resistance is 100,000 ohms in a healthy, balanced person. These points correspond to the acupuncture points."[3]

The impetus for Dr. Voll's research was an attempt to reverse his own bladder cancer; he integrated this new research with his own medical training in acupuncture and came up with EAV point testing (Electro-Acupuncture according to Voll).[4] Specifically, Dr. Voll established a scale of 0 to 100, with 45-55 being "normal" or "balanced." Readings above 55 indicate an inflammation of the organ associated with the meridian, while readings below 45-50 suggest organ stagnation and degeneration.[5]

The key idea is that an energetic event transfers its signal through a meridian to the nervous system, with the end result being a cellular pathology. "Every inflammatory alteration of a cell starts with an increased energy production," says Clark. He adds that EDS is a "data acquisition process" in which the trained practitioner conducts an "interview" with the patient's organs and tissues, gathering information about their basic functional status and their energy pathways. As such, EDS is an investigational, not diagnostic, device because it requires the physician's knowledge of acupuncture, physiology, and therapeutic substances to interpret the energy

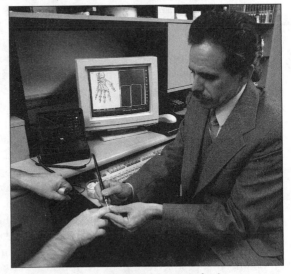

James H. Clark, the "Father of Computerized Electrodermal Screening (CEDS)" technology, takes a reading using the portable LISTEN System.

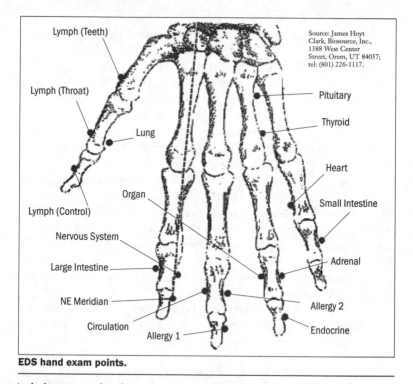

Source: James Hoyt Clark, Biosource, Inc., 1388 West Center Street, Orem, UT 84057; tel: (801) 226-1117.

Lymph (Teeth)

Lymph (Throat)

Lung

Lymph (Control)

Organ

Nervous System

Large Intestine

NE Meridian

Circulation

Allergy 1

Pituitary

Thyroid

Heart

Small Intestine

Adrenal

Allergy 2

Endocrine

EDS hand exam points.

imbalances and select the most appropriate therapeutic response. Another way of explaining it, says Clark, is that EDS "like a thermometer, measures energy. The thermometer measures heat while the typical electrodermal screening device measures electric flow. In either case, if the optimal reading is not measured, an energy imbalance has been detected."

Of even keen interest to EDS operators is a phenomenon called the Indicator Drop (ID). Soon after the initial reading is registered, the value may suddenly drop off; this is interpreted as an imbalance while a reading that does not include an ID is a sign of energy balance. "When an ID is present, it is considered the most important part of the reading," explains EDS researcher Julia J. Tsuei, Ph.D., founder of the Foundation for East-West Medicine in Taipei, Taiwan. The EDS operator can use the ID to determine the nature and cause of an imbalance, Dr. Tsuei explains. Various substances can then be tested against the points that produced an ID. The physician's task is to find a single substance or combination of substances that will balance the point. Researchers at the University of California at Los Angeles and the University of Southern California demonstrated an 87% correlation between an electrodermal screening diagnosis of lung cancer and a standard X-ray diagnosis.[6]

According to Douglas Lieber, L.Ac., director of Computronix Electro-Medical Systems in Argyle, Texas, Dr. Voll identified approximately 1,050 electrodermal screening points during his 35 years of research. Lieber reports that he has identified more than 400 additional points that are valuable EDS testing nodes. Since 1983, Lieber has performed EDS testing on thousands of individuals with cancer. He finds that there are seven basic underlying contributors to the development and perpetuation of cancer.

According to Lieber, these are: 1) geopathic stress; 2) parasites present in the body; 3) a degenerative toxic focus, most commonly from chronic dental infections in the jaw where teeth have been extracted or root canals have been installed, but sometimes also in the tonsils, fallopian tubes, appendix, gallbladder, liver, or pancreas; 4) unresolved emotional trauma, often involving subconscious issues from childhood; 5) miasmic (SEE QUICK DEFINITION) influences passed from parent to child for several generations, usually the *Tubercular* miasm (as in lung cancer) and the *Syphilitic* miasm in other cancers; 6) radiation and/or electromagnetic exposure; and 7) chemical toxins, especially nickel, cadmium, mercury, aflatoxins (from molds and fungi), pesticides, benzene, toluene, xylene, formaldehyde, isopropyl alcohol, and autotoxins (produced mostly from toxic intestines). In conducting follow-up EDS research on cancer patients who have identified and removed these cancer-contributing factors, Lieber has usually found dramatic improvement in the general condition of the patients, according to subsequent medical history, conventional tests, and EDS indicators.

For information about the **LISTEN System and EDS seminars**, contact: Biosource, Inc., 1388 West Center Street, Orem, UT 84057; tel: 801-226-1117. For the **Omega Acubase system**, contact: Digital Health, Inc., 1770 East Fort Union Blvd., No. 101, Salt Lake City, UT 84121; tel: 801-944-4070; fax: 801-944-4067. For **Computronix and Acupro**, contact: Douglas Lieber, L.Ac., Computronix Electro-Medical Systems, 145 Canyon Oaks Drive, Argyle, TX 76226; tel: 817-241-2768; fax: 817-455-2605.

QUICK DEFINITION

A homeopathic **miasm**, as originally described by Samuel Hahnemann, the 19th-century German founder of homeopathy, is a subtle taint or energy residue of previous illness, even across the generations. As an inherited predisposition for chronic disease that is far more subtle than anything genetic, miasms are broad-focused, predisposing individuals and families to specific illnesses, such as tuberculosis or cancer. According to Hahnemann, three miasms underlie all chronic illness and parallel broad stages in the history of human experience with primary disease states. They are the *Psoric* miasm, the *Syphilitic* miasm (deriving from syphilis), and the *Sycotic* miasm (arising as a residue of gonorrhea). Some homeopaths add a fourth *Cancer* miasm, and a fifth *Petroleum* miasm.

Success Story: Electrodermal Screening Identifies a Hidden Dental Problem

Judy, 58, consulted with Anthony J. Scott-Morley, H.M.D. (honorary), Ph.D., D.Sc., of Dorset, England, regarding small tumors on her right breast. At the time of her initial visit, Judy did not know if the tumors were malignant. Instead of taking a biopsy of the breast tissue, which could perhaps spread any existing cancer cells in the region, he performed an EDS analysis.

During the course of Dr. Scott-Morley's EDS assessment, a chronic dental focus became evident. This means that, somewhere in Judy's teeth or jaw, a source of untreated infection was disturbing the energy and thus the structure and function of the body, in this case, Judy's breast. EDS practitioners call this a "focal point" of toxicity; specifically in Judy's case, it was detected in the lower right second premolar. Troubles in this tooth "focused" toxicity and imbalanced energy through the acupuncture meridians to her breast. EDS indicated that the cause of this toxic focus was a mercury amalgam filling. At this point, Judy became irritated and told Dr. Scott-Morley that she felt this was wasting her time and money. "I do not have any teeth of my own. I am wearing full dentures, so there cannot be any filling material in my teeth."

This was potentially confusing, even for an EDS expert such as Dr. Scott-Morley. He had never physically looked inside her mouth. He rechecked the EDS results and again concluded that it was amalgam toxicity. At this point, he suggested to Judy that she receive a dental X ray of the tooth socket. He trusted in the outcome so much that he told her he would pay for it if nothing was found. She remained skeptical but agreed to see a dentist.

For more on **dental factors**, see Chapter 2: Cancer and Its Causes, pp. 48-93; Chapter 9: Physical Support Therapies, pp. 254-297.

For information about **electrodermal screening, energy medicine, and devices**, contact: America Association of Acupuncture and Bio-Energetic Medicine, 2512 Manoa Road, Honolulu, HI 96822; tel: 808-946-2069; fax: 808-946-0378.

After chastising Judy for seeing an alternative physician, the dentist agreed to take the X ray if only to confirm what he deemed to be nonsense. But when the X ray was processed, he apologized to Dr. Scott-Morley and congratulated him on the diagnosis. "There was a large amalgam fragment embedded in the socket, which he thought must have fallen into the socket when the tooth was extracted," says Dr. Scott-Morley. "He estimated that this had been there for at least ten years."

Arrangements were made to have the amalgam fragment carefully removed and Dr. Scott-Morley prescribed appropriate homeopathic medicines to desensitize Judy against the amalgam and also to support her immune system. "Within ten weeks of taking these steps, all breast nodules had disappeared and no further treatment was necessary," Dr. Scott-Morley reports.

Other Energy Medicine–Based Devices

TENS—The Transcutaneous Electrical Nerve Stimulator, or TENS, is widely used for pain relief in doctors' offices and physiotherapy clinics, and can be used at home as well. It works by applying an electrical current to the affected nerves, causing nerve conduction to be blocked and pain to be relieved. TENS units are also believed to stimulate the production of endorphins (a type of brain chemical or neurotransmitter), the body's natural painkillers. Many physicians have found TENS useful in pain reduction for cancer patients, who typically respond positively after 2-3 TENS treatments; a considerable reduction in pain and discomfort is often reported within two weeks of regular TENS use.

Cold Laser Therapy—According to Marvin Prescott, D.M.D., of Los Angeles, California, cold laser therapy uses a beam of low-intensity laser light to initiate a series of enzymatic reactions and bioelectric events that stimulate the natural healing process at the cellular level. "Cold laser therapy has been successfully applied to pain control, orthopedic myofascial syndrome (inflammation of the muscles and their surrounding membranes), neurology, trauma, dermatology, and dentistry," says Dr. Prescott. "The effects on microcirculation, increased synthesis of collagen in the skin, production of neurotransmitters, and pain relief have all been documented."

Cell Com System—Hugo Nielsen, a Danish acupuncturist, spent 25 years investigating alternative treatments for cancer. On the basis of his research, he devised a cell energy system that enhances communication among the cells. It is a form of cellular biofeedback called the Cell Com System.

Nielsen's Cell Com System uses a small instrument run by a 9-volt battery to measure the energies represented on the surface of the skin at a given time; the amount of energy detected is transferred to the instrument, where it is displayed digitally. The instrument uses electrodes that are connected to acupuncture points on the skin enabling the physician to locate the exact position of these points on the body. Once the information is recorded by the instrument, it is altered and fed back to the brain. The brain then reads the altered signals, and controls and maintains the resulting pain-free situation.

Following operations for lung, kidney, and other cancers, patients visiting the Hugo Nielsen Institute in Gram, Denmark, have reported significant pain relief from Cell Com. "Nielsen believes that the electrical status of each cell's sodium/potassium balance controls overall health and enables the body to regulate its production of natural painkillers, such as the endorphins," says Etienne Callebout, M.D. Moreover, the benefits may extend beyond pain relief to

For information about the **Cell Com System**, contact: Hugo Nielsen, Kirkealle 14, 6510 Gram, Denmark; tel: 45-74-822233; fax: 45-74-822065.

include direct therapeutic effects: when used in conjunction with conventional acupuncture treatment, a regression in lung cancer has been achieved. Since the potential toxicity of pain-killing drugs or medications is avoided, the individual's cancer-fighting resources can be more readily strengthened.

Magnetic Field Therapy

Electromagnetic energy is an integral part of the human body. It can help produce illness and help bring healing, depending on its type and strength. The world is surrounded by magnetic fields: some are generated by the Earth's magnetism, others by solar storms and changes in the weather. Magnetic fields are also created by everyday electrical devices: motors, televisions, office equipment, computers, electrically heated water beds, electric blankets, microwave ovens, the electrical wiring in homes, and the power lines that supply them.

Recently, scientists have discovered that external magnetic fields can affect the body's functioning in both positive and negative ways, and this observation has led to the development of magnetic field therapy. The use of magnets and electrical devices to generate controlled magnetic fields has many medical applications and has proven to be one of the most effective means available for diagnosing human illness.

Magnets and electromagnetic therapy devices are now being used to relieve symptoms and reverse degenerative diseases, eliminate pain, facilitate the healing of broken bones, counter the effects of stress, and address the reversal of cancer. In 1974, researcher Albert Roy Davis noted that positive and negative magnetic energies have different effects upon the biological systems of animals and humans. Davis concluded that negative magnetic fields have a beneficial effect, whereas positive magnetic fields have a stressful effect. He found that magnets could be used to arrest and kill cancer cells in animals and could also be used in the treatment of arthritis, glaucoma, infertility, and diseases related to aging.[7]

Magnetic Field Therapy:
Changing Energy at the Cellular Level
"The healing potential of magnets is possible because the body's nervous system is governed, in part, by varying patterns of ionic currents and electromagnetic fields," reports John Zimmerman, Ph.D., president of the Bio-Electro-Magnetics Institute in Reno, Nevada. There are numerous forms of magnetic field therapy, including static field magnets and pulsating magnetic fields generated by electrical devices,

which are able to penetrate the human body and therapeutically affect the functioning of the nervous system, organs, and cells.

According to William Philpott, M.D., a magnetic therapy pioneer of Choctaw, Oklahoma, when used properly, magnetic field therapy has no known harmful side effects. Dr. Philpott has found that the negative magnetic field can even reverse cancer. "Whether it is a cut, bruise, broken bone, infection, or cancer, it is the negative magnetic energy that heals," Dr. Philpott states. He also points out that magnetic energy is capable of countering the toxic effects of poisonous chemicals, addictive drugs, and other potentially harmful substances.

CAUTION

Magnetic therapy should be administered only under the close supervision of a trained physician. Only the negative magnetic field should contact the subject's skin.

The therapy is based on the fact that the body is surrounded by a magnetic field and is composed of numerous smaller magnetic fields, which become disturbed in the course of illness. When positive magnetic energy is stronger than the negative magnetic energy in a living organism, the system has a tendency to develop acidity, lack of cellular oxygen, accumulation of toxins, increased microbial growth, and the uncontrolled cell division that leads to cancer.[8] Clinical research indicates that magnetic therapy can restore the body's healthy magnetic fields and thereby promote recovery from cancer, says Dr. Philpott. "The body, through the cells that surround the nervous system, concentrates the negative electromagnetic field at the site of injury for healing," says Dr. Philpott.

The key to how magnetic fields can help in reversing cancer has to do with its effect on oxygen, says Dr. Philpott. Magnetic fields can stimulate metabolism and increase the amount of oxygen available to cells. "Oxygen deficiency coupled with acidity are unique characteristics of all cancer cells and are the two main causes of cancer. From the standpoint of the physics and chemistry of life, the difference between normal cells and cancer cells is so great that one can hardly picture a greater contrast." The more alkaline pH (SEE QUICK DEFINITION) produced by a negative magnetic field is necessary for healing, as cancer cannot grow in an alkaline environment, Dr. Philpott explains. "It is the negative field that maintains the alkaline state. You can take an external magnetic field, place it over the body area, and get a bodily response as if the energy came from itself."

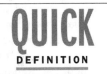

QUICK

DEFINITION

The term **pH**, which means "potential hydrogen," represents a scale for the relative acidity or alkalinity of a solution. Acidity is measured as 0.1 to 6.9, alkalinity is 7.1 to 14, and neutral is about 7.0. The numbers refer to how many hydrogen atoms are present compared to an ideal or standard solution. Normal blood is slightly alkaline, at 7.35 to 7.45; urine pH can range from 4.8 to 7.5, although normal is closer to 7.0.

A Quick Review of Magnet Basics

Magnets have two poles, positive and negative. There are conflicting methods of naming the pole of a magnet, so a magnetometer should be used to determine which side of the magnet is negative (north) or positive (south). If you're using a compass to locate the poles, the arrowhead of the needle marked "N" or "North" will point to the magnet's negative pole. A magnetometer reads magnetic poles as negative and positive, which is the electromagnetic definition and identification of magnetic polarity.

Many researchers claim that the negative pole generally has a calming effect and helps to normalize metabolic functioning. The positive pole, on the other hand, has a stressful effect—prolonged exposure interferes with metabolic functioning, produces acidity, reduces cellular oxygen, and encourages the replication of microorganisms.

The strength of a magnet is measured in units of gauss (a measurement of the intensity of magnetic flux) or Tesla (1 Tesla=10,000 gauss), and every magnet or magnetic device carries a manufacturer's gauss rating. The actual strength of the magnet at the skin surface, however, is less than this number. For example, a 4,000-gauss magnet transmits only about 1,200 gauss to the patient. Magnets placed in bed pads will render even lower amounts of field strength, because a magnet's strength decreases with the distance from the subject.

According to Dr. Philpott, cancer only develops in acid-hypoxia cellular tissue. This refers to a cellular condition of acidity and low oxygen status. Numerous precipitating factors, such as carcinogens, excess free radicals, maladaptive reactions to foods, geopathic stress, and aberrant electromagnetic energy, can produce acid-hypoxia. The conversion of normal cells to cancerous cells is the next step.

A normal cell is alkaline, he explains, because otherwise oxygen could not be available for the cell to make its energy. A key chemical called adenosine triphosphate (ATP) is made by cells as a biological energy source through the use of oxygen; it is central to the way energy is released and transported. This process is called oxidative phosphorylation. Normal, healthy human cells use oxygen to produce ATP as an energy source. Infectious microorganisms (bacteria, fungi, and some parasites) and cancer cells have a different way of producing energy; it is called fermentative phosphorylation. Here, under conditions of acidity and low or no oxygen, ATP is made through the fermentation of glucose (blood sugar) instead of oxygen. "In fact, if there were a lot of oxygen present, it would not work. Oxygen and the alkaline pH would inhibit this fermentation process," explains Dr. Philpott.

These two mechanisms of making energy are incompatible and thus are never working at the same time. In fact, oxidative phosphorylation actually blocks the fermentative. "The human energy system is able to defeat the energy system of cancer cells," he says. "This is because our oxidative method is ten times more efficient than the fermentation method used by cancer cells." The normal human cell (running on oxidative phosphorylation) has a lot of molecular oxygen and a normal alkaline pH, but the cancer cell (running on fermentation phosphorylation) has an acid pH and lack of oxygen.

"The way we can defeat cancer," says Dr. Philpott, "is to change the cellular conditions so that cancer cannot exist under them. To do this, raise the alkalinity and oxygen level of the cells with a negative magnetic field." Cancer cells cannot thrive in an area dominated by negative magnetic fields. The same principle also makes this approach an ideal preventive measure. "An effective method of preventing cancer is through the daily application of negative magnetic energy to the body."

Dr. Philpott relates the following cases from his clinical files to demonstrate how magnetic therapy works in treating cancer:

■ Melanoma: Roberta, 75, suddenly developed a rapidly growing invasive melanoma on her forehead. "This had the clinical appearance of a serious malignant melanoma," Dr. Philpott says. However, after three months of continuous treatment with a negative magnetic field, the melanoma dried up and peeled off and new skin appeared. Following three more weeks of negative magnetic field exposure, the depressed area in Roberta's forehead (where the melanoma had been situated) filled in, leaving no evidence of a scar. "There is now no way to tell where the tumor was," Dr. Philpott notes.

■ Prostate Cancer: After Thomas was diagnosed as having prostate cancer with bone metastasis, he underwent magnetic treatment. "He was treated continuously over the sacral and lower abdominal areas, so that the magnetic energy would radiate into the pelvic area," Dr. Philpott says. Three months later, there was no evidence of bone cancer on Thomas' X ray and his prostate specific antigen (PSA, a marker for prostate cancer) had reverted from an abnormal 28 to a normal level of 2.

■ Spinal Cancer: After Patricia had a benign tumor removed from her spine, she could not walk without dragging her feet. When Dr. Philpott placed a positive magnetic pole over the area where the tumor had been removed, Patricia could walk perfectly. Practicing walking while the positive magnetic field was being applied to her spine restored her ability to walk. These practice sessions were three minutes each, followed by application of the negative magnetic field. The positive field stimulated the nonfunctioning neurons while the negative field restored oxygen and alkalinity to the tissues after each use of the positive field.

■ In addition, magnetic field therapy can reduce the side effects of chemotherapy. Mark had been treated with chemotherapy for his cancer prior to seeing Dr. Philpott. Two years later, as the cancer was still present, Mark's oncologist advised a second course of chemotherapy. During his first chemotherapy treatment, Mark had lost his hair, fingernails, and toenails; during the second course, he did not lose them. The oncologist asked Mark what he had done differently this time. Mark told him he was sleeping on a negative-poled magnetic bed pad. "It may be that the entrance of magnetic therapy into oncology will be furthered by this example, in which a patient's exposure to a negative magnetic field reduced the harsh side effects of chemotherapy," says Dr. Philpott.

Guidelines for Treating Cancers with Magnetic Therapy

Dr. Philpott states, "I do not claim a cure for any degenerative disease or even guarantee relief of pain or insomnia by means of magnetics. My only claim is that there is evidence justifying a definitive controlled research project following FDA guidelines to determine the value and limitations of magnetic therapy." The application of magnetic fields to humans has been approved by the FDA and, based on toxicity studies, classified as "not essentially harmful." Magnetic therapy for cancer must still be considered an experimental approach warranting controlled studies, Dr. Philpott advises. The clinical guidelines that follow are based on protocols that produced recoveries from cancer in patients treated by Dr. Philpott.

Prostate Cancer—Always use a negative magnetic field, negative pole side facing the body. For local treatment, sit on a chair pad (containing 1⅞" x ⅞" x ⅜" magnets placed 1½" apart throughout the seat and back of the pad) with a 4" x 6" x ½" ceramic magnet (3,950 gauss) under the pad directly beneath the genital-rectal area. The more hours of treatment, the better.

For systemic treatment, use a magnetic bed pad (containing 1⅞" x ⅞" x ⅜" magnets, 3,950 gauss, placed ½" apart throughout the pad). Place a 5" x 12" multi-magnet (2,450 gauss) flexible mat crosswise on the lower abdomen–pubic area. In the center of this, place a 4" x 6" x ½" ceramic magnet lengthwise. This can be held in place with a body band. Also use four magnets (6" x 4" x 1", 5,000 gauss) at the crown of the head, placed ¾" apart in a wooden carrier on the headboard. The

Success Story: Brain Tumor Treated with Magnetic Energy

Here is a case from Michael B. Schachter, M.D., of the Schachter Center for Complementary Medicine, in Suffern, New York, where magnetic therapy is used as part of a multimodal cancer treatment program.

At 31, Rafael's left cheek began to tingle. Soon after, he lost his ability to talk and his left arm moved uncontrollably. This episode lasted for about a minute. EEG and a CT scan of the brain were both negative. Doctors informed Rafael that the episode was probably migraine related. Five months later, he had a similar episode except, this time, he lost consciousness. It was now clear that Rafael was experiencing seizures. An MRI showed a tumor on the right side of his brain, which a biopsy revealed to be malignant.

The expected survival for individuals with malignancies of the brain is from six to 18 months. Due to its location, the tumor was considered inoperable. A cancer specialist offered Rafael immediate radiation therapy or the option of waiting until he became more symptomatic before undergoing radiation. Rafael decided to wait because of the risks associated with radiation to the brain, which include stroke and radiation-induced tumors. Instead, he sought alternative cancer therapy with Dr. Schachter. His neurologists and his sister, who was a nurse, thought this decision was a mistake.

After conducting a comprehensive laboratory evaluation to measure immune system function and check for vitamin and mineral deficiencies, hormonal imbalances, and toxic metabolite exposure, Dr. Schachter started Rafael on intravenous vitamin C and amygdalin, intravenous hydrogen peroxide on different days, and a host of oral agents including shark cartilage, amygdalin, antioxidant and immune-enhancing vitamins, minerals, and natural herbs.

Magnetic energy therapy was also incorporated into the treatment protocol throughout this time period. Here, a small, but powerful magnet (more than 12,000 gauss) was placed on Rafael's head, the negative pole against the skin, over the area of the tumor and kept in place with a headband for several hours each day. The only conventional treatment Rafael continued was anti-seizure medication to treat the epileptic episodes that accompanied the tumor.

Over 4½ years later, Rafael is doing well. He has a new baby and has worked almost continuously during this period. Repeated MRIs have revealed no further growth in the tumor. Rafael's sister and neurologists were so impressed by the results of the alternative treatment that they wrote letters on his behalf to keep his insurance company from ending compensation for these therapies. Rafael has survived well beyond the expected six to 18 months and looks forward to many more years with his family.

holder can be raised or lowered depending on the height of the pillow. The magnets should be slightly lower than the back of the head and no closer than three inches to the top of the head.

Squamous Cell Carcinoma of the Lips and Mouth–Always use a negative magnetic field, negative pole side facing the body. Place a 5" x 6" multi-magnet (2,450 gauss) flexible mat across the mouth to cover the lips, chin, and the area between the upper lip and the nose. Place a 4" x 6" x ½" ceramic magnet (3,950 gauss) on each side of the face, extending sufficiently forward for the magnetic field to cover the nose. This local treatment is a necessity and should be kept in place continuously, except for the brief periods of washing or eating. The minimum duration is three months. Systemic treatment is optional (see Prostate Cancer, above).

Malignant Melanoma–Always use a negative magnetic field, negative pole side facing the body. Tape a cushion (with a hole in the middle, as those used for bunions) over the malignant mole to prevent pressure on it; use hypoallergenic tape. Tape a 1" x ¼" superneodymium disc magnet (12,300 gauss) on the cushion. The magnet needs to be larger than the lesion being treated. For systemic treatment, see Prostate Cancer above. In addition, sleep with magnets on the front and back of the chest. Use a 5" x 12" x ⅛" multi-magnet (2,450 gauss) flexible mat held in place with a body wrap supported by shoulder straps. This accomplishes negative magnetic poling of the oxygen in the lungs, which then circulates throughout the body and prevents metastatic spread. During waking hours, wear a 5" x 6" multi-magnet (2,450 gauss) flexible mat over the heart with the negative pole facing the heart. Eliminating a malignant melanoma may take three to four months of these treatments.

For more on **electro-magnetic energy**, see Chapter 2: Cancer and Its Causes, pp. 48-93.

See "Magnetic Therapy," pp. 330-338.

For more about **magnetic therapy**, contact: William H. Philpott, M.D., 17171 SE 29th Street, Choctaw, OK 73020; tel: 405-390-3009.

Magnetic Therapy for Pain Relief

Pain is the body's signal of injury, which registers both locally and in the brain as a positive magnetic field. Therefore, the solution for pain is to provide a negative magnetic field both at the site of pain and to the brain.

Place a magnet of suitable size over the pain site, negative pole side facing the body. The magnetic field must be larger than the site. Pain is frequently relieved in 10-15 minutes, only occasionally taking up to 30 minutes. However, the longer the period of exposure the better, since the negative magnetic field also governs the healing process. Some common magnets used are: the 1½" x ⅜" ceramic disc magnet (3,950 gauss); 1" x ¼" neodymium magnet (12,300 gauss); 4" x 6" x ½" ceramic magnet (3,950 gauss), often used for treatment of body organs; and flexible plastiform magnets (2,450 gauss) in 2"-4" widths and as long as needed.

Science Demonstrates the Power of Magnetic Therapy

The French Academy of Sciences published a report in March, 1965 on the magnetic treatment of mice with lymphosarcoma. Every mouse in the untreated or control group died within 15 to 18 days. In three other groups, mice began magnetic treatment at different points in time, but with the same strength and duration of magnetic treatment: 620 gauss for two hours a day.

The first group received magnetic treatment within five days of starting the test and recovered quickly; all tumors and metastases disappeared. The second group began treatment on day seven and showed the same recovery as the first group; a third group of mice was treated from the tenth day on, but did not recover. These mice all died in 19 to 22 days, just after the untreated mice had died.[9]

These findings were compelling enough to encourage the French Academy of Sciences to conduct another experiment, this time testing the effect of the daily dosage given. In the first group, the mice were treated from the fifth day, with 620 gauss one hour a day; in the second group, the mice were treated with 620 gauss two hours a day, also from the fifth day. Once again, the results were striking. As expected, all the mice in the untreated (control) group died within 15 days; all the mice in the first test group died after 19 days. Meanwhile, the mice in the second test group—they received twice the magnetic treatment per day as the first group—all survived and showed no signs of cancer.[10]

To treat the brain, place 1½" x ⅜" ceramic disc magnets on each temple along with a 5" x 6" x ⅛" multi-magnet flexible mat, both held in place by an adjustable elastic headband. This is valuable in treating brain lesions or increasing depth of sleep. Systemic treatment when sleeping (see Prostate Cancer, above) is particularly helpful for people with generalized body pain.

Light Therapy

Many health disorders can be traced to problems with the daily night-and-day rhythms called circadian. These rhythms are the body's inner clock and govern the timing of sleep, hormone production, body temperature, and many key biological functions. Disturbances in circadian rhythm can lead to health problems such as depression and sleep disorders. Natural sunlight and various forms of light therapy can help reestablish the body's natural rhythms. The ability of light to activate certain chemicals has become the basis of treatment for certain forms of cancer.

Here is how light can be therapeutic. When light enters the eye, millions of light- and color-sensitive cells called photoreceptors convert it into electrical impulses. These impulses travel along the optic nerve to the brain, where they trigger the hypothalamus gland to send chemical messengers (neurotransmitters) to regulate the autonomic functions of the body. The hypothalamus is part of the endocrine system, whose secretions govern most bodily functions, including blood pressure, body temperature, breathing, digestion, sexual function, moods, and the immune system. Full-spectrum light (containing all wavelengths) sparks the delicate impulses that regulate these functions and maintain health.

Poor light poses a serious threat to health, according to the numerous published studies of photobiologist John Nash Ott, D.Sc.[11] He contends that the kind of light adequate for maintaining health must contain the full wavelength spectrum found in natural sunlight. In contrast, most artificial lighting, both incandescent and fluorescent, lacks the complete balanced spectrum of sunlight and, as Dr. Ott discovered, interferes with the body's optimal absorption of certain nutrients. He calls this condition "malillumination"—malnutrition of the nutrient called light.

Many products we commonly rely on in daily life—windows, windshields, eyeglasses, suntan lotions—filter out parts of the light spectrum (as does smog) and contribute to malillumination. Research reveals that if certain wavelengths are absent in light, the body cannot fully absorb all dietary nutrients.[12] Malilllumination contributes to fatigue, depression, hostility, suppressed immune function, strokes, skin damage, and cancer.[13]

According to John Downing O.D., Ph.D., of Santa Rosa, California, "By spending 90% of our lives indoors, under inadequate lighting conditions, we cause or worsen a wide range of health problems, including depression, heart disease, hyperactivity, osteoporosis, and lowered resistance to infection."[14] To maintain health, it is important to be exposed to light containing the full wavelength spectrum found in natural sunlight, says Dr. Downing. While many people associate an overexposure to sunlight with melanoma or other skin cancers, the research of Drs. Downing, Ott, and others suggests that an underexposure to sunlight may also be involved in producing cancer.

See "Light Therapy," pp. 319-329.

Full-Spectrum Light Therapy

A ten-year epidemiological study conducted at Johns Hopkins University Medical School in Baltimore, Maryland, showed that exposure to full-spectrum light is positively related to the prevention of breast, colon, and rectal cancers.[15] In Russia, a full-spectrum lighting system was installed in factories where colds and sore throats had become commonplace among workers. This system lowered the bacterial contamination of the air by 40% to 70%. Workers who did not receive the full-spectrum light were absent twice as many days as those who did, strongly suggesting that the lights performed a health-protective role.[16] In a recent study undertaken by Dr. Ott and his associates, full-spectrum lighting was tested on first-grade students in Sarasota, Florida. Using four classrooms, two as a control with standard fluorescent lighting and two outfitted with full-spectrum lights, the researchers tracked the students' behavior for a full semester. Their results demonstrated that the students exposed to the full-spectrum lighting had less absenteeism and a higher academic achievement record when compared with classes conducted under ordinary fluorescent lighting.[17]

Ultraviolet Light Therapy

Nobel Prize winner and Danish physician Niels Finsen, M.D., observed that tubercular lesions occurred commonly during the winter but only rarely in the summer. Dr. Finsen suspected a lack of sunlight to be the cause of the lesions and successfully treated skin tuberculosis with ultraviolet light. Today, ultraviolet light therapies are used to treat diseases ranging from high cholesterol to premenstrual syndrome to cancer. Hemo-irradiation or photophoresis involves the removal of up to a pint of a patient's blood from the body, irradiating it with ultraviolet light, and reinfusing it back into the patient's circulation. William Campbell Douglass, M.D., of Clayton, Georgia, a practitioner of photophoresis, reports that irradiating blood with ultraviolet light produces the following results: calcium metabolism improves, body toxins become inert, bacteria are killed either directly or indirectly (by increased systemic resistance), biochemical balances are restored, and oxygen absorption is increased. He has successfully used ultraviolet light therapy to treat asthma and various immune-related disorders.[18]

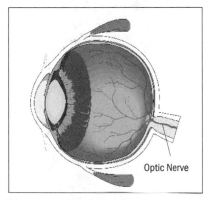

Optic Nerve

The eye and the optic nerve.

Photodynamic Therapy for Cancer

Photodynamic therapy (PDT) has been demonstrated effective as a cure for cancers of the lung, esophagus, stomach, and cervix,[19] resulting in complete remission in 90% of patients.[20] Denis Cortese, M.D., of Jacksonville, Florida, found that 43% of early-stage lung cancer patients treated with PDT stayed disease free for at least five years.[21]

In PDT, dyes or medications that absorb light are absorbed by tumors then exposed to specific types of light. "Light photons are absorbed by the pigment of the dye, which becomes chemically reactive and causes the cancer cells to die," says Meyrick Peak, Ph.D., a senior scientist at the Center of Mechanistic Biology and Biotechnology at Argonne National Laboratory in Argonne, Illinois. "This therapy has been used in China for over 20 years and has been successful in eliminating some types of tumors."

With the use of anti-malignin antibody screen (AMAS) and other early detection strategies, PDT could become a powerful form of medicine. Particularly with respect to lung cancer, the combination of aggressive AMAS screening and PDT could reduce mortality in one of the nation's top killers.

Nicholas J. Lowe, M.D., Clinical Professor of Dermatology at the UCLA School of Medicine in Los Angeles and director of the Skin Research Foundation of California, concurs with Dr. Peak: "Photodynamic therapy is currently being tested on basal and squamous cell cancer (skin cancers). However, the concern with some of these treatments is unwanted phototoxicity—some treatments are likely to make the patient sensitive to sunlight."

Warren Grundfest, M.D., of Cedars-Sinai Medical Center in Los Angeles, is using a type of photodynamic therapy called light-activated chemotherapy to treat patients with lung and bladder cancer. "We're using light to cause a chemical change in the drug. Because it is located only (or predominantly) in the cancer tissue, it causes only the cancer cells to die." Dr. Grundfest reports that, after 18 months of treatment, bladder tumors showed an 85% successful response.

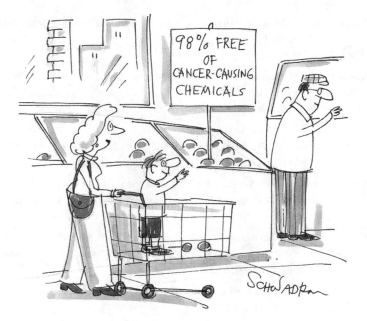

98% FREE
OF
CANCER-CAUSING
CHEMICALS

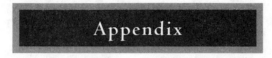

Appendix

RESOURCES FOR CANCER PATIENTS

Selected Alternative Medicine Physicians and Clinics

*For additional information on cancer clinics,
visit our website at www.alternativemedicine.com and follow the Clinics link.*

Advanced Medical Group, 5862 Cromo Drive, Suite 100, El Paso, TX 79912; tel: 800-621-8924 or 915-581-2273.

American Biologics, Azucena #15 La Mesa, T.J., B.C., Mexico; fax: 52-66-816435; for mailing: AB-Mexico, 1180 Walnut Avenue, Chula Vista, CA 91911; tel: 800-227-4458 or 619-429-8200; fax: 619-429-8004.

American Asian Medical Institute S.A. de C.V., 970 Broadway, Suite 103, Chula Vista, CA 91911; tel: 800-381-5888 or 619-585-2988; fax: 619-585-2980. Address in Mexico: Paseo Playas # 400, Playas De Tijuana, Mexico; tel; 011-526-630-0700; fax: 011-526-630-0319.

Robert C. Atkins, M.D., The Atkins Center, 152 East 55th Street, New York, NY 10022; tel: 212-758-2110; fax: 212-754-4284.

Biomedics Institute, Medi Systems, S.A. de C.V., Av. General Ferreira, No. 2250 Col. Juarez, C.P. 22150, Tijuana, B.C., Mexico; tel: 888-626-8067 or 011-526-684-8154; fax: 011-526-684-8159.

The BioPulse Rejuvenation Center is located in Tijuana, Mexico. For more information, call 888-552-2855 (from U.S.), 801-233-9094 (outside U.S.), or 011-526-686-1880 (international direct); fax: 801-233-9089.

Keith I. Block, M.D., Block Medical Center, 1800 Sherman Avenue, Suite 515, Evanston, IL 60201; tel: 847-492-3040; fax: 847-492-3045.

Burzynski Research Institute, Inc., 9432 Old Katy Road, Suite 200, Houston, TX 77055; tel: 713-335-5697; fax: 713-935-0649.

Etienne Callebout, M.D., 10 Harley Street, London, England W1N1AA; tel: 44-171-467-8300; fax: 44-171-467-8312 or 44-158-276-9832.

Center for Cell Specific Cancer Therapy, Avenida Palacio de los Deportes 121, Esq. G. Mejia Ricart, El Millon Santo Domingo, DN, Dominican Republic; tel: 877-741-2728 or 809-534-2090; fax: 809-534-3089.

Ernesto R. Contreras, M.D., Oasis Hospital, Organizacion Avanzada en Sistemas Integrales Para la Salud, S.C., Paseo Playas de Tijuana No. 19, Apartado Postal No. 179, Playas de Tijuana, B.C. 22700 Mexico; tel: 5266-80-18-50; fax: 5266-80-18-55. U.S. address: P.O. Box 43-9045, San Ysidro, CA 92143, or 4630 Border Village

Road, Suite 203, San Ysidro, CA 92173; tel: 800-700-1850.

Serafina Corsello, M.D., The Corsello Centers, 200 West 57th Street, New York, NY 10019; tel: 212-399-0222; fax: 212-399-3817. Also: 175 East Main Street, Huntington, NY 11743; tel: 516-271- 0222; fax: 516-271-5992.

W. Lee Cowden, M.D., Conservative Medicine Institute, P.O. Box 832087, Richardson, TX 75083-2087; fax: 214-238-0327.

Ravi Devgan, M.D. In Mexico: tel: 011-526-634-2933; fax: 011-526-634-6087. In Canada: tel: 416-487-0882; fax: 416-487-9164; website: www.ravidevganmd.com.

W. John Diamond, M.D., Triad Medical Center, 4600 Kietzke Lane, M-242, Reno, NV 89502; tel: 702-829-2277; fax: 702-829-2365.

Patrick Donovan, N.D., University Health Clinic, 5312 Roosevelt Way NE, Seattle, WA 98105; tel: 206-525-8015; fax: 206-525-8014.

Stephen B. Edelson, M.D., F.A.A.F.P., F.A.A.E.M., 3833 Roswell Road, Suite 110, Atlanta, GA 30342; tel: 404-841-0088; fax: 404-841-6416.

James W. Forsythe, M.D., H.M.D., Cancer Screening and Treatment Center of Nevada, 521 Hammill Lane, Building B, Reno, NV 89509; tel: 775-827-0707. Also: Century Wellness Center. 380 Brinkby Avenue, Reno, NV 89509; tel: 702-826-9500; fax: 702-329-6219.

The Gerson Research Organization, 7807 Artesian Road, San Diego, CA, 92127-2117, tel: 800-759-2966; fax: 619-759-2967. Max Gerson Memorial Cancer Center of CHIPSA, 670 Nubes, Playas de Tijuana, Mexico. The Gerson Institute, P.O. Box 430, Bonita, CA 91908-0430; tel: 619-585-7600; fax: 619-585-7610.

Joseph M. Gold, M.D., Syracuse Research Institute, 600 East Genesee Street, Syracuse, NY 13202; tel: 315-472-6616.

Nicholas Gonzalez, M.D., 36A East 36th Street, Suite 204, New York, NY 10016; tel: 212-213-3337; fax: 212-213-3414.

Abram Hoffer, M.D., Ph.D., F.R.C.P., 2727 Quadra, Suite 3, Victoria, British Columbia, Canada V8T 4E5; tel: 250-386-8756; fax: 250-386-5828.

Tori Hudson N.D., A Woman's Time—Menopause Options and Natural Medicine, 2067 N.W. Lovejoy, Portland, OR 97209; tel: 503-222-2322; fax: 503-222-0276.

Wolfgang Kostler, M.D., Sofienalpanstrasse 17, A-1140 Vienna, Austria.

Dan Labriola, N.D., P.O. Box 99157, Seattle, WA 98199; tel: 206-285-4993; fax: 206-285-0085.

Livingston Foundation Medical Center, 3232 Duke Street, San Diego, CA 92110; tel: 888-777-7321 or 619-224-3515; fax: 619-224-6253.

Victor A. Marcial-Vega, M.D., 4037 Poinciana Avenue, Coconut Grove, FL 33133; tel: 305-442-1233; fax: 305-445-4504.

Martin Milner, N.D., Center for Natural Medicine, Inc., 1330 SE 39th Avenue, Portland OR 97214; tel: 503-232-1100; fax: 503-232-7751.

New Hope Clinic, SA de CV, Blvd. Agua Caliente #4558-607, 22420 Tijuana, B.C., Mexico; tel: 888-532-0897 or 011-526-686-4936; e-mail: newhope@newhopeclinic.com.

The Revici Life Science Center, Inc., Kenneth Korins, M.D., 200 West 57th Street, Suite 402, New York, NY 10019; tel: 212-246-5122; fax: 212-246-5711.

Robert C. Rountree, M.D., Helios Health Center, 4150 Darley Avenue, Suite 1, Boulder, CO 80303; tel: 303-499-9224; fax: 303-499-9593.

Geronimo Rubio, M.D., American Metabolic Institute, 555 Saturn Blvd., Building B, M/S 432, San Diego, CA 92154; tel: 619-267-1107, 619-229-3003, or 800-388-1083; fax: 619-267-1109. In Mexico, tel: 52-6621-7602 or 52-6621-7603.

San Diego Clinic, 555 Saturn Blvd., Suite B-452, San Diego, CA 92154; tel: 619-778-6828; e-mail: info@sdclinic.com. In Mexico: Circuito Bursátil #9031, Edificio Terra Zona Rio - Suite 306, C.P. 22320 Tijuana, B.C., Mexico; tel: 011-526-683-13-98 or 011-526-683-6055; fax: 011-526-683-6055.

Michael B. Schachter, M.D., Schachter Center for Complementary Medicine, Two Executive Boulevard, Suite 202, Suffern, NY 10901; tel: 914-368-4700; fax: 914-368-4727.

Charles B. Simone, M.MS., M.D., Simone Protective Cancer Center, 123 Franklin Corner Road, Lawrenceville, NJ 08648; tel: 609-896-2646.

Vincent Speckhart, M.D., P.C., 902 Graydon Avenue, No. 2, Norfolk, VA 23507; tel: 757-622-0014; fax: 757-622-9808.

Jesse Stoff, M.D., IntegraMed Clinic, 3402 E. Broadway Blvd., Tucson, AZ 85716; tel: 520-740-1315; fax: 520-319-9074.

Jack O. Taylor, M.S., D.C., CASS Professional Center, 7702 S. Cass Avenue, Suite 115, Darien, IL 60561; tel: 630-493-9516.→ Judy (nurse)

Lawrence H. Taylor, M.D., Advanced Medicine and Research Center, 1000 Cordova Court, Chula Vista, CA 91910; tel: 888-422-7434; fax: 619-656-1916. (Patients are treated at Allen W. Lloyd Building, Second Floor, Paseo, Tijuana, #406-201, Tijuana, B.C., Mexico.)

Organizations

Cancer Control Society, 2043 North Berendo Street, Los Angeles CA 90027; tel: 213-663-7801. Provides listings and information on alternative cancer treatment centers and patients who have recovered from various cancers using alternative therapies. Particular emphasis on metabolic therapies. Also sponsors an annual convention showcasing 40-50 alternative practitioners who treat cancer.

Foundation for Advancement in Cancer Therapy, P.O. Box 1242, Old Chelsea Station, New York, NY 10113; tel: 212-741-2790. A clearinghouse for information regarding alternative cancer therapies, emphasising nutritional and metabolic approaches.

People Against Cancer, P.O. Box 10, Otho, Iowa 50569; tel: 515-972-4444. A nonprofit, grassroots membership organization dedicated to cancer prevention and medical freedom of choice. Provides counseling and information on alternative cancer treatments.

World Research Foundation, 15300 Ventura Boulevard, Suite 405, Sherman Oaks, CA 91403; tel: 818-907-5483. Large research library of alternative medicine. Library is open to the public. Provides a computer search and printout of specific health issues for a nominal fee.

Information Resources on the Internet

http://www.alternativemedicine.com

This site, maintained by AlternativeMedicine.com (the publisher of this book), offers access to all issues and contents of *Alternative Medicine*, an Interactive Index enabling users to research health conditions, and other practical features central to alternative medicine.

http://cancerguide.org

Developed by kidney cancer survivor Steve Dunn, this site reviews the clinical merits and research regarding numerous alternative cancer therapies and substances, such as bovine cartilage, Essiac, and antineoplastons.

http://www.graylab.ac.uk/cancerweb

This is an England-based multimedia information resource for oncology, providing data on conventional approaches mostly with links to other sites and bibliographic resources.

http://cancer.med.upenn.edu

Also known as OncoLink, this site provides information on types of cancer, treatment options, clinical trials, and online patient support services; it offers extensive information-searching tools.

http://www.healthy.net

Sponsored by HealthWorld Online, this site provides information on both conventional and natural health (alternative medicine) through 11 information centers (e.g., health clinics, books, professional association network, library of health and medicine) and 15,000 electronic pages of health data.

http://www.allabouthealth.com

This site features the latest research findings, events, trends, books, software, products, articles, commentaries, and numerous links to other relevant web sites.

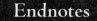

Endnotes

Chapter I: The Road to Recovery

1. Atkins, Robert C., M.D. *Dr. Atkins' Health Revolution: Cancer Therapy* (Boston, MA: Houghton Mifflin Co., 1988), 324.

2. Eysenck, H. "Psychosocial Factors, Prognosis, and Prevention of Cancer." *Coping With Cancer and Beyond* (Berwyn, PA: Swets and Zeitlinger, The Helen Dowling Institute, 1991), 35.

3. Levy, S.M. et al. "Survival Hazards Analysis in First Recurrent Breast Cancer Patients: Seven-Year Follow-Up." *Psychosomatic Medicine* 50 (1988), 520-528.

4. Shekelle, R.B. et al. "Psychological Depression and 17-Year Risk and Death From Cancer." *Psychosomatic Medicine* 43 (1981), 117-125.

5. William, Redford B., M.D. "Hostility and the Heart." In: Daniel Goleman, Ph.D., and Joel Gurin, eds. *Mind/Body Medicine* (Yonkers, NY: Consumer Reports Books, 1993), 66-67.

6. Jenkins, C. David. "The Mind and the Body." *World Health* 47:2 (March/April 1994), 6-7.

7. Stanwyck and Anson. MMPI study of five cluster groups. Georgia State University.

8. Dossey, Larry, M.D. *Healing Words: The Power of Prayer and the Practice of Medicine* (San Francisco: HarperCollins, 1993), 268.

9. Elias, Marilyn. "Attending Church Found Factor in Longer Life." *USA Today* (August 8, 1999), 1A.

10. Greer, S. et al. "Psychological Response to Breast Cancer: Effects on Outcome." *The Lancet* 2 (1979), 785-787. See also: G. Rogentine et al. "Psychological Factors in the Prognosis of Malignant Melanoma: A Prospective Study." *Psychosomatic Medicine* 41 (1979), 647-655.

11. Goodkin, K. et al. "Stress and Hopelessness in the Promotion of Cervial Intraepithelial Neoplasia in Invasive Squamous Cell Carcinoma of the Cervix." *Journal of Psychosomatic Research* 30:1 (1986), 67-76. See also: Schmale, A.H., and H. Iker. "The Effect of Hopelessness in the Development of Cancer I: Identification of Uterine Cervical Cancer in Women With Atypical Cytology." *Psychosomatic Medicine* 28 (1966), 714-721.

12. Ramirez, A.J. et al. "Stress and Relapse of Breast Cancer." *British Medical Journal* 298 (1989), 291-293.

13. Berkman, L.F., and S.L. Syme. "Social Networks, Host Resistance, and Mortality: A Nine-Year Follow-Up Study of Alameda County Residents." *American Journal of Epidemiology* 109:2 (1979), 189-204.

14. Spiegel, D. et al. "Effect of Psychosocial Treatment on Survival of Patients with Metastatic Breast Cancer." *The Lancet* 2:8668 (1989), 888-891.

15. J.W. Shaffer et al. "Clustering Personality Traits in Youth and the Subsequent Development of Cancer Among Physicians." *Journal of Behavioral Medicine* 10:5 (1987), 441-448. Cited in: B. Bower. "The Character of Cancer." *Science News* 131 (1987), 120-121.

16. Geffen, Jeremy, M.D. *The Journey Through Cancer* (New York: Crown, 2000), 76.

17. Schlessel Harpham, Wendy, M.D. *Diagnosis: Cancer—Your Guide Through the First Few Months* (New York: W.W. Norton, 1992), 163-164.

18. Wilkens, Cheryl. "Daring to Heal My Cancer with Nutrition." *Alternative Medicine Digest* 6 (1995), 4-7.

19. Eisenberg, David M. et al. "Unconventional Medicine in the United States: Prevalence, Costs, and Patterns of Use." 328:4 *The New England Journal of Medicine* (January 28, 1993), 246-252.

20. "Government Data Proves It: Alternative Medicine Is Growing." *Alternative Medicine Digest* 9 (1995), 42.

21. "Patients Want Alternative Medicine—Their Office Visits Prove It." *Alternative Medicine Digest* 6 (1995), 32.

22. "Alternative Medicine Thrives in Bay Area." *San Francisco Chronicle* (May 17, 1995). See also: "Acceptance of Acupuncture Grows." *Marin Independent Journal* (July 3, 1995).

23. Kennedy, B.J. "Use of Questionable Methods and Physician Education." 8:2 *Journal of Cancer Education* (1993), 129-131.

24. Hauser, S.P. "Unproven Methods in Cancer Treatment." *Current Opinions in Oncology* 5:4 (1993), 646-654.

25. Office of Alternative Medicine. *Office of Alternative Medicine Workshop on the Collection of Clinical research Data Relevant to Alternative Medicine and Cancer* (Bethesda,

MD: Office of Alternative Medicine, 1994).

26. McGinnis, L.S. "Alternative Therapies, 1990. An Overview." *Cancer* 67: Suppl 6 (1991), 1788-1792.

27. Guzley, G.J. "Alternative Cancer Treatments: Impact of Unorthodox Therapy on the Patient with Cancer." *Southern Medical Journal* 85(5):5 (1992), 19-23.

28. Boik, John. *Cancer & Natural Medicine. A Textbook of Basic Science and Clinical Research* (Princeton, MN: Oregon Medical Press, 1995), 3.

29. Nash, J. Madeleine. "The Enemy Within." *Time* (Fall 1996), 20.

30. American Cancer Society. *Facts about Cancer* (Atlanta, GA: American Cancer Society, 1996).

31. Bailar, J.S., and E.M. Smith. "Progress Against Cancer?" *New England Journal of Medicine* 314 (1986), 1226.

32. Hankey, B. Chief of the Cancer Statistics Branch, National Cancer Institute. Personal communications (1994). The incidence of all cancers combined for the total population increased 13% from 1975 to 1989, from 332 per 100,000 to 376 per 100,000. The mortality rate rose 7%, from 162 deaths per 100,000 to 173 per 100,000.

33. National Cancer Institute. *Cancer Statistics Review*, 1973-1989 (Washington, DC: National Institutes of Health, Office of Cancer Communications, 1992).

34. Henderson, B.E. et al. "Toward the Primary Prevention of Cancer." *Science* 254 (1991), 1131-1138. Cited in: McAllister, R.M. et al. *Cancer: What Cutting-Edge Science Can Tell You and Your Doctor about the Causes of Cancer and the Impact of Diagnosis and Treatment* (New York: HarperCollins, 1993), 3-4.

35. Meredith, Nikki. "Medical Dilemma." *Pacific Sun* (July 24-30, 1996), 11.

36. Nash, J. Madeleine. "The Enemy Within." *Time* (Fall 1996), 20.

37. Hankey, B. Chief of the Cancer Statistics Branch, National Cancer Institute. Personal communications (1994).

38. Beardsley, Tim. "A War Not Won." *Scientific American* (January 1994), 130-138.

39. Hankey, B. Chief of the Cancer Statistics Branch, National Cancer Institute. Personal communications (1994).

40. Schuette, et al. "The Costs of Cancer Care in the United States: Implications for Action." *Oncology* 9:11S (1995), 19-22.

41. Ibid. These costs include the estimates of the value of lost days of work due to illness, as well as the costs reflected in premature death of workers.

42. Hankey, B. Chief of the Cancer Statistics Branch, National Cancer Institute. Personal communications (1994).

43. Page, H.S., and A.J. Asire. *Cancer Rates and Risks* 3rd Edition. (Washington, DC: National Institutes of Health, 1985), 11. Cited by: Prescott, D.M., and A.S. Flexer. *Cancer: The Misguided Cell* 2nd Edition. (Sunderland, MA: Sinauer Associates, 1986), 224.

44. Rennie, John, and Ricki Rusting. "Making Headway Against Cancer." *Scientific American* (September 1996), 56-58.

45. Foster, H. "Lifestyle Changes and the Spontaneous Regression of Cancer: An Initial Computer Analysis." *International Journal of Biosocial Research* 10:1 (1988), 17-33.

Chapter 2: Cancer and Its Causes

1. Zajicek, G. "A New Cancer Hypothesis." *Medical Hypotheses* 47 (1996), 111-115.

2. Dr. Zajicek suggests that carcinogens deplete a vital metabolic substance, as yet not precisely identified; this depletion induces a state of progressive wasting and deterioration (called cachexia) and eventually the emergence of a tumor. Dr. Zajicek further suggests that the tumor arises as a self-protective mechanism of the body to replenish the missing substance; over time, the tumor worsens and begins to seriously compromise the entire organism.

3. Dermer, G.B. "Contradictions of Stability and Differentation." *The Immortal Cell* (Garden City Park, NY: Avery Publishing, 1994), 47.

4. Blackburn, G. et al. "Developing Strategies for Intervention/Prevention Trials of Individuals at Risk of Hereditary Colon Cancer." *Journal of the National Cancer Institute Monographs* 17 (1995), 107-110.

5. Gerson, Max, M.D. *A Cancer Therapy. Results of Fifty Cases* (Bonita, CA: Gerson Institute, 1958), 102.

6. Becker, Robert O., M.D. *Cross Currents: The Promise of Electromedicine, The Perils of Electropollution* (Los Angeles: Jeremy P. Tarcher, 1990), 206.

7. Pizzorno, Joseph, N.D. *Total Wellness* (Rocklin, CA: Prima Publishing, 1996), 24.

8. Weinberg, Robert A. *Racing to the Beginning of the Road: The Search for the Origin of Cancer* (New York: Harmony Books, 1996), 252.

9. Macek, C. "Of Mind and Morbidity: Can Stress

and Grief Depress Immunity?" *Journal of the American Medical Association* 248:4 (1982), 405-407.

10. Havlik, R.J., A.P. Vukasin and S. Ariyan. "The Impact of Stress on the Clinical Presentation of Melanoma." *Plastic and Reconstructive Surgery* 90:1 (1992), 57-61.

11. Greene, M.H., T.I. Young and W.H. Clark. "Malignant Melanoma in Renal Transplant Recipients." *The Lancet* 1 (1981), 1196.

12. Herberman, R.B., and J.R. Ortaldo. "Natural Killer Cells: Their Role in Defenses Against Disease." *Science* 214 (1981), 24.

13. Calabrese, J.R. et al. "Alterations in Immunocompetence during Stress, Bereavement, and Depression: Focus on Neuroendocrine Regulation." *American Journal of Psychiatry* 144 (1987), 1123.

14. Adams, D.O. "Molecular Biology of Macrophage Activation: A Pathway Whereby Psychosocial Factors Can Potentially Affect Health." *Psychosomatic Medicine* 56 (1994), 316-327.

15. Boik, J. "The Immune System: Monocyte-macrophages." *Cancer and Natural Medicine* (Princeton, MN: Oregon Medical Press, 1996), 63.

16. Leffell, David J., and Douglas E. Brash. "Sunlight and Skin Cancer." *Scientific American* (July 1996), 52-59.

17. Mugh, T.H., II. "Studies Stir Fears over Cancer Risks for Children." *The Los Angeles Times* (November 8, 1992), A1.

18. Holmberg, B. "Magnetic Fields and Cancer: Animal and Cellular Evidence—An Overview." *Environmental Health Perspectives* 103:Suppl 2 (1995), 63-67.

19. Feychting, M., and A. Ahlbom. "Childhood Leukemia and Residential Exposure to Weak Extremely Low Frequency Magnetic Fields." *Environmental Health Perspectives* Suppl 2 (1995), 59-62. See also: Savitz, D.A. "Overview of Epidemiologic Research on Electric and Magnetic Fields and Cancer." *American Industrial Hygiene Association Journal* 54:4 (1993), 197-204.

20. Savitz, D.A., and D.P. Loomis. "Magnetic Field Exposure in Relation to Leukemia and Brain Cancer Mortality Among Electric Utility Workers." *American Journal of Epidemiology* 141:2 (1995), 123-134. See also: Loomis, D.P., and D.A. Savitz. "Mortality from Brain Cancer and Leukemia among Electrical Workers." *British Journal of Industrial Medicine* 47:9 (1990), 633-638.

21. Loomis, D.P. et al. "Breast Cancer Mortality among Female Electrical Workers in the United States." *Journal of the National Cancer Institute* 86:12 (1994), 921-925.

22. Edwards, R. "Leak Links Power Lines to Cancer." *New Scientist* (October 7, 1995), 4.

23. U.S. Department of Health, Education, and Welfare. *Geomagnetism, Cancer, Weather, and Cosmic Radiation* (Salt Lake City, UT: 1979).

24. Steinman, D. *Diet for a Poisoned Planet* (New York: Ballantine, 1992), 265.

25. Simone, C. B., M.D. *Cancer and Nutrition* (Garden City Park, NY: Avery Publishing, 1992), 20-21.

26. Wing, S. et al. "Mortality among Workers at Oak Ridge National Laboratory: Evidence of Radiation Effects in Follow-up Through 1984." *Journal of the American Medical Association* 265:11 (1991), 1397-1402.

27. Cancer Prevention Coalition. *Breast Cancer Deaths Linked to Nuclear Emissions* (New York: Cancer Prevention Coalition, 1994). This press release cites a 1991 article in the *Journal of the American Medical Association*, which claims "if...any excess cancer risk was present in U.S. counties with nuclear facilities, it was too small to be detected with the methods employed." This study raises serious questions about the particular statistical methods used by NCI in that they used inappropriate controls based on small populations that were also exposed to nuclear emissions.

28. Sternglass, E.J., and J.M. Gould. "Breast Cancer: Evidence for a Relation to Fission Products in the Diet." *International Journal of Health Services* 23:4 (1993), 783-804.

29. "Changing Profile of Pesticide Poisonings." *New England Journal of Medicine* 316:13 (1987), 807-809.

30. Sewell, B.H. "The Littlest Consumers: Exposure to Pesticide Residues in Childhood May Pose Lifelong Risks." *American Health* (May 1988).

31. Wasserman, M. et al. "Organochlorine Compounds in Neoplastic and Adjacent Apparently Normal Breast Tissue." *Bulletin of Environmental Contaminants and Toxicology* 15 (1976), 478-484.

32. Westin, J., and E. Richter. "Israeli Breast Cancer Anomaly." *Annals of the New York Academy of Sciences* 609 (1990), 269-279.

33. *National Academy of Sciences 1984 Report on Pesticides and Cancer*. Note: These findings are based on the highest pesticide levels found in produce and assumes that consumers will not wash or cook their food.

34. Lowengart, R. A. et al. "Childhood Leukemia and

Parents' Occupational and Home Exposures." *Journal of the National Cancer Institute* 79:1 (July 1987), 39-46.

35. Davis, J. R. et al. "Family Pesticide Use and Childhood Brain Cancer." *Archives of Environmental Contamination and Toxicology* 24:1 (1993), 87-92.

36. Trichopoulos, Dimitrios, Frederick P. Li and David J. Hunter. "What Causes Cancer?" *Scientific American* (September 1996), 84.

37. Simone, Charles B., M. D. *Cancer & Nutrition* (Garden City Park, NY: Avery Publishing Group, 1992), 18, 21.

38. The Burton Goldberg Group. *Alternative Medicine: The Definitive Guide* (Tiburon, CA: Future Medicine Publishing, 1995), 186.

39. Ibid.

40. Ibid., 185.

41. Ibid.

42. Maugh, T.H., II. "Experts Downplay Cancer Risk of Chlorinated Water." *The Los Angeles Times* (July 2, 1992).

43. Judd, G.J. "Mass Fluoridation Causes Alarming Rise in Cancer Deaths." *Health Freedom News* (May 1995), 10.

44. Trichopoulos, Dimitrios, Frederick P. Li and David J. Hunter. "What Causes Cancer?" *Scientific American* (September 1996), 80-87.

45. American Cancer Society. *Cancer Facts & Figures* (Atlanta, GA: ACS. 1993). See also: Dreher, H. Your Defense against Cancer (New York: Harper & Row, 1988), 149-150.

46. Simone, C.B. "Carcinogens in Tobacco Smoke." *Breast Health* (Garden City, NY: Avery Publishing, 1995), 134.

47. Dreher, H. *Your Defense Against Cancer* (New York: Harper & Row, 1988), 200.

48. Weinstein, A.L. et al. "Breast Cancer Risk and Oral Contraceptive Use: Results from a Large Case-Control Study." *Epidemiology* 2:5 (September 1991), 353-358.

49. Minkin, Mary Jane, M.D., and Carol V. Wright. *What Every Woman Needs to Know about Menopause* (New Haven, CT: Yale University Press, 1996), 111-112.

50. Mayell, M. "Zapping Your Daily Diet: The Risks of Irradiated Foods." *EastWest: The Journal of Natural Living* (February 1986), 36.

51. Ibid.

52. The Burton Goldberg Group. *Alternative Medicine: The Definitive Guide* (Tiburon, CA: Future Medicine Publishing, 1995), 170.

53. Ibid.

54. Rosenberg, B. "A Diner's Guide to Irradiation."

Science Digest (September 1986), 30.

55. Dreher, H. *Your Defense Against Cancer* (New York: Harper & Row, 1988), 113.

56. Isaac, K., and S. Gold. "Some Chemicals Found in Food." *Eating Clean: Overcoming Food Hazards* (Washington, DC: Center for the Study of Responsive Law, 1990), 16.

57. Jacobson, M. F. "Undoing Delaney: FDA Allows Free Use of Dangerous Additives." *Eating Clean: Overcoming Food Hazards* (Washington, DC: Center for the Study of Responsive Law, 1990), 48-49.

58. Royal, Daniel F., DO. "Health Hazard in Your Teeth." *Alternative Medicine Digest* 13 (1996), 40-44.

59. The Burton Goldberg Group. *Alternative Medicine: The Definitive Guide* (Tiburon, CA: Future Medicine Publishing, 1995), 7.

60. Ibid., 8.

61. Ibid., 9.

62. Committee on Diet, Nutrition and Cancer. Assembly of Life Sciences, National Research Council. *Diet, Nutrition and Cancer* (Washington, DC: National Academy Press, 1982).

63. Toniolo, P. et al. "Consumption of Meat, Animal Products, Protein and Fat and Risk of Breast Cancer: A Prospective Cohort Study in New York." *Epidemiology* 5:4 (1994), 391.

64. Giovannucci, E. et al. "A Prospective Study of Dietary Fat and Risk of Prostate Cancer." *Journal of the National Cancer Institute* 85:19 (1993), 1571.

65. Giovannucci, E. et al. "Intake of Fat, Meat and Fiber in Relation to Risk of Colon Cancer in Men." *Cancer Research* 54:9 (1994), 2390.

66. The Burton Goldberg Group. *Alternative Medicine: The Definitive Guide* (Tiburon, CA: Future Medicine Publishing, 1995), 171.

67. Committee On Diet, Nutrition and Cancer. Assembly of Life Sciences, National Research Council. *Diet, Nutrition and Cancer* (Washington, DC: National Academy Press, 1982).

68. Simone, C.B., M.D. *Cancer and Nutrition* (Garden City Park, NY: Avery Publishing, 1992), 15.

69. Enig, M.G. et al. "Dietary Fat and Cancer Trends." *Federation Proceedings* 37 (1978), 2215-2220.

70. Simone, C.B. *Cancer and Nutrition* (Garden City Park, NY: Avery Publishing, 1992), 99.

71. Boik, J. "Humoral Factors that Affect Neoplasia: Eicosanoids." *Cancer and Natural Medicine*

(Princeton, MN: Oregon Medical Press, 1995), 46-49.

72. Bougnoux, P. et al. "Alpha-linolenic Acid Content of Adipose Breast Tissue: A Host Determinant of the Risk of Early Metastasis in Breast Cancer." *British Journal of Cancer* 70:2 (1994), 330-334.

73. Bristol, J.B. "Colorectal Cancer and Diet: A Case-Control Study with Special Reference to Dietary Fibre and Sugar." *Proceedings of the American Association of Cancer Research* 26 (March 1985), 206. See also: Bristol, J.B. et al. "Sugar, Fat and the Risk of Colorectal Cancer." *British Medical Journal Clinical Research Edition* 291:6507 (November 1985), 1467-1470.

74. Pizzorno, Joseph, N.D. *Total Wellness* (Rocklin, CA: Prima Publishing, 1996), 39-40.

75. Hsing, A.W. et al. "Cancer Risk Following Primary Hemochromatosis: A Population-based Cohort Study in Denmark." *Journal of Cancer* (1995), 160-162.

76. Knekt, P. et al. "Body Iron Stores and Risk of Cancer." *International Journal of Cancer* 56 (1994), 379-382. See also: Sevenes, R.G. et al. "Moderate Elevation of Body Iron Level and Increased Risk of Cancer Occurrence and Death." *Journal of Cancer* 56 (1994), 364-369.

77. Giovannucci, E., and W.C. Willett. "Dietary Lipids and Colon Cancer." *PPO Updates: Principles and Practice of Oncology* 9:5 (1995), 1-12.

78. Sandler, R.S. "Diet and Cancer: Food Additives, Coffee, and Alcohol." *Nutrition and Cancer* 4:4 (1983), 273-278. See also: "Beer Drinking and the Risk of Rectal Cancer." *Nutrition Reviews* 42:7 (July 1984), 244-247. See also: Potter, J.D., and A.J. McMichael. "Alcohol, Beer and Lung Cancer: A Meaningful Relationship?" *International Journal of Epidemiology* 13:2 (June 1984), 240-242.

79. Simone, C.B. *Breast Health* (Garden City Park, NY: Avery Publishing, 1995), 143.

80. Simon, D. et al. "Coffee Drinking and Cancer of the Lower Urinary Tract System." *Journal of the National Cancer Institute* 54:3 (1975), 587.

81. Mulvihill, J. "Caffeine as a Teratogen and Mutagen." *Teratology* 8:69 (1973). See also: Weinstein, D. et al. "The Effects of Caffeine on Chromosomes of Human Lymphocytes." *Mutation Research* 16 (1972), 391.

82. Schleifer, S.J., S.E. Keller and M. Stein. "Central Nervous System Mechanisms and Immunity: Implications for Tumor Reponse." Cited in: Levy, S.M. *Behavior and Cancer* (San Francisco: Jossey-Bass, 1985), 130-133. See also: Borysenko, M., and J. Borysenko. "Stress, Behavior and Immunity." *General Hospital Psychiatry* 4 (1985), 59-67.

83. Pettingale, K.W. "Towards a Psychobiological Model of Cancer: Biological Considerations." *Social Science & Medicine* 20 (1985), 179-187. See also: Lippman, M.E. "Psychosocial Factors and the Hormonal Regulation of Tumor Growth." *Behavior and Cancer*, edited by Levy, S.M. (San Francisco: Jossey-Bass, 1985), 134-147.

84. Forsen, A. "Psychosocial Stress as a Risk for Breast Cancer." *Psychotherapy and Psychosomatics* 55 (1991), 176-185.

85. Northrup, Christiane, M.D. *Women's Bodies, Women's Wisdom* (New York: Bantam, 1994), 35-40.

86. Greer, S. "Psycho-Oncology: Its Aims, Achievements and Future Tasks." *Psycho-Oncology* 3 (1994), 87-101. Eight prospective studies are cited: Schmale and Iker, 1971. Wiesman and Worden, 1977. Greer, et al., 1979. Di Clemente and Temoshok, 1985. Goodkin, et al., 1986. Jensen, 1987. Wirsching, et al., 1988. Morris, et al., 1992.

87. Ader, R. et al. *Psychoneuroimmunology* 2nd edition. (San Diego, CA: Academic Press, 1991), xxv.

88. Ader, R., and N. Cohen. "Behaviorally Conditioned Immunosuppression." *Psychosomatic Medicine* 37 (1975), 333. Borysenko, M., and J. Borysenko. "Stress, Behavior and Immunity." *General Hospital Psychiatry* 4 (1985), 59-67.

89. Grossarth-Maticek, R. et al. "Interpersonal Repression as a Predictor of Cancer." *Social Science & Medicine* 16 (1982), 493-498.

90. Dattore, P. et al. "Premorbid Personality Differentiation of Cancer and Non-cancer Groups." *Journal of Counseling and Clinical Psychology* 48:3 (1980), 388-394.

91. Shaffer, J.W. et al. "Clustering of Personality Traits in Youth and the Subsequent Development of Cancer among Physicians." *Journal of Behavioral Medicine* 10:5 (1987), 441-448. See also: Graves, P.L. et al. "Familial and Psychological Predictors of Cancer." *Cancer Detection and Prevention* 15:1 (1991), 59-64.

92. Davies, Daniel T., and James T.G. Illtyd. "An Investigation into the Gastric Secretion of a Hundred Normal Persons over the Age of Sixty." *Quarterly Journal of Medicine* 24 (1930), 1-4. See also: Rafsky, Henry A., and Michael Weingarten. "A Study of Gastric Secretory Response in the Aged." *Gastroenterology* 8 (1947), 348-352. See also: Montgomery, R.D. et al. "The Aging Gut: A Study of Intestinal Absorption in Relation to Nutrition in the

Elderly." *Quarterly Journal of Medicine* 47 (1978), 197-211.

93. Gittleman, Ann Louise. *Guess What Came to Dinner: Parasites and Your Health* (Garden City, NY: Avery Publishing, 1993).

94. Clark, Hulda Regehr, Ph.D., N.D. *The Cure for All Cancers* (San Diego, CA: ProMotion Publishing, 1993), 1-20.

95. Trichopoulos, Dimitrios, Frederick P. Li, and David J. Hunter. "What Causes Cancer?" *Scientific American* (September 1996), 82-83.

96. Warburg, O. "On the Origin of Cancer Cells." *Science* 123 (1956), 309-315.

97. Thomas, Gordon. *Dr. Issels and His Revolutionary Cancer Treatment* (New York: Peter H. Wyden, 1973), 137-138.

98. Perera, F.P. "Uncovering New Clues to Cancer Risk." *Scientific American* (May 1996), 54-62.

Chapter 3: Early Detection and Prevention

1. Morra, M., and E. Potts. "Diagnostic Tests." *Choices: Realistic Alternatives in Cancer Treatment* (New York: Avon, 1987), 97.

2. Scardino, P.T. "Early Detection of Prostate Cancer." *Urologic Clinics of North America* 16 (1989), 635-655.

3. McDonagh, E.W. "Detecting Cancer." *Townsend Letter for Doctors & Patients* (February/March 1996), 108-110.

4. Skerrett, P.J. "Screening for Prostate Cancer." *Technology Review* 8-9 (1994), 16-17.

5. Garnick, M.B. "The Dilemmas of Prostate Cancer." *Scientific American* (April 1994), 72.

6. Editorial. "The PSA Debate Continues." *Johns Hopkins Medical Letter* (February 1995), 2.

7. Waterbor, J.W., and A.J. Bueschen. "Prostate Cancer Screening." *Cancer Causes and Control* 6 (1995), 267-274.

8. Skerrett, P.J. "Screening for Prostate Cancer." *Technology Review* 8-9 (1994), 16-17.

9. American Cancer Society. *Prostate Cancer Information* (Atlanta, GA: ACS, 1995).

10. Baran, G.W. et al. "Biological Aggressiveness of Palpable and Nonpalpable Prostate Cancer: Assessment with Endosonography." *Radiology* 178 (1991), 201-206.

11. Catalona, W.J. "Management of Cancer of the Prostate." *New England Journal of Medicine* 331:15 (1994), 996-1003.

12. Fowler, F.J. "Prostate Conditions, Treatment Decisions, and Patient Preferences." *Journal of the American Geriatrics Society* 43:9 (1995), 1058-1060.

13. Mills, P.K. et al. "Cohort Study of Diet, Lifestyle and Prostate Cancer in Adventist Men." *Cancer* 64 (1989), 598-604. See also: Oishi, K. et al. "A Case-Control Study of Prostatic Cancer with Reference to Dietary Habits." *The Prostate* 12 (1988), 179-190.

14. "Tomatoes Prevent Cancer." Associated Press (December 6, 1995). Commentary on a report that appeared in the Journal of the National Cancer Institute.

15. Wynder, E. L. "Research on Omega-3 Fatty Acids." Cited by: Challem, J. "Prevent Prostate Cancer and Other Male Problems" *Let's Live* (July 1995), 14-26.

16. Karmah, R. et al. "The Effects of Dietary Omega-3 Fatty Acids on DU-145 Transplantable Human Prostate Tumors." *Antioxidant Research* 7 (1987), 1173-1179.

17. Webber, M.M. "Inhibitory Effects of Selenium on the Growth of DU-145 Human Prostate Carcinoma Cells In Vitro." *Biochemical and Biophysical Research Communications* 130:2 (1985), 603-609.

18. Webber, M.M. "Selenium Prevents the Growth Stimulatory Effects of Cadmium on Human Prostatic Epithelium." *Biochemical and Biophysical Research Communications* 127:3 (1985), 871-877.

19. Aldercreutz, H. et al. "Plasma Concentrations of Phyto-estrogens in Japanese Men." *The Lancet* 342:8881 (1993), 1209-1210.

20. Linehan, W. "Inhibition of Prostate Cancer Metastasis: A Critical Challenge Ahead." *Journal of the National Cancer Institute* 87 (1995), 348-352.

21. Oliveria, S.A. et al. "The Association between Cardiorespiratory Fitness and Prostate Cancer." *Medicine and Science in Sports and Exercise* 28:1 (1996), 97-104.

22. Nelson, et al. *Proceedings of the National Academy of Sciences USA* 91 (1994), 11733-11737.

23. Schardt, D. "The Cancer Men Don't Talk About." *Nutrition Action* 20:1 (1993), 1-6.

24. Whittemore, A. S. et al. "Prostate Cancer in Relation to Diet, Physical Activity, and Body Size in Blacks, Whites, and Asians in the United States and Canada." *Journal of the National Cancer Institute* 87:9 (1995), 652-661.

25. Gann, P.H. et al. "Prospective Study of Plasma Fatty Acids and Risk of Prostate Cancer." *Journal of the National Cancer Institute* 86 (1994), 281-286.

26. Parker, S.L. et al. "Cancer Statistics 1996." *CA: A Cancer Journal for Clinicians* 46 (1996), 5-27.

27. Meyskens, F.L., and A. Manetta. "Prevention of Cervical Intraepithelial Neoplasia and Cervical Cancer." *American Journal of Clinical Nutrition* 62:Suppl (1995), 1417S-1419S.

28. Passwater, R.A. "Cervical Cancer." *Cancer Prevention and Nutritional Therapies* (New Canaan, CT: Keats Publishing, 1993). This conclusion is based on Dr. Passwater's assessment of nine studies published in peer-review journals, all listed on page 184.

29. Butterworth, C.E. "Effect of Folate on Cervical Cancer: Synergism among Risk Factors." *Annals of the New York Academy of Sciences* 669 (1992), 293-299.

30. Licciardone, J.C. et al. "Cigarette Smoking and Alcohol Consumption in the Etiology of Uterine Cervical Cancer." *International Journal of Epidemiology* 18:3 (1989), 533-537. Graham, I.T. et al. "Cigarette Smoking and the Incidence of Cervical Intraepithelial Neoplasia, Grade III, and Cancer of the Cervix Uteri." *American Journal of Epidemiology* 135:4 (1992), 341-346.

31. Szarewski, A. "Effect of Smoking Cessation on Cervical Lesion Size." *The Lancet* 347:9006 (1996), 941-943.

32. Parker, S.L. et al. "Cancer Statistics 1996." *CA: A Cancer Journal for Clinicians* 46 (1996), 5-27.

33. Petrek, J.A., and A.I. Holleb. "The Foremost Cancer—Revisited." *CA: A Cancer Journal for Clinicians* 45:4 (1995), 197-243.

34. Ernster, Virginia L., et al. "Incidence of and Treatment for Ductal Carcinoma in Situ of the Breast." *Journal of the American Medical Association* 275 (March 27, 1996), 913-918.

35. Wright, C.J., and C.B. Mueller. "Screening Mammography and Public Health Policy: The Need For Perspective." *The Lancet* 346 (July 1995), 29-32.

36. Plotkin, D. "Good News and Bad News About Breast Cancer." *The Atlantic Monthly* (June 1996), 82.

37. Helvie, M.A., et al. "Mammographic Follow-up of Low-Suspicion Lesions: Compliance Rate and Diagnostic Yield." *Radiology* 178 (1991), 155-158.

38. National Women's Health Network Position Paper. *Mammography in Women Before Menopause* (Washington, DC: National Women's Health Network, 1993).

39. Ibid..

40. Breen, Nancy, and Brown, Martin L. "The Price of Mammography in the U.S.. Data from the National Survey of Mammography Facilitators." *The Milbank Quarterly* 72:3 (1994).

41. Wright, C.J. and C.B. Mueller. "Screening Mammography and Public Health Policy: The Need for Perspective." *The Lancet* 346 (July 1995), 29-35.

42. Bogoch, S., and E.S. Bogoch. "A Checklist for Suitability of Biomarkers as Surrogate Endpoints in Chemoprevention of Breast Cancer." *Journal of Cellular Biochemistry* Suppl 19 (1994), 173-185.

43. Bogoch, S. et al. *Return of Elevated Antimalignin Antibody to Normal Indicates Remission of Breast Cancer* (Boston: Foundation for Research on the Nervous System and Oncolab, 1996). Unpublished manuscript.

44. Sox, H. "Screening Mammography in Women Younger Than 50 Years of Age." *Annals of Internal Medicine* 122:7 (1995), 550-552.

45. For an excellent review of the literature on the relationship between low-fat diet and low breast cancer incidence, please refer to: Pelton, R. et al. "Dietary Fat—The 20 Percent Solution." *How to Prevent Breast Cancer* (New York: Simon & Schuster, 1995), 145-158.

46. Pelton, R. et al. "The Pros and Cons of Hormone Replacement Therapy." *How to Prevent Breast Cancer* (New York: Simon & Schuster, 1995), 11-12.

47. Ibid., 104-116.

48. Wolff, M.S. et al. "Blood Levels of Organochlorine Residues and Risk of Breast Cancer." *Journal of the National Cancer Institute* 85 (1993), 648-652. See also: Falck, F. et al. "Pesticides and Polychlorinated Biphenyl Residues in Human Breast Lipids and Their Relation to Breast Cancer." *Archives of Environmental Health* 47 (1992), 143-146.

49. Krieger, N. et al. "Breast Cancer and Serum Organochlorines: A Prospective Study among White, Black, and Asian Women." *Journal of the National Cancer Institute* 86:8 (1994), 589-599.

50. Falck, F., Jr. et al. "Pesticides and Polychlorinated Biphenyl Residues in Human Breast Lipids and Their Relation to Breast Cancer." *Archives of Environmental Health* 47:2 (1992), 143-146.

51. Hayes, W.J., and E.R. Laws. *Handbook of Pesticide Toxicology* (San Diego, CA: Academic Press, 1991).

52. Raloff, J. "Pesticides May Challenge Human Immunity." *Science News* 149 (1996), 149.

53. Bock, S., and M. Boyette. *Stay Young the Melatonin Way* (New York: Dutton, 1995). Excellent discussion of factors affecting the body's melatonin supply, and possible health

consequences. Many of these factors overlap with risk factors for breast cancer.

54. Morra, M., and E. Potts. "Diagnostic Tests." *Choices: Realistic Alternatives in Cancer Treatment* (New York: Avon, 1987), 86.

55. Giovannucci, E., and W. Willett. "Dietary Factors and Risk of Colon Cancer." *Annals of Medicine* 26 (1994), 443-452.

56. Steinmetz, K.A. et al. "Vegetables, Fruit, and Colon Cancer in the Iowa Women's Study." *American Journal of Epidemiology* 139 (1994), 1-15.

57. Sandler, R.S. et al. "Cigarette Smoking, Alcohol, and the Risk of Colorectal Adenomas." *Gastroenterology* 104 (1993), 1445-1451.

58. Flaten, T.P. "Chlorination of Drinking Water and Cancer Incidence in Norway." *International Journal of Epidemiology* 21 (1992), 6-15.

59. J.L. Marx. "The Immune System 'Belongs to the Body'." *Science* 277 (1985), 1190-1192.

60. R. Dilts and T. Hallbom. *Beliefs: Pathways to Health and Well-Being* (Portland, OR: Metamorphous Press, 1990), 1-2.

61. The Burton Goldberg Group. *Alternative Medicine: The Definitive Guide* (Tiburon, CA: Future Medicine Publishing, 1993), 245.

62. Springer, G.F. "Blood Group MN Antigens and Precursors in Normal and Malignant Human Breast Glandular Tissues." *Journal of the National Cancer Institute* 40 (1975), 183-192.

63. Studies reviewed in: Springer, G.F. "T and Tn Pancarcinoma Markers: Autoantigenic Adhesion Molecules in Pathogenesis, Prebiopsy Carcinoma Detection, and Long-Term Breast Carcinoma Immunotherapy." *Critical Reviews in Oncogenesis* 6:1 (1995), 57-85.

64. Coulter, H.L. Proposals for the Immunological Diagnosis and Treatment of Patients (Washington, DC: V.I. Govallo Center for Empirical Medicine, 1996).

Chapter 4: Nutrition as Cancer Medicine

1. The Burton Goldberg Group. *Alternative Medicine: The Definitive Guide* (Tiburon, CA: Future Medicine Publishing, 1995), 385.

2. Ibid.

3. Ibid.

4. Ibid.

5. Ibid.

6. Djuric, Z., and D. Kritchevsky. "Modulation of Oxidative DNA Damage Levels by Dietary Fat and Calories." *Mutation Research* 295 (1993), 181-190.

7. Colditz, G.A. et al. "Increased Green and Yellow Vegetable Intake and Lowered Cancer Deaths in an Elderly Population." *American Journal of Clinical Nutrition* 41:1 (January 1985), 32-36.

8. La Vecchia, C. et al. "Dietary Vitamin A and the Risk of Invasive Cervical Cancer." *International Journal of Cancer* 34:3 (1984), 319-322.

9. Menkes, M.S. et al. "Serum Beta-Carotene, Vitamins A and, Selenium and the Risk of Lung Cancer." *New England Journal of Medicine* 315 (1986), 1250.

10. "Dietary Aspects of Carcinogenesis." (September 1983).

11. Ramaswany, P., and R. Natarajan. "Vitamin B-6 Status in Patients with Cancer of the Uterine Cervix." *Nutrition and Cancer* 6 (1984), 176-180.

12. Stahelin, H. B. et al "Cancer, Vitamins, and Plasma Lipids: Prospective Basel Study." *Journal of the National Cancer Institute* 73 (1984), 1463-1468.

13. Ibid.

14. Willett, W.C., and B. MacMahon. "Prediagnostic Serum Selenium and the Risk of Cancer." *The Lancet* 2:8342 (July 1983), 130-134.

15. Butterworth, C.E. et al. "Improvement in Cervical Dysplasia Associated with Folic Acid Therapy in Users of Oral Contraceptives." *American Journal of Clinical Nutrition* 35:1 (1982), 73-82.

16. Slattery, M. L., A.W. Sorenon, and M.H. Ford. "Dietary Calcium Intake as a Mitigating Factor in Colon Cancer." *American Journal of Epidemiology* 128:3 (1988), 504-514.

17. Stadel, V.W. "Dietary Iodine and the Risk of Breast, Endometrial, and Ovarian Cancer." *The Lancet* 1:7965 (1976), 890-891.

18. Blondell, J. M. "The Anticarcinogenic Effect of Magnesium." *Medical Hypothesis* 6:8 (1980), 863-871.

19. Whelen, P., B.E. Walker and J. Kelleher. "Zinc, Vitamin A and Prostatic Cancer." *British Journal of Urology* 55:5 (1983), 525-528.

20. Kroning, F. "Garlic as an Inhibitor for Spontaneous Tumors in Mice." *Acta—Unio Internationalis Contra Cancrum* 20:3 (1964), 855.

21. You, W.C. et al. "Allium Vegetables and Reduced Risk of Stomach Cancer." *Journal of the National Cancer Institute* 81:2 (1989), 162-164.

22. Wynder, E.L. et al. "Diet and Breast Cancer in Causation and Therapy." *Cancer* 58:8 Suppl (1986), 1804-1831

23. Greenward, P., and E. Lanze. "Dietary Fiber and

Colon Cancer." *Contemporary Nutrition* 11:1 (1986).

24. "Risk Reduction Objectives." *Healthy People 2000* (Washington, DC: U.S. Public Health Service, U.S. Dept. of Health and Human Services, 1990), 425.

25. The Burton Goldberg Group. *Alternative Medicine: The Definitive Guide* (Tiburon, CA: Future Medicine Publishing, 1995), 385.

26. Emerich, Monica. "Industry Growth: 22.6%." *Natural Foods Merchandiser* XVII:6 (June 1996).

27. Newberne, P.M., and M. Locniskar. "Roles of Micronutrients in Cancer Prevention: Recent Evidence from the Laboratory." *Progress in Clinical and Biological Research* 346 (1990), 119-134.

28. Petrie, H.T. "Differential Regulation of Lymphocyte Functional Activities by Selenium." University of Nebraska Medical Center Dissertation, 1988.

29. Aso, H. et al. "Induction of Interferon and Activation of NK Cells and Macrophages in Mice by Oral Administration of Ge-132, an Organic Germanium Compound." *Journal of Microbiology and Immunology* 29 (1985), 65-74. See also: Kumano, N. et al. "Antitumor Effect of Organogermanium Compound Ge-132 on the Lewis Lung Carcinoma (3LL) in C57 BL (B6) Mice." *Tohoku Journal of Experimental Medicine* 146 (1985), 97-104.

30. Vojdani, A., and M. Ghoneum. "In Vivo Effect of Ascorbic Acid on Enhancement of Human Natural Killer Cell Activity." *Nutrition Research* 13 (1993), 753-754.

31. Malter, M. et al. "Natural Killer Cells, Vitamins, and Other Blood Components of Vegetarian and Omnivorous Men." *Nutrition and Cancer* 12:3 (1989), 271-278.

32. Bougnoux, P. et al. "Alpha-Linolenic Acid Content of Adipose Breast Tissue: A Host Determinant of the Risk of Early Metastasis in Breast Cancer." *British Journal of Cancer* 70:2 (1994), 330-334.

33. Baronzio, G.F. et al. "Adjuvant Therapy with Essential Fatty Acids (EFAs) for Primary Liver Tumors." *Medical Hypotheses* 44 (1995), 149-154.

34. Barnes, S. et al. "Soybeans Inhibit Mammary Tumors in Models of Breast Cancer." *Mutagens and Carcinogens in the Diet*, edited by Pariza, M. (New York: Alan R. Liss, 1990), 239-257.

35. Messina, M.J. et al. "Soy Intake and Cancer Risk: A Review of the In Vitro and In Vivo Data." *Nutrition & Cancer* 21:2 (1994), 113-131.

36. Haag, J.D. et al. "Enhanced Inhibition of Protein Isoprenylation and Tumor Growth by Perillyl Alcohol, an Hydroxylated Analog of d-limonene." *Proceedings of the American Association of Cancer Research* 33 (1992), 524.

37. Rhee, Y.H. et al. "Inhibition of Mutagenesis and Transformation by Root Extracts by Panax Ginseng In Vitro." *Planta Medica* 57 (1991), 125-128.

38. Clifford, C., and B. Kramer. "Diet as Risk and Therapy for Cancer." *Medical Clinics of North America* 77:4 (1993), 725-744.

39. Harman, D. "Nutritional Implications of the Free-radical Theory of Aging." *Journal of the American College of Nutrition* 1:1 (1982), 27-34.

40. Grimble, R.F. "Nutritional Antioxidants and the Modulation of Inflammation: Theory and Practice." *New Horizons* 2:2 (1994), 175-185.

41. Chaitow, L., and N. Trenev. "The Role and Nature of Friendly Bacteria." *Probiotics* (Prescott, AZ: Hohm Press, 1995), 11-18.

42. Chaitow, L., and N. Trenev. "The Lactobacilli and Bifidobacteria." *Probiotics* (Prescott, AZ: Hohm Press, 1995), 24-25.

43. Aso, Y. et al. "Preventive Effect of *Lactobacillus casei* Preparation on the Recurrence of Superficial Bladder Cancer in a Double-blind Trial." *European Urology* 27 (1995), 104-109.

44. Gogdanov, I.G. et al. "Antitumor Glycopeptides from *Lactobacillus bulgaricus* Cell Wall." *FEBS Letters* 57 (1975), 259-261. Cited by Moss, R. *Cancer Therapy* (New York: Equinox Press, 1992), 239.

45. Reynolds, J.V. et al. "Immunomodulatory Mechanisms of Arginine." *Surgery* 104:2 (1988), 142-151.

46. Akimoto, M. et al. "Modulation of the Antitumor Effect of BRM under Various Nutritional or Endocrine Conditions." *Gan To Kagaku Ryoho* 13 (1986), 1270-1276.

47. Tachibana, K. et al. "Evaluation of the Effect of Arginine-Enriched Amino Acid Solution on Tumor Growth." *Japanese Journal of Parenteral and Enteral Nutrition* 9 (1985), 428-434.

48. Newberne, P.M. et al. "Inhibition of Hepatocarcinogenesis in Mice by Dietary Methyl Donors Methionine and Choline." *Nutrition and Cancer* 14 (1990), 175-181.

49. Palermo, M.S. et al. "Immunomodulation Exerted by Cyclophosphamide Is Not Interfered by N-acetyl cysteine." *International Journal of Immunopharmacology* 8:6 (1986), 651-655. See also: Schmitt-Graff, A., and M.E. Scheulen. "Prevention of Adriamycin Cardiotoxicity by Niacin, Isocitrate or N-acetyl-cysteine in Mice: A Morphological Study." *Pathology Resident*

Practice 181:2 (1986), 168-174. See also: Kim, J.A. et al. "Topical Use of N-acetyl cysteine for Reduction of Skin Reaction to Radiation Therapy." *Seminars in Oncology* 10:Suppl 1 (1983), 86.

50. Kuroda, M. et al. "Decreased Serum Levels of Selenium and Glutathione Peroxidase Activity Associated with Aging, Malignancy and Chronic Hemodialysis." *Trace Elements in Medicine* 5:3 (1988), 97-103.

51. Strong, Gary. *Does Mercury from Dental Amalgams Influence Systemic Health?* (Billings, MT: Strong Health Publications, 1995).

52. Boit, J. "Amino Acids." *Cancer and Natural Medicine: A Textbook of Basic Science and Clinical Research* (Princeton, MN: Oregon Medical Press, 1995), 139-140.

53. Palermo, M.S. et al. "Immunomodulation Exerted by Cyclophosphamide is Not Interfered by N-acetyl cysteine." *International Journal of Immunopharmacology* 8:6 (1986), 651-655. See also: Schmitt-Graff, A., and M.E. Scheulen. "Prevention of Adriamycin Cardiotoxicity by Niacin, Isocitrate or N-acetyl-cysteine in Mice: A Morphological Study." *Pathology Resident Practice* 181:2 (1986), 168-174. See also: Kim, J.A. et al. "Topical Use of N-acetyl-cysteine for Reduction of Skin Reaction to Radiation Therapy." *Seminars in Oncology* 10:Suppl 1 (1983), 86.

54. Goldfarb, R.H., and R.B. Herberman. "Natural Killer Cell Reactivity: Regulatory Interactions among Phorbol Ester, Interferon, Cholera Toxin and Retinoic Acid." *Journal of Immunology* 126 (1981), 21-29. Dennert, G., and R. Lotan. "Effects of Retinoic Acid on the Immune System: Stimulation of T-killer Cell Induction." *European Journal of Immunology* 8 (1978), 23. Dennert, G. et al. "Retinoic Acid Stimulation of the Induction of Mouse Killer T-cell in All Ogeneic and Syngeneic Systems." *Journal of the National Cancer Institute* 62 (1979), 89.

55. Machlin, L.J., and A. Bendich. "Free Radical Tissue Damage: Protective Role of Antioxidant Nutrient." *FASEB Journal* 1:6 (1987), 441-445.

56. Bendich, A. "Carotenoids and the Immune Response." *Journal of Nutrition* 119:1 (1989), 112-115.

57. Garland et al. "Dietary Vitamin D and Calcium and Risk of Colorectal Cancer: A 19-year Prospective Study in Men." *The Lancet* i (1985), 307.

58. Wargovich, M.J. et al. "Modulating Effects of Calcium in Animal Models of Colon Carcinogenesis and Short-Term Studies in Subjects at Increased Risk for Colon Cancer." *American Journal of Clinical Nutrition* 54 (1991), 202S-205S. See also: Wargovich, M.J. "New Dietary Anticarcinogens and Prevention of Gastrointestinal Cancer." *Diseases of the Colon and Rectum* 31 (1988), 72-75.

59. Underwood, E. *Trace Elements in Human and Animal Nutrition* 4th ed. (New York: Academic Press, 1977), 267.

60. Todd, Gary P. "The Trace Elements." *Nutrition, Health, & Disease* (Norfolk, VA: Donning, 1985), 183.

61. Bliznakov, Emile, and Gerald Hunt. *The Miracle Nutrient Coenzyme Q10* (New York: Bantam, 1987).

62. Leibovitz, B. et al. "Dietary Supplements of Vitamin E, Beta-carotene, Coenzyme Q10, and Selenium Protect Tissues Against Lipid Peroxidation in Rat Tissue Slices." *Journal of Clinical Nutrition* 120 (1990), 97-104.

63. Folkers, K. et al. "Survival of Cancer Patients on Therapy with CoQ10." *Biochemical and Biophysical Research Communications* 192:1 (1993), 241-245.

64. Lockwood, K. et al. "Partial and Complete Regression of Breast Cancer in Relation to Dosage of Coenzyme Q10." *Biochemical and Biophysical Research Communications* 199 (1994), 1504-1508.

65. Lockwood, K. et al. "Progress on Therapy of Breast Cancer with CoQ10 and the Regression of Metastases." *Biochemical and Biophysical Research Communications* 212:1 (1995), 172-177.

66. Gershwin, M.E. et al. "The Potential Impact of Nutritional Factors on Immunological Responsiveness." *Nutrition and Immunity* (Orlando, FL: Academic Press, 1985), 222.

67. Beach, R.S. et al. "Zinc, Copper and Manganese in Immune Function and Experimental Oncogenesis." *Nutrition and Cancer* 3 (1982), 172-191.

68. Murray, Michael T., N.D. *Encyclopedia of Nutritional Supplements* (Rocklin, CA: Prima Publishing, 1996), 237-278. See also Barilla, Jean, ed. *The Nutrition Superbook* (New Canaan, CT: Keats Publishing, 1996) 261-263.

69. Sakaguchi, M. et al. "Reduced Tumor Growth of the Human Colonic Cancer Cell Lines COLO-320 and HT-29 In Vivo by Dietary n-3 Lipids." *British Journal of Cancer* 62:5 (1990), 742-747.

70. Reich, R. et al. "Eicosapentanoic Acid Reduces the Invasive and Metastatic Activities of Malignant Tumor Cells." *Biochemical & Biophysical Research Communications* 160:2

(1989), 59-564.

71. Burns, C.P., and A.A. Spector. "Effects of Lipids on Cancer Therapy." *Nutrition Reviews* 48:6 (1990), 233-240.

72. Man-Fan, W.J. et al. "Omega-3 fatty Acids and Cancer Metastasis in Humans." *World Review of Nutrition and Dietetics* 66 (1991), 477-487.

73. Erasmus, U. "Fatty Degeneration: Cancer." *Fats and Oils: The Complete Guide to Fats and Oils in Health and Nutrition* (Vancouver, Canada: Alive Books, 1988), 303-304.

74. Budwig, Johanna. *Flax Oil as a True Aid Against Arthritis, Heart Infarction, Cancer, and Other Diseases* (Vancouver, Canada: Apple Publishing, 1992).

75. Van Der Merwe, C.F. et al. "Oral Gamma-Linolenic Acid in 21 Patients with Untreatable Malignancy: An Ongoing Pilot Open Clinical Trial." *British Journal of Clinical Practice* 41:9 (1987), 907.

76. Van Der Merwe, C.F. "The Reversibility of Cancer." *South African Medical Journal* 65:18 (1984), 712.

77. Begin, M.E. et al. "Differential Killing of Human Carcinoma Cells Supplemented with n-3 and n-6 Polyunsaturated Fatty Acids." *Journal of the National Cancer Institute* 77:5 (1986), 1053-1062.

78. Erasmus, U. "Oil of Evening Primrose." *Fats and Oils: The Complete Guide to Fats and Oils in Health and Nutrition* (Vancouver, Canada: Alive Books, 1986), 251.

79. Ibid.

80. Kidd, P. "Germanium-132: Homeostatic Normalizer and Immunostimulant: A Review of Its Preventive and Therapeutic Efficacy." *International Clinical Nutrition Review* 7:1 (1987), 11-20.

81. Itoh, K. and K. Kumagai. "Augmentation of NK Activity by Several Anti-inflammatory Agents." Proceedings of the International Symposium on Natural Killer Cell Activity and its Regulation, Fifth International Congress of Immunology (1983).

82. Gerson, Max, M.D. *A Cancer Therapy: Results of Fifty Cases* (Bonita, CA: Gerson Institute, 1958), 7-10.

83. Ibid., 124.

84. Hildenbrand, G., and S. Cavin. "Five-Year Survival Rates of Melanoma Patients Treated by Diet Therapy after the Manner of Gerson: A Retrospective Review." *Alternative Therapies in Health and Medicine* 1:4 (1995), 29-37.

85. Ibid.

86. Steinmetz, K.A., and J.D. Potter. "Vegetables, Fruit and Cancer II Mechanisms." *Cancer Causes and Control* (1991), 427-442.

87. Murray, Michael T., N.D. *Encyclopedia of Nutritional Supplements* (Rocklin, CA: Prima Publishing, 1996).

88. Kutsky, R. "Iodine." *Handbook of Vitamins, Minerals, and Hormones* (New York: Van Nostrand Reinhold, 1981), 138.

89. Stadel, V.W. "Dietary Iodine and the Risk of Breast, Endometrial and Ovarian Cancer." *The Lancet* 1:7965 (1976), 890-891.

90. Langer, S.E. et al. *Solved: The Riddle of Illness* (New Canaan, CT: Keats, 1984). Shoden, R.J. and S. Griffin. "Iodine." *Fundamentals of Clinical Nutrition* (New York: McGraw Hill, 1980), 97.

91. Quillan, P. "Nutrients Have a Profound Impact on the Immune System." *Beating Cancer with Nutrition* (Tulsa, OK: Nutrition Times Press, 1994), 214.

92. Kutsky, R. "Iodine." *Handbook of Vitamins, Minerals, and Hormones* (New York: Van Nostrand Reinhold, 1981), 125.

93. Gershwin, M.E. et al. "The Potential Impact of Nutritional Factors on Immunological Responsiveness." *Nutrition and Immunity* (Orlando, FL: Academic Press, 1985), 201-204.

94. Kutsky, R. "Iodine." *Handbook of Vitamins, Minerals, and Hormones* (New York: Van Nostrand Reinhold, 1981), 167.

95. Todd, G.P. "The Trace Elements." *Nutrition, Health and Disease* (Norfolk, VA: Donning, 1985), 183.

96. The Burton Goldberg Group. *Alternative Medicine: The Definitive Guide* (Tiburon, CA: Future Medicine Publishing, 1995), 398.

97. Schrauzer, G.N. "Selenium in Nutritional Cancer Prophylaxis: An Update." *Vitamins, Nutrition and Cancer*, edited by Prosad, K.N. (Basel, Switzerland: Karger, 1984).

98. Schrauzer, G.N. "Selenium for the Cancer Patient." Adjuvant Nutrition in Cancer Treatment Symposium. Tampa, Florida (September 29, 1995). Dr. Schrauzer is based at the Biological Trace Element Research Institute, San Diego, CA.

99. Petrie, H.T. "Differential Regulation of Lymphocyte Functional Activities by Selenium." (University of Nebraska Medical Center, 1988).

100. Ip, C. "Prophylaxis of Mammary Neoplasia by Selenium Supplementation in the Initiation and Promotion Phases of Carcinogenesis." *Cancer Research* 41 (1981), 4386-4393.

101. Schrauzer, G.N. "Selenium in Nutritional Cancer Prophylaxis: An Update." *Vitamins, Nutrition and Cancer*, edited by Prosad, K.N. (Basel, Switzerland: Karger, 1984).

102. Goldfarb, R.H., and R.B. Herberman. "Natural Killer Cell Reactivity: Regulatory Interactions among Phorbol Ester, Interferon, Cholera Toxin and Retinoic Acid." *Journal of Immunology* 126 (1981), 2129. Dennert, G., and R. Lotan. "Effects of Retinoic Acid on the Immune System: Stimulation of T-killer Cell Induction." *European Journal of Immunology* 8 (1978), 23. Dennert, G. et al. "Retinoic Acid Stimulation of the Induction of Mouse Killer T-cell in Allogeneic and Syngeneic Systems." *Journal of the National Cancer Institute* 62 (1979), 89.

103. Hong, W.K. et al. "Prevention of Second Primary Tumors with Isotreninoin in Squamous-cell Carcinoma of the Head and Neck." *New England Journal of Medicine* 323 (1990), 795-801.

104. Miscksche, M. et al. "Vitamin A in the Treatment of Metastatic Unresectable Squamous Cell Carcinoma of the Lung." *Oncology* 34 (1977), 234.

105. Panush, R.S., and J.C. Delafuente. "Vitamins and Immunocompetence: Group B Vitamins. World Review." *Nutrition Digest* 45 (1985), 97-132. Posner, B.M. et al. "Nutrition in Neoplastic Disease." *Advances in Modern Human Nutrition and Dietetics* 29 (1980), 130-169.

106. Ibid.

107. Beisel, W.R. et al. "Single Nutrients and Immunity." *American Journal of Clinical Nutrition* 35 Suppl (1982), 417-468.

108. Basu, T.K. "Significance of Vitamins in Cancer." *Oncology* 33 (1976), 183.

109. Hoffer, A. "Vitamin B-3: Niacin and Its Amide." *Townsend Letter for Doctors & Patients* (October 1995), 35.

110. Gridley, D.S. et al. "In Vivo and In Vitro Stimulation of Cell-Mediated Immunity by Vitamin B6." *Nutrition Research* 8:2 (1988), 201-207.

111. Posner, B.M. et al. "Nutrition in Neoplastic Disease." *Advances in Modern Human Nutrition and Dietetics* 29 (1980), 130-169.

112. DiSorbo, D.M., and G. Litwack. "Vitmain B6 Kills Hepatoma Cells in Culture." *Nutrition and Cancer* 3:4 (1982), 216-222.

113. Byar, D., and C. Blackard. "Comparisons of Placebo, Pyridoxine, and Topical Thiopepa in Preventing Recurrence of Stage I Bladder Cancer." *Urology* 10:6 (1977), 556-561.

114. Ladner, H.A. et al. *Nutrition, Growth & Cancer* (New York: Alan Liss, 1988), 273. Cited in: Quillan, P. *Beating Cancer With Nutrition* (Tulsa, OK: Nutrition Times Press, 1994).

115. Stahelin, H.B. et al. "Cancer, Vitamins and Plasma Lipids. Prospective Basel Study." *Journal of the National Cancer Institute* 73 (1984), 1463-1468. See also: Cameron, E., and L. Pauling. *Cancer and Vitamin C* (Menlo Park, CA: Linus Pauling Institute of Science and Medicine, 1979).

116. Cameron, E.T. et al. "Ascorbic Acid and Cancer: A Review." *Cancer Research* 39 (1979), 663-681.

117. Yonemoto, R.H. "Vitamin C and Immunological Response in Normal Controls and Cancer Patients." *Medico Dialogo* 5 (1979), 23-30.

118. Siegel, B.V., and J.I. Morton. "Vitamin C and the Immune Response." *Experientia* 33 (1977), 393-395.

119. Riordan, D. "Nutrition Therapy for Cancer Patients." Adjuvant Nutrition in Cancer Treatment Symposium. Tampa, Florida (September 30, 1995).

120. Tschetter, L. et al. "A Community-based Study of Vitamin C (Ascorbic Acid)—Therapy in Patients with Advanced Cancer." *Proceedings of the American Society of Clinical Oncology* 2 (1983), 92. See also: Cameron, E., and L. Pauling. "Vitamin C and Cancer." *International Journal of Environmental Studies* 75 (1977), 4538-4542.

121. Veltri, R.W. et al. "L-ascorbic acid (vitamin C) Augmentation of Anticancer Activity of Methoxy-substituted Benzoquinones, Adriamycin, and a Dihydroxyulated Amino Substituted Quinone (DHAQ)." Unpublished. Cited in: Pelton, R., and L. Overholser. *Alternatives in Cancer Therapy* (New York: Fireside/Simon & Schuster, 1994).

122. Koch, C.J., and J.E. Bigalow. "Toxicity Radiation Sensitivity Modification, and Metabolic Effects of Dehydroscorbate and Ascorbate in Mammalian Cells." *Journal of Cell Physiology* 94 (1978), 299-306. See also: Okunieff, P. "Ascorbic Acid: Biologic Functions and Relation to Cancer." Symposium in Bethesda, MD (September 1989). Cited in Pelton, R. and L. Overholser. *Alternatives in Cancer Therapy* (New York: Fireside/Simon & Schuster 1994).

123. Riordan , N.H. et al. "Intravenous Ascorbate as a Tumor Cytotoxic Chemotherapeutic Agent." *Medical Hypotheses* 44:3 (1995), 205.

124. Poydock, M.E. "Effect of Combined Ascorbic Acid and B12 on Survival of Mice with Implanted Ehrlich Carcinoma and L1210 Leukemia." *American Journal of Clinical Nutrition* 54:Suppl 6 (1991), 1261S-1265S.

125. Cameron, E., and L. Pauling. *Proceedings of*

the *National Academy of Sciences* 75:9 (1978), 4538.

126. The Burton Goldberg Group. *Alternative Medicine: The Definitive Guide* (Tiburon, CA: Future Medicine Publishing, 1995), 9.

127. Block, G. "Vitamin C and Cancer Prevention: The Epidemiologic Evidence." *American Journal of Clinical Nutrition* 53 (1991), 270S.

128. Cameron, E. "Protocol for the Use of Vitamin C in the Treatment of Cancer." *Medical Hypotheses* 36 (1991), 190-194.

129. Park, C.H. "Vitamin C in Leukemia and Preleukemia Cell Growth." *Nutrition, Growth and Cancer*, edited by Tryfiates and Prasad. (New York: Alan R. Liss, 1988), 321-330.

130. Good, R.A. et al. "Nutrition, Immunity and Cancer—A Review." *Clinical Bulletin* 9 (1979), 3-12, 63-75.

131. Boik, J. "Conducting Research on Natural Agents: Vitamin D Metabolites." *Cancer and Natural Medicine* (Princeton, MN: Oregon Medical Press, 1995), 181.

132. Martin, Wayne. "Anti-Cancer Effect of Vitamin D." *Townsend Letter for Doctors & Patients* (October 1996), 111.

133. "The Effect of Vitamin E on Immune Responses." *Nutrition Reviews* 45:1 (1987), 27.

134. Benner, S.E. et al. "Regression of Oral Leukoplakia with Alpha-Tocopherol: A Community Clinical Oncology Program Chemoprevention Study." *Journal of the National Cancer Institute* 85:1 (1993), 44-47. Note: The subjects in this study were all in the early stages of oral cancer (premalignant oral leukoplakia lesions).

135. Cook, M.G., and P. McNamara. "Effect of Dietary Vitamin E on Dimethyl-Hydrazine-Induced Colonic Tumors in Mice." *Cancer Research* 40:4 (1980), 1329-1331.

136. Shklar, G. et al. "Regression by Vitamin E of Experimental Oral Cancer." *Journal of the National Cancer Institute* 78:5 (1987), 987-992.

137. Prasad, K.N. et al. "Vitamin E Increases the Growth Inhibitory and Differentiating Effects of Tumor Therapeutic Agents on Neuroblastoma and Glioma Cells in Culture." *Proceedings of the Society for Experimental Biology and Medicine* 164:2 (1980), 158-163.

138. Svingen, B.A. et al. "Vitamin E Deficiency Accentuates Adriamycin Cardiotoxicity." *Cancer Research* 41 (1981), 3395.

139. Myers, C.E. et al. "Effect of Tocopherol and Selenium on Defenses Against Reactive Oxygen Species and Their Effect on Radiation Sensitivity." *Annals of the New York Academy of Sciences* 393 (1982), 419-425.

140. Quillan, P. "Vitamin K." *Beating Cancer With Nutrition* (Tulsa, OK: Nutrition Times Press, 1994), 216-217.

141. Good, R.A. et al. "Nutrition, Immunity and Cancer: A Review." *Clinical Bulletin* 9 (1979), 3-12, 63-75.

142. Boik, J. "Zinc: Dietary Micronutrients and Their Effects on Cancer." *Cancer and Natural Medicine* (Princeton, MN: Oregon Medical Press, 1995), 147.

143. Gershwin, M.E. et al. "The Potential Impact of Nutritional Factors on Immunological Responsiveness." *Nutrition and Immunity* (Orlando, FL: Academic Press, 1985), 222.

Chapter 5: Herbs for Cancer

1. Duke, J.A. "Weeds? Or Wonder Drugs?" *Organic Gardening* (July/August 1994), 38-40.

2. Tyler, V.E. "Significant Anticancer Herbs." *Herbs of Choice: The Therapeutic Use of Phytomedicinals* (New York: Pharmaceutical Products Press, 1994), 178-179.

3. Pisha, E. et al. "Discovery of Betulinic Acid as a Selective Inhibitor of Human Melanoma that Functions by Induction of Apoptosis." *Nature Medicine* 10 (1995), 1046-1051.

4. Centofanti, M. "Birch Bark Has Anticancer Bite." *Science News* 148 (1995), 231. Original report appeared in *Nature Medicine* (October 1995).

5. Cook, B. "Tree of Life Helps in Advanced Cancer." *International Journal of Alternative & Complementary Medicine* (January 1992), 23.

6. "Cancer Patients Should Eat Pineapples." *International Journal of Alternative & Complementary Medicine* (January 1992), 23. Original report appeared in *Planta Medica* 54:5 (1988), 377-378.

7. Duke, J.A. "Weeds? Or Wonder Drugs?" *Organic Gardening* (July/August 1994), 39.

8. Tenney, L. "Gotu kola." *Today's Herbal Health* (Provo, UT: Woodland Books, 1992), 78.

9. Babu, T.D. et al. "Cytotoxic and Antitumor Properties of Certain Taxa of Umbelliferae with Special Reference to Centella asiatica." *Journal of Ethnopharmacology* 48 (1995), 53-57.

10. Haag, J.D. et al. "Enhanced Inhibition of Protein Isoprenylation and Tumor Growth by Perillyl Alcohol, an Hydroxylated Analog of d-limonene." *Proceedings of the American Association of Cancer Research* 33 (1992), 524.

11. Brown, R. *Bee Hive Product Bible* (Garden City Park, NY: Avery Publishing, 1994), 47.

12. Ibid., 116-117.

13. Ibid., 49.

14. Johnson, T. "Herbs for Cancer." Personal communications (1996).

15. Chang, M. *Preface to Anticancer Medicinal Herbs* (Hunan Changsha, China: Hunan Science and Technology Press, 1992), ii.

16. Zhuang, H. et al. "Effects of Radix Slaviae Mlltlorrhizae Extract Injection on Survival of Allogenic Heart Transplantation." *Journal of Traditional Chinese Medicine* 10:4 (1990), 276-281.

17. Liu, F. "Application of Traditional Chinese Drugs in Comprehensive Treatment of Primary Liver Cancer." *Journal of Traditional Chinese Medicine* 10:1 (1990), 54-60. This study showed that TCM diagnosis could enhance the prognosticative accuracy of survival of patients with primary liver cancer and that Chinese herbal medicine enabled patients to recuperate to a point where they could successfully undergo surgery and complete regimens of chemotherapy, thus prolonging survival.

18. Dharmananda, S. *Chinese Herbal Therapies for Immune Disorders* (Portland, OR: Institute for Traditional Medicine, 1988), 9-25.

19. "Special Hearing on Alternative Medicine." Report of the Subcommittee of the Committee on Appropriations, U.S. Senate (June 24, 1993), 65.

20. Liu, X.Y., and N.Q. Ang. "Effect of Liu Wei Di Huang or Jin Gui Shen Qi Decoction as an Adjuvant Treatment in Small Cell Lung Cancer." *Chung Hsi I Chieh Ho Tsa Chih* 10 (1990), 720-722.

21. Wang, R.L. et al. "Potentiation by Rabdosia rubescens on Chemotherapy of Advanced Esophageal Carcinoma." *Chung Hua Chung Liu Tsa Chih* 8 (1986), 297-299.

22. Cheng, J.H. "Clinical Study on Prevention and Treatment to Chemotherapy Caused Nephrotoxicity with Jian-pi Yi-qi Li-shui." *Chung-Kuo Chung Hsi Chieh Ho Tsa Chih* 14:6 (1994), 331-333.

23. You, J.S. et al. "Combined Effects of Chuling (Polyporous umbellatus) Extract and Mitomycin C on Experimental Liver Cancer." *American Journal of Chinese Medicine* 22:1 (1994), 19-28.

24. Ji, Y.B. et al. "Effects of buzhong yiqi Decoction on the Anticancer Activity and Toxicity Induced by Cyclophosphamide." *Chung Kuo Chung Yao Tsa Chih* 14 (1989), 48-51.

25. Lin, P.F. "Antitumor Effect of Actinidia Chinensis Polysaccharide on Murine Tumor." *Chung Hua Chung Liu Tsa Chih* 10 (1988), 441-444. See also: Franz, G. "Polysaccharides in Pharmacy: Current Application and Future Concepts." *Planta Medica* 55 (1989), 493-497.

26. Chang, M. *Preface to Anticancer Medicinal Herbs* (Hunan Changsha, China: Hunan Science and Technology Press, 1992), ii.

27. Konoshima T. et al. "Antitumor Promoting Activities and Inhibitory Effects on Epstein Barr Virus Activation of Shi-un-kou and Its Constituents." *Yakugaku Zasshi* 109 (1989), 843-846.

28. Okamoto, T. et al. "Clinical Effects of Juzen-taiho-to on Immunologic and Fatty Metabolic States in Postoperative Patients with Gastrointestinal Cancer." *Gan To Kagaku Ryoho* 16 (1989), 1533-1537. See also: Kiyohara, H. et al. "Characterization of Mitogenic Pectic Polysaccharides from Kampo Medicine Juzen-taiho-to." *Planta Medica* 57 (1991), 254-259.

29. Nagatsu, Y. et al. "Modification of Macrophage Functions by Shosaikoto (Kampo Medicine) Leads to Enhancement of Immune Response." *Chemical and Pharmaceutical Bulletin* 37 (1989), 1540-1542.

30. Ning, C. et al. "Therapeutic Effects of Jian Pi Yi Shen Prescription on the Toxicity Reactions of Postoperative Chemotherapy in Patients with Advanced Gastric Carcinoma." *Journal of Traditional Chinese Medicine* 8:2 (1988), 113-116.

31. Guo, Z.H. et al. "Chinese Herb Destagnation Series 1: Combination of Radiation with Destagnation in the Treatment of Nasopharyngeal Carcinoma (NPC), a Prospective Randomized Trial on 188 Cases." *International Journal of Radiation Oncology, Biology and Physics* 16 (1989), 297-300. See also: Sun, Y. "The Role of Traditional Chinese Medicine in Supportive Care of Cancer Patients." *Recent Results in Cancer Research* 108 (1988), 327-344.

32. Shiu, W.T.C. et al. "A Clinical Study of PSP on Peripheral Blood Counts during Chemotherapy." *Phytotherapy Research* 6 (1992), 217-218.

33. Sharma, H.M. et al. "Marharish Ayur-veda: Modern Insights into Ancient Medicine." *Journal of the American Medical Association* 265 (1991), 2633-2634. Published erratum appears in *Journal of the American Medical Association* 266 (1991), 798.

34. Prasad, G.C. "The Use of Ayurvedic Drugs in the Management of Cancer." *World Congress on*

Cancer. Sydney, Australia (April 1994), 315-319.

35. "Greater Health and Longevity: Chlorella, the Green Algae Superfood, May be the Answer." *Alternative Medicine Digest* 12 (1996), 56.

36. Wilner, J. "Suggested Nutritional Supplements: Algae." *The Cancer Solution* (Boca Raton, FL: Peltec Publishing, 1994).

37. Beim, A. "Algae May Curb Mouth Cancer." *American Health* (June 1996), 29.

38. Yamamoto, I. et al. "Antitumor Effect of Seaweeds." *Japanese Journal of Experimental Medicine* 44 (1974), 543-546.

39. Yamamoto, I. et al. "Antitumor Effect of Seaweeds." *Japanese Journal of Experimental Medicine* 47:3 (1977), 133-140.

40. Teas, J. et al. "Dietary Seaweed (Laminaria) and Mammary Carcinogenesis in Rats." *Cancer Research* 44:7 (1984), 2758.

41. Tanaka, Y. et al. "Studies on Inhibition of Intestinal Absorption of Radioactive Strontium." *Canadian Medical Association Journal* 99 (1968), 169-175.

42. Ibid.

43. "The Super Vitamin: 2 Ways to Go Green." *Alternative Medicine Digest* 11 (1996), 58-59.

44. Ibid.

45. Kupchan, S.M., and A. Karim. "Tumor Inhibitors. Aloe Emodin: Antileukemic Principle Isolated from Rhamnus Frangula L." *Lloydia* 39 (1976), 223-224.

46. Ralamboranto, L. et al. "Immunomodulating Properties of an Extract Isolated and Partially Purified from Aloe Vahombe. Study of Antitumoral Properties and Contribution to the Chemical Nature and Active Principle." *Archives de l'Institut Pasteur de Madagascar* 50 (1982), 227-256.

47. Grivel, N.V., and V.G. Pashinskii. "Antimetastatic Properties of Aloe Juice." *Voprosy Onkologii* 32 (1986), 38-40.

48. Harris, C. et al. "Efficacy of Acemannan in Treatment of Canine and Feline Spontaneous Neoplasms." *Molecular Biotherapy* 3:2 (1991), 207-213. Peng, S.Y. et al. "Decreased Mortality of Norman Murine Sarcoma in Mice Treated with Immunomodulator, Acemannan." *Molecular Biotherapy* 3:2 (1991), 79-87.

49. Moss, R.W. *The Cancer Industry: Unraveling the Politics* (New York: Paragon House, 1989).

50. Rubin, D. "Dosage Levels for Laetrile." *Choice* 3:6 (1977), 8-9.

51. Tatsumura, T. et al. "Antitumor Effect of 4, 6 ben-zylidene-D-glucose in Clinical Studies." *Proceedings of the Annual Meeting of the American Society of Clinical Oncologists* 6

(1987), A559.

52. Kochi, M. et al. "Antitumor Activity of Benzaldehyde Derivative." *Cancer Treatment Report* 69:5 (1985), 533-537.

53. Zhang, Z.L. et al. "Hepatoprotective Effects of Astragalus Root." *Journal of Ethnopharmacology* 30 (1990), 145-149.

54. Chan, T. "Ancient Remedies Clues to Cancer Cures." *Health Freedom News* 3:5 (1984), 12-13.

55. Tani, T. et al. "Biphasic Action of Rikkunshi-to and Hochu-ekki-to (GAC)." *Japanese Journal of Allergy* 37:2 (1988), 107-114.

56. Sugiyama, K. et al. "Protective Effects of Kampo Medicine Against Cis-diaminedischloroplatinum Induced Nephrotoxicity and Bone Marrow Toxicity in Mice." *Wakan Iyaku Gakkaishi* 10:1 (1993), 76-85.

57. Yang, Y.Z. et al. "Effect of *Astragalus mem-branaceus* on Natural Killer Cell Activity and Induction of Alpha- and Gamma-Interferon in Patients with Coxsackie B Viral Myocarditis." *Chinese Medical Journal* 103:4 (1990), 304-307.

58. U.S. Patent No. 4,844,901. Oxindole alkaloids, from uña de gato (cat's claw), have immune-stimulating properties.

59. "Uña de Gato: Its Therapeutic Characteristics, History and Clinical Effectiveness." *Wellness Advocate* 5:1 (1995), 1-5.

60. Ibid.

61. Lersch, C. et al. "Simulation of Immunocompetent Cells in Patients with Gastrointestinal Tumors During an Experimental Therapy with Low-dose Cyclophophamide, Thymostimulin, and Echinacea purpurea Extract (Echinacin)." *Tumordiagen Therapy* 13 (1992), 115-120. Cited in: Werbach, M., and M. Murray. *Botanical Influences on Illness* (Tarzana, CA: Third Line Press, 1994), 94-95.

62. Lersch, C. et al. "Stimulation of the Immune Response in Outpatients with Hepatocellular Carcinomas by Low Doses of Cyclophopsphamide (LDCY), *Echinacea pur-purea* Extracts (Echinacin) and Thymostimulin." *Arch Geschhwulstforsch* 60:5 (1990), 379-383.

63. Luettig, B. et al. "Macrophage Activation by the Polysaccharide Arabinogalactan Isolated from Plant Cell Cultures of Echinacea purpurea." *Journal of the National Cancer Institute* 81:9 (1989), 669-675.

64. Thomas, R. *The Essiac Report* (Los Angeles: Alternative Treatment Information Network, 1993).

65. Moss, R. "Essiac." *Cancer Therapy: The Independent Consumer's Guide* (New York: Equinox Press, 1992), 146-147. Moss reviews the technical cancer-related research on Essiac; many substances isolated from the herbs in Essiac show specific kinds of anti-cancer activity.

66. Chen, Q.H. et al. "Studies on Chinese Rhubarb XII. Effect of Anthraquinone Derivatives on the Respiration and Glycolysis of Ehrlich Ascites Carcinoma Cells." *Acta Pharmaceutica Sinica* 15 (1980), 65-70. See also: Kawai, K. et al. "A Comparative Study on Cytotoxicities and Biochemical Properties of Anthraquinone Mycotoxins Emodin and Skyrin from Penicillium Islandium Sopp." *Toxicology Letters* 20 (1984), 155-160.

67. Lu, M., and Q.H. Chen. "Biochemical Study of Chinese Rhubarb XXIX. Inhibitory Effects of Anthraquinone Derivatives on P338 Leukemia in Mice." *Journal of China Pharmacology University* 20 (1989), 155-157.

68. Morita, K. et al. "A Desmutagenic Factor Insolated from Burdock (*Arctium lappa linne*)." *Mutation Research* 129 (1984), 25-31.

69. Walters, R. "Essiac." *Options: The Alternative Cancer Therapy Book* (Garden City, NY: Avery Publishing, 1993), 110.

70. Yoshida, M. et al. "The Effect of Quercetin on Cell Cycle Progression and Growth of Human Gastric Cancer Cells." *FEBS Letters* 260 (1990), 10-13.

71. Morazzoni, P., and S. Malandrino. "Anthocyanins and Their Aglycons as Scavengers of Free Radicals and Antilipoperoxidant Agents." *Pharmacology Rees Commission* 20:2 Suppl (1988), 254. See also: Meunier, M.T. et al. "Free Radical Scavenger Activity of Procyanidolic Oligomers and Anthocyanocides with Respect to Superoxide Anion and Lipid Peroxidation." *Plantes Medicinales et Phytotherapies* XXIII (1989), 267.

72. Lau, B.H.S. et al. "Allium sativum (Garlic) and Cancer Prevention." *Nutrition Research* 10 (1990), 937-948.

73. Lin, R.S. *Garlic and Health: Recent Advances in Research* (Irvine, CA: International Academy of Health and Fitness, 1994), 23.

74. Bennett, S.A. et al. "Platelet Activating Factor, an Endogenous Mediator of Inflammation, Induces Phenotypic Transformation of Rat Embryo Cells." *Carcinogenesis* 14:7 (1993), 1289-1296.

75. Nigam, S. et al. "Elevated Plasma Levels of Platelet-activating Factor (PAF) in Breast Cancer Patients with Hypercalcemia." *Journal of Lipid Mediators and Cell Signalling* 1:6 (1989), 323-328. See also: Pitton, C. et al. "Presence of PAF-acether in Human Breast Carcinoma: Relation to Axillary Lymph Node Metastasis." *Journal of the National Cancer Institute* 81:17 (1989), 1298-1302.

76. Wilford, J.N. "Ancient Tree Yields Secrets of Potent Healing Substance." *The New York Times* (March 1, 1988), C3. Cited in: Murray, F. *Ginkgo Biloba* (New Canaan, CT: Keats Publishing, 1993).

77. Rong, Y. et al. "*Ginkgo Biloba* Attenuates Oxidative Stress in Macrophages and Endothelial Cells." *Free Radical Biology & Medicine* 20:1 (1996), 121-127.

78. *Ginkgo Biloba Extract (EGb 761) in Perspective* (Auckland, New Zealand: ADIS Press, 1990), 3. Cited in: Murray, F. *Ginkgo Biloba* (New Canaan, CT: Keats Publishing, 1993), 37-38.

79. Hu, S.Y. "The Genus Panax (Ginseng) in Chinese Medicine." *Economic Botany* 30:1 (1976), 11-28.

80. Hou, J.P. "Chemical Constituents of Ginseng Plants." *American Journal of Chinese Medicine* 5:2 (1977), 123-145.

81. Boik, J. "Effect of *Panax Ginseng* (ren shen)." *Cancer and Natural Medicine* (Princeton, MN: Oregon Medical Press, 1995), 73.

82. Zhang, D. et al. "Ginseng Extract Scavenges Hydroxyl Radical and Protects Unsaturated Fatty Acids from Decomposition Caused by Iron-mediated Lipid Peroxidation." *Free Radical Biology and Medicine* 20:1 (1996), 145-150.

83. Ng, T.B., and H.W. Yeung. "Scientific Basis of the Therapeutic Effects of Ginseng." *Folk Medicine: The Art and the Science*, edited by Steiner, R.P. (Washington, DC: American Chemical Society, 1986), 139-151. See also: Zhang, D. et al. "Ginseng Extract Scavenges Hydroxyl Radical and Protects Unsaturated Fatty Acids from Decomposition Caused by Iron-mediated Lipid Peroxidation." *Free Radical Biology & Medicine* 20:1 (1996), 145-150.

84. Yun, Taik-koo et al. "Anticarcinogenic Effect of Long-term Oral Administration of Red Ginseng on Newborn Mice Exposed to Various Chemical Carcinogens." *Cancer Detection and Prevention* 6 (1983), 515-525.

85. Tode, T. et al. "Inhibitory Effects of Oral Administration of Ginsenoside Rh2 on Tumor Growth in Nude Mice Bearing Serous Cyst Adenocarcinoma of the Human Ovary." *Acta*

Obstetrica et Gynaecologica Japonica 45 (1993), 1275-1282.

86. Yun, Taik-koo, and Soo-yong Choi. "Preventive Effect of Ginseng Intake against Various Human Cancers: A Case-control Study on 1987 Pairs." *Cancer Epidemiology, Biomarkers & Prevention* 4 (1995), 401-408.

87. Kim, J.Y. et al. "Panax Ginseng as a Potential Immunomodulator: Studies in Mice." *Immunopharmacology and Immunotoxicology* 12:2 (1990), 257-276.

88. Meunier, M.T. et al. "Free Radical Scavenger Activity of Procyanidolic Oligomers and Anthocyanocides with Respect to Superoxide Anion and Lipid Peroxidation." *Plantes Medicinales et Phytotherapies* XXIII (1989), 267.

89. Chisaka, T. et al. Chemical and Pharmaceutical Bulletin (1988). Cited in: Wilner, J. "Green Tea." *The Cancer Solution* (Boca Raton, FL: Peltec Publishing, 1994), 75.

90. Bu-Abbas, A. et al. "Marked Antimutagenic Potential of Aqueous Green Tea Extracts: Mechanism of Action." *Mutagenesis* 9 (1994), 325-331.

91. Mukhtar, H. et al. "Green Tea and Skin—Anticarcinogenic Effects." *Journal of Investigative Dermatology* 102 (1994), 3-7.

92. Klaunig, J.E. "Chemopreventive Effects of Green Tea Components on Hepatic Carcinogenesis." *Preventative Medicine* 21 (1992), 510-519. See also: Gao, Y.T. et al. "Reduced Risk of Esophageal Cancer Associated with Green Tea Consumption." *Journal of the National Cancer Institute* 86 (1994), 855-858.

93. "The Role of Haelan Nutrition in Enhancing the Anti-cancer Effect of Chemotherapeutic Drugs in Mice with HAC Cell Liver Cancer." Report #110. *The Therapeutic of Soybean Phytochemicals* (Metairie, LA: U.S. Research Reports, 1995).

94. "Gastric Cancer in vivo Study." Report #112. "Anti-Lipid Peroxidation and Improvement of Lung Function." Report #108. "Relieving Leukopenia in Liver Cancer." Report #109. *The Therapeutic of Soybean Phytochemicals* (Metairie, LA: U.S. Research Reports, 1995).

95. "A Clinical Study of Haelan 851 Concentrated Nutritional Oral Liquid in Supporting Healthy Energy and Lowering Toxic Effects of Radiation and Chemotherapy on Cancer Patients." Report #103. *The Therapeutic of Soybean Phytochemicals* (Metairie, LA: U.S. Research Reports, 1995).

96. Walker, Morton. "Anticancer Attributes of Modified Citrus Pectin." *Townsend Letter for Doctors & Patients* (August/ September 1996), 85.

97. Office of Technology Assessment. *Unconventional Cancer Treatments* (Washington, DC: U.S. Government Printing Office, 1990).

98. Kazuyoshi, M. et al. "A Desmutagenic Factor Isolated from Burdock. *Arctium lappa linne.*" *Mutation Research* 129 (1984), 25-31.

99. Dhawan, B.N. et al. "Screening of Indian Plants for Biological Activity: VI." *Indian Journal of Experimental Biology* 15 (1977), 208. See also: Hoshi, A. et al. "Anti-tumor Activity of Berberine Derivatives." *Japanese Journal of Cancer Research* 67 (1976), 321-325.

100. Messina, M.J. et al. "Soy Intake and Cancer Risk: A Review of in vitro and in vivo Data." *Nutrition and Cancer* 21:2 (1994), 113-131.

101. Boik, J. "Conducting Research on Natural Agents: A Summary of Effects of *Glycyrrhiza uralensis.*" *Cancer and Natural Medicine* (Princeton, MN: Oregon Medical Press, 1995), 179.

102. Pierson, H. "Designer Foods and Cancer." World Congress on Cancer. Sydney, Australia (April 1994), 25.

103. Austin, S. et al. "Long-term Follow-up of Cancer Patients Using Contreras, Hoxsey, and Gerson Therapies." *Journal of Naturopathic Medicine* 5:1 (1994), 74-76. Given the small size of this study, and the fact that many different cancers were involved, at different stages and with different treatments used for each cancer, it is impossible to draw statistically meaningful conclusions from this study. However, the results at least suggest a benefit for cancer patients receiving the Hoxsey formula. In no way should the reader assume that the Gerson or Contreras clinics are failing to help patients based on the results of this study. Remember, these were advanced-stage cancer patients, many of whom had undergone conventional therapies first.

104. Office of Technology Assessment. *Unconventional Cancer Treatments* (Washington, DC: U.S. Government Printing Office, 1990), 83. Iscador with copper is used for primary tumors of the liver, gallbladder, stomach, and kidneys; Iscador with mercury is used to treat tumors of the intestine and lymphatic system; Iscador with silver is used to treat cancers of the breast and urogenital tract; and Iscador without any added metals is used to treat most other cancers. The OTA report notes that this form, *Viscum album,* differs

markedly from mistletoe found in the U.S.

105. Kiene, H. "Clinical Studies on Mistletoe Therapy for Cancerous Diseases: A Review." *Therapeutikon* 3:6 (1989), 347-350.

106. Hajito, T., and C. Lanzrein. "Natural Killer and Antibody-Dependent Cell-mediated Cytotoxicity and Large Granular Lymphocyte Frequencies in Viscum album-Treated Breast Cancer Patients." *Oncology* 43 Suppl 1 (1986), 93-97. See also: Hajito, T. "Immunomodulatory Effects of Iscador: A Viscum album Preparation." *Oncology* 43 Suppl 1 (1986), 51-65.

107. Nienhaus, J. "Tumor Inhibition and Thymus Stimulation with Mistletoe Preparations." *Elemente Naturowissenschaft* 13 (1970), 45-54. See also: Salzer, G., and H. Muller. "Local Treatment of Malignant Pleural Effusions with Mistletoe Preparation Iscador." *Praxix Pneumologia* 32 (1978), 721-729. See also: Linder, M. "Mistletoe Preparations Prevent Changes in Copper Metabolism." American Association of Cancer Researchers, Annual Meeting. Saint Louis, Missouri (1982).

108. Leroi, R. "Fundamentals of Mistletoe Therapy." *Krebsgeschehen* 5 (1979), 145-146. Kiene, H. "Clinical Studies on Mistletoe Therapy for Cancerous Diseases: A Review." *Therapeutikon* 3:6 (1989), 347-533.

109. Studies on clinical effects of Iscador were all cited in *Journal of Anthroposophical Medicine* 11:2 (1994), 20-26; and in Heiligtag, R. *Anthroposophical Medicine and Therapies for Cancer* (Spring Valley, NY: Mercury Press, 1994).

110. *Unconventional Cancer Treatments; Herbal Treatments: Mistletoe* (Washington, DC: Office of Technology Assessment, U.S. Congress, 1990), 84.

111. Egert, D., and N. Beuscher. "Studies on Antigen Specificity of Immunoreactive Arabinogalactan Proteins Extracted from *Baptisia tinctoria* and *Echinacea purpurea*." *Planta Medica* 58:2 (1992), 163-165.

112. Ibid.

113. D'Adamo, P. "Larch Arabinogalactan is a Novel Immune Modulator." *Townsend Letter for Doctors & Patients* (April 1996), 42-46.

114. Kiyohara, H. et al. "Relationship between Structure and Activity of an Anti-complementary Arabinogalactan from the Roots of *Angelica Autiloba Kitagawa*." *Carbohydrate Research* 193 (1989), 193-200.

115. Gonda, R. et al. "Arabinogalactan Core Structure and Immunological Activities of Ukonana C, an Acidic Polysaccharide from the Rhizome of *Curcuma longa*." *Biological & Pharmaceutical Bulletin* 16:3 (1993), 235-238.

116. D'Adamo, P. "Larch Arabinogalactan is a Novel Immune Modulator." *Townsend Letter for Doctors & Patients* (April 1996), 42-46.

117. Hagmar, B. et al. "Arabinogalactan Blockade of Experimental Metastases to Liver by Murine Hepatoma." *Invasion Metastasis* 11:6 (1991), 348-355. See also: Beuth, J. et al. "Inhibition of Liver Metastasis in Mice by Blocking Hepatocyte Lectins with Arabinogalactan Infusions and D-galactose." *Journal of Cancer Research and Clinical Oncology* 113:1 (1987), 51-55.

118. Beuth, J. et al. "Inhibition of Liver Tumor Cell Colonization in Two Animal Tumor Models by Lectin Blocking with D-galactose or Arabinogalactan." *Clinical and Experimental Metastasis* 6:2 (1988), 115-120.

119. Hauer, J., and F.A. Anderer. "Mechanism of Stimulation of Human Natural Killer Cytotoxicity by Arabinogalactan from Larix Occidentalis." *Cancer Immunology and Immunotherapy* 36 (1993), 237-244.

120. Note: In some of the blood donors, the lack of NK activity was likely traced to an increase in a "bad eicosanoid" (PGE2) from immune cells (monocytes). This undesirable effect could perhaps be inhibited by fish oils and certain other nontoxic agents, though this has yet to be studied.

121. Chang, R. Personal communications (1995). New York-based Raymond Chang, M.D., formerly at Memorial Sloan-Kettering Cancer Center, is an expert on medicinal mushrooms.

122. Adachi, K. et al. "Potentiation of Host-mediated Antitumor Activity in Mice by Beta-Glucan Obtained from *Grifola frondosa* (Maitake)." *Chemical & Pharmacological Bulletin* 35:1 (1987), 262-270.

123. Nanba, H. "Maitake Mushroom: Immune Therapy to Prevent Cancer Growth and Metastasis." *Explore* 6:1 (1995), 17.

124. Nanba, H. "Antitumor Activity of Orally Administered 'D-fraction' from Maitake Mushroom (*Grifola frondosa*)." *Journal of Naturopathic Medicine* 1:4 (1993), 10-15.

125. Rao, K.V. "Quinone Natural Products. Streptonigrin (NSC-45383) and Lapachol (NSC-11905) Structure-activity Relationships." *Cancer Chemotherapy Reports* (Part 2) 4:4 (1974), 11-17. See also: Rao, K.V. et al. "Recognition and Evaluation of Lapachol as an Antitumor Agent." *Cancer Research* 28 (1968), 1952-1954.

126. Santana, C.F. et al. "Preliminary Observations with the Use of Lapachol in Human Patients Bearing Malignant Neoplasms." *Revista de Instituto de Antibioticos* 20 (1980/1981), 61-68. Cited in: Werbach, M.R., and M.T. Murray. *Botanical Influences on Illness* (Tarzana, CA: Third Line Press, 1994).

127. Linardi, M.D.C. et al. "A Lapachol Derivative Active against Mouse Lymphocyte Leukemia P-388." *Journal of Medicinal Chemistry* 18:11 (1975), 1159-1162.

128. Block, J.B. et al. "Early Clinical Studies with Lapachol (NSC-11905)." *Cancer Chemotherapy Reports* (Part 2) 4:4 (1978), 27-28.

129. Zollner, T.M. et al. "Induction of NK-like Activity in T cells by ILs/anti-CD3 Is Linked to Expression of a New Antitumor Receptor with Specificity for Acetylated Mannose." *Anticancer Research* 13:4 (1993), 923-930.

130. Zhu, H.G. et al. "Activation of Human Monocyte/Macrophage Cytotoxicity by IL-2/IFN Gamma is Linked to Increased Expression of an Antitumor Receptor with Specificity for Acetylated Mannose." *Immunology Letters* 38:2 (1993), 111-119.

131. Pienta, K.J. et al. "Inhibition of Spontaneous Metastases in a Rat Prostate Cancer Model by Oral Administration of Modified Citrus Pectin." *Journal of the National Cancer Institute* 87:5 (1995), 348-353.

132. "Cardui Mariae Fructus: Silybum marianum." Monograph of the German Health Authorities (BGA). *Bundesanzeiger* 13:3 (1986).

133. Hikino, H., and Y. Kiso. *Natural Products for Liver Disease*, edited by Wagner, H. (New York: Academic Press, 1988). See also: *Economic and Medicinal Plant Research* 2 (1988), 39-72.

134. Feher, H. et al. "Hepatoprotective Activity of Silymarin Therapy in Patients with Chronic Alcoholic Liver Disease." *Orvosi Hetilap* 130 (1990), 51.

135. Nagabhushan, M., and S.V. Bhide. "Curcumin as an Inhibitor of Cancer." *Journal of the American College of Nutrition* 11:2 (1992), 192-198.

136. Polasa, K. et al. "Effect of Turmeric on Urinary Mutagens in Smokers." *Mutagen* 7:2 (1992), 107-109.

137. Azuine, M.A., and S.V. Bhide. "Protective Single/Combined Treatment with Betel Leaf and Turmeric Against Methyl (acetoxymmethyl) Nitrosamine-induced Hamster Oral Carcinogenesis." *International Journal of Cancer* 51:3 (1992), 412-415.

138. Kakar, S.S., and D. Roy. "Curcumin Inhibits TPA Induced Expression of C-fos, C-jun and C-myc Proto-oncogene Messenger RNAs in Mouse Skin." *Cancer Letters* 87:1 (1995), 85-89.

139. Kuttan, R. et al. "Turmeric and Curcumin as Topical Agents in Cancer Therapy." *Tumori* 73 (1987), 29-31.

140. Nagabhushan, M. and S.V. Bhide. "Curcumin as an Inhibitor of Cancer." *Journal of the American College of Nutrition* 11:2 (1992), 192-198.

Chapter 6: The New Cancer Pharmacology

1. The exception to this statement concerns the use of hormones, which in any case may be deemed a different form of therapy.

2. Reich, R., and J. Metcalf. *Dealing with Side-Effects: The Facts About Chemotherapy* (Mount Vernon, NY: Consumer Reports Books, 1991), 161.

3. Greenwald, H. "Cancer Treatment: The Industry of Hope." *Who Survives Cancer?* (Berkeley, CA: University of California Press, 1992), 46.

4. Abel, U. *Cytostatic Therapy of Advanced Epithelial Tumors: A Critique* (Stuggart, Germany: Hippocrates Verlag, 1990).

5. Powles, T.J. "Failure of Chemotherapy to Prolong Survival in a Group of Patients with Metastatic Breast Cancer." *The Lancet* (March 15 1980), 580.

6. Lucien, I. *Conquering Cancer* (New York: Random House, 1978), 95.

7. Lazlo, J. *Understanding Cancer* (New York: Harper and Row, 1987).

8. Schmahl, D. "Experimental Development of Anticancer Drugs—Problems and Objectives, Strategies and Results." *Current Cancer Research* (New York: Springer, 1989), 157-243.

9. Ibid.

10. Eidem, William Kelley. *The Man Who Cures Cancer* (Bethesda, MD: Be Well Books, 1996).

11. Pace, J.C. "Oral Ingestion of Encapsulated Ginger and Reported Self-care Actions for the Relief of Chemotherapy-Associated Nausea and Vomiting." *Dissertation Abstracts International* 8 (1987), 3297.

12. Kolata, G. "New Finding Offers Insights into How Cancer Develops: Why Tumors Resist Chemotherapy and Radiation." *The New York Times* (January 4, 1996).

13. Greenwald, H. "Cancer Treatment: The Industry of Hope." *Who Survives Cancer?* (Berkeley, CA: University of California Press, 1992), 45.

14. Abel, U. *Cytostatic Therapy of Advanced Epithelial Tumors: A Critique* (Stuggart, Germany: Hippocrates Verlag, 1990).

15. Silberstein, S. "German Biostatistician Cites Chemotherapy's Failures." *Health News & Views* 1:2 (1992), 1.

16. Malins, D.C. et al. "Progression of Human Breast Cancer to the Metastatic Stage is Linked to Hydroxyl Radical Induced DNA Damage." *Proceedings of the National Academy of Sciences* 93:6 (1996), 2557-2563.

17. Lockwood, K. et al. "Apparent Partial Remission of Breast Cancer in "High Risk" Patients Supplemented with Nutritional Antioxidants, Essential Fatty Acids and Co-enzyme Q10." *Molecular Aspects of Medicine* 15 (1994), 231-240.

18. Lamm, D.L. et al. "Megadose Vitamins in Bladder Cancer: A Double-blind Clinical Trial." *Journal of Urology* 151 (1994), 21-26.

19. Boyar, A.P. et al. "Response to a Diet Low in Total Fat in Women with Postmenopausal Breast Cancer: A Pilot Study." *Nutrition and Cancer* 11 (1988), 3-99.

20. Newberne, P.M., and M. Locniskar. "Roles of Micronutrients in Cancer Prevention: Recent Evidence from the Laboratory." *Progress in Clinical and Biological Research* 346 (1990), 119-134.

21. Ning, C. et al. "Therapeutic Effects of jian pi yi shen Prescription on the Toxicity Reactions of Postoperative Chemotherapy in Patients with Advanced Gastric Carcinoma." *Journal of Traditional Chinese Medicine* 8:2 (1988), 113-116.

22. Guo, Z.H. et al. "Chinese Herb Destagnation Series 1: Combination of Radiation with Destagnation in the Treatment of Nasopharyngeal Carcinoma (NPC), a Prospective Randomized Trial on 188 Cases." *International Journal of Radiation Oncology, Biology and Physics* 16 (1989), 297-300. See also: Sun, Y. "The Role of Traditional Chinese Medicine in Supportive Care of Cancer Patients." *Recent Results in Cancer Research* 108 (1988), 327-344.

23. Shiu, W.T.C. et al. "A Clinical Study of PSP on Peripheral Blood Counts during Chemotherapy." *Phytotherapy Research* 6 (1992), 217-218.

24. Boice, J.D., and L.B. Travis. "Body Wars: Effect of Friendly Fire (Cancer Therapy)." *Journal of the National Cancer Institute* 87:10 (1995), 732-741.

25. Kostler, W. Personal communications (June 1996).

26. Ibid.

27. Brohult, A. "Effect of Alkoxyglycerols on the Frequency of Injuries Following Radiation Therapy for Carcinoma of the Uterine Cervix." *Acta Obstetrica et Gynecologica Scandinavica* 56:4 (1977), 441-448. See also: Brohult A. "Effect of Alkoxyglycerols on the Frequency of Injuries Following Radiation Therapy." *Experientia* 29 (1973), 81-82.

28. Hallgren, B., and S. Larsson. "The Glycerol Ethers in the Liver Oils of Elasmobranch Fish." *Lipid Research* 3 (1962), 31-38.

29. Ibid., 39-43.

30. Berdel, W.E. et al. "Antitumor Action of Alkyl-lysophospholipids." *Anticancer Research* 1:6 (1981), 345-352.

31. Diamoede, L. "Increased Ether Lipid Cytotoxicity by Reducing Membrane Cholesterol Content." *International Journal of Cancer* 49:3 (1991), 409-413.

32. Brohult, A. et al. "Regression of Tumor Growth after Administration of Alkoxyglycerols." *Acta Obstetrica et Gynecologica Scandinavica* 57 (1978), 79-83.

33. Brohult, A. "Alkoxyglycerols and Their Use in Radiation Treatment." *Acta Radiologica* 223 (1963), 7-99.

34. "Burzynski's Antineoplastons Increase Activity of Tumor Suppressor Genes." *Options* 2 (June 1995).

35. Pelton, R., and L. Overholser. "Antineoplastons." *Alternatives in Cancer Therapy* (New York: Simon & Schuster, 1994), 192.

36. Tsuda, H. et al. "The Inhibitor Effect of Antineoplaston A10 on Breast Cancer Transplanted to Athymic Mice and Human Hepatocellular Carcinoma Cell Lines." *Kurume Medical Journal* 37 (1990), 97-104.

37. Wiewel, F. "Burzynski's Antineoplastons Increase Activity of Tumor Suppressor Genes." *Options* 1:4 (1995), 2.

38. Krishnaswamy, M., and K.K. Purushothaman. "Plumbagin: A Study of Its Anticancer, Antibacterial, and Antifungal Properties." *Indian Journal of Experimental Biology* 18 (1980), 876-877. See also: Chandrasekaran, B. et al. "New Methods for Urinary Estimation of Antitumor Compounds Echitamine and Plumbagin." *Indian Journal of Biochemistry and Biophysics* 19 (1982), 48-149.

39. Melo, A.M. et al. "First Observations on the Topical Use of Primin, Plumbagin, and Maytenin in Patients with Skin Cancer." *Revista de Instituto de Antibioticos* 14:1-2 (1974), 9-16.

40. Prudden, J. "The Treatment of Human Cancer with Agents Prepared from Bovine Cartilage." *Journal of Biological Response Modifiers* 4:6 (1985), 590-595.

41. Prudden, J. "Use of Cartilage in Cancer Treatment" Adjuvant Nutrition for Cancer Treatment Symposium. Tampa, Florida (September 30, 1995).

42. Lane, I. William. "Shark Cartilage Therapy Results and Research Today." Physician Information Package. Cartilage Consultants (Spring 1995). Contact LaneLabs at 201-391-8601.

43. Lane, I.W. *Shark Cartilage Update Newsletter* 1:3 (1994), 1.

44. Oikawa, T. et al. "A Novel Angiogenic Inhibitor Derived from Japanese Shark Cartilage. Extraction and Estimation of Inhibitory Activities toward Tumor and Embryonic Angiogenesis." *Cancer Letters* 51 (1990), 181-186.

45. Altman, L. "Tumor Growth Is Controlled by Substance Found in Sharks." *The New York Times* (May 1, 1996).

46. Moss, R. "Cesium and Rubidium." *Cancer Therapy: The Independent Consumer's Guide* (New York: Equinox Press, 1992), 91-95.

47. Sartori, H.E. "Nutrients and Cancer: An Introduction to Cesium Therapy." *Pharmacology, Biochemistry and Behavior* 1 (1984), 7-10.

48. Sartori, H.E. "Cesium Therapy in Cancer Patients." *Pharmacology, Biochemistry and Behavior* 1 (1984), 11-13.

49. Messha, F.S., and D.M. Stocco. "Effect of Cesium and Potassium Salts on Survival of Rats Bearing Novikoff Hepatoma." *Pharmacology, Biochemistry and Behavior* 1 (1984), 31-34.

50. El Domeiri, A. et al. "Effect of Alkali Metalsalts on Sarcoma I in A/J mice." *Journal of Surgical Oncology* 18 (1981), 423-429.

51. Moss, R. "Cesium and Rubidium." *Cancer Therapy: The Independent Consumer's Guide* (New York: Equinox Press, 1992), 91-95.

52. Neulieb, R. "Effects of Oral Intake of Cesium Chloride: A Single Case Report." *Pharmacology, Biochemistry and Behavior* 21 (1984), 15-16.

53. Moss, R.W. "DMSO." *Cancer Therapy: The Independent Consumer's Guide* (New York: Equinox Press, 1992), 301.

54. De la Torre, J.C. "Biological Actions and Medical Applications of Dimethyl Sulfoxide." *Annals of the New York Academy of Sciences* (1983). See also: Spremulli, E.N., and D.L. Dexter. "Polar Solvents: A Novel Class of Antineoplastic Agents." *Journal of Clinical Oncology* 2:3 (1984), 227-241.

55. Toren, A., and G. Rechavi. "What Really Cures in Autologous Bone Marrow Transplantation? A Possible Role for Dimethylsulfoxide." *Medical Hypotheses* 41:6 (1993), 495-498.

56. "DMSO Report." *Urology Times* (April 1987). Cited by: Walters, R. "DMSO Therapy." *Options: The Alternative Cancer Therapy Book* (Garden City Park, NY: Avery Publishing, 1993), 249. Stanley, J.W., and R. Herschler. "Pharmacology of DMSO." *Cryobiology* 23 (1986), 14-27. Pommier, R.F. et al. "Synergistic Cytotoxicity between DMSO and Antineoplastic Agents Against Ovarian Cancer In Vitro." *American Journal of Obstetrics and Gynecology* 159 (1988), 848-852. McCabe, D. et al. "Polar Solvents in the Chemoprevention of Dimethylbenzanthracene-induced Rat Mammary Cancer." *Archives of Surgery* 121 (1986). Volden, D.G. et al. "Inhibition of Methyl-cholanthrene-induced Skin Carcinogenesis in Hairless Mice by Membrane-Labelizing Agent DMSO." *British Journal of Dermatology* 109:225S (1983), 133-136.

57. Marks, P.A., and R.A. Rifkind. "Erythroleukemic Differentiation." *Annual Review of Biochemistry* 47 (1990), 419-448.

58. Wilner, J. "DMSO." *The Cancer Solution* (Boca Raton, FL: Peltec Publishing, 1994), 76.

59. Pommier, R.F. et al. "Cytotoxicity of DMSO and Antineoplastic Combinations Against Human Tumors." *American Journal of Surgery* 155 (1988), 672-676.

60. Walters, R. "DMSO Therapy." *Options: The Alternative Cancer Therapy Book* (Garden City Park, NY: Avery Publishing, 1993), 249.

61. Walker, M. *DMSO—Nature's Healer* (Garden City Park, NY: Avery Publishing, 1993), 177-207.

62. Kuroda, M. et al. "Decreased Serum Levels of Selenium and Glutathione Peroxidase Activity Associated with Aging, Malignancy and Chronic Hemodialysis." *Trace Elements in Medicine* 5:3 (1988), 97-103.

63. Boit, J. "Amino Acids." *Cancer and Natural Medicine* (Princeton, MN: Oregon Medical Press, 1995), 139-140.

64. Palermo, M.S. et al. "Immunomodulation Exerted by Cyclophosphamide is Not Interfered by N-Acetyl-Cysteine." *International Journal of Immunopharmacology* 8:6 (1986), 651-655. See also: Schmitt-Graff, A., and M.E. Scheulen. "Prevention of Adriamycin Cardiotoxicity by Niacin, Isocitrate or N-Acetyl-Cysteine in Mice: A Morphological Study." *Pathology Resident Practice* 181:2 (1986), 168-174. See also: Kim, J.A. et al. "Topical Use of N-Acetyl-Cysteine for Reduction of Skin Reaction to Radiation Therapy." *Seminars in Oncology* 10:Suppl 1 (1983), 86.

65. Filov, V.A. et al. "Results of Clinical Evaluation of

Hydrazine Sulfate." *Voprosy Onkologii* 36:6 (1990), 721-726. See also: Gershanovich, M.L. et al. "Results of Clinical Study of Antitumor Action of Hydrazine Sulfate." *Nutrition and Cancer* 3 (1981), 7-12.

66. Chlebowski, R.T. et al. "Hydrazine Sulfate's Influence on Nutritional Status and Survival in Non-small-cell Lung cancer." *Journal of Clinical Oncology* 8:1 (1990), 9-15. Note: This was a randomized, placebo-controlled clinical trial—the gold standard of modern medical research.

67. Filov, V. et al. "Results of Clinical Evaluation of Hydrazine Sulfate." *Voprosy Onkologii* 36 (1990), 721-726.

68. Pitard, C.E. "Protocol for Combined Immunologic/Pharmacologic Therapy: Indocin." Personal communications with Etienne Callebout, M.D. Knoxville, TN (1996).

69. Pollard, M., and P. Luckert. "Indomethacin Treatment of Rats with Dimethylhydrazine-induced Intestinal Tumors." *Cancer Treatment and Research* 64 (1980), 1323-1327. See also: Kudo, T. et al. "Antitumor Activity of Indomethacin on Methylazoxy-Methanol-Induced Bowel Tumors in Rats." *Gann* 71 (1980), 260-264. See also: Pollard, M., and P. Luckert. "Treatment of Chemically-induced Intestinal Cancers with Indomethacin." *Proceedings of the Society for Experimental Biology and Medicine* 167 (1981), 161-164.

70. Beckman, M.D. "The Latest Buzz on Cancer Cures." *The Natural Way* (June/July 1995), 6.

71. Callebout, E., M.D. Personal communications (1996).

72. Patte, M. "Communication et Information Medicales." Twenty-one case histories in French (April 19, 1996). Contact: LaboLife, La Rambourgere Sainte Marie, 79160, La Chapelle Thireuil, France.

73. Naessens, G. "Béchamp's Microzyma to the Somatid Theory: 714X, a Highly Promising Non-toxic Treatment for Cancer and Other Immune Deficiencies." (Unpublished manuscript.) Symposium. Quebec, Canada (1991).

74. Ibid.

75. Anger, G. et al. "Treatment of Multiple Myeloma with New Cytostatic Agent: Gamma-1-methyl-5-bis-(beta-chloroethyl)-amyino-benzimidazolyl-(2)-butyric Acid Hydrochloride." *Deutsche Medizinische Wochenschrift* 94 (1969), 2495-2500. See also: Finklestine, J.Z. et al. "Unorthodox Therapy for Murine Neuroblastoma with 6-Hydroxydomapine (NSC-233898), Bretylium Tocylate (NSC-62164), Papaverine (NSC-35443), and Butyric Acid (NSC-8415)." *Cancer Chemotherapy Reports* 59 (1975), 571-574.

76. Marks, P.A., and R.A. Rifkind. "Differentiating Factors." *Biologic Therapy of Cancer*, edited by DeVita, V.T. et al. (Philadelphia: J.B. Lippincott, 1991).

77. Freeman, J.H. "Effects of Differing Concentrations of Sodium Butyrate on 1,2-Dimethylhydrazine-Induced Rat Intestinal Neoplasia." *Gastroenterology* 91 (1986), 596-602.

78. Pitard, C.E. "Protocol for Combined Immunologic/Pharmacologic Therapy." Personal communications to Etienne Callebout, M.D. Knoxville, TN (1996).

79. Pitard, C.E. "Cancer Combination Therapy Utilizing Licensed, Low-cost, Effective and Universally Available Members of That Class of Biologicals and Biological Response Modifiers Constituting the Fourth Conventional Modality of Cancer Treatment." University of Tennessee School of Medicine. Unpublished manuscript (1987), 1-18.

80. Esber, H.J. et al. "Specific and Nonspecific Immune Resistance Enhancement Activity of Staphage Lysate." *Journal of Immunopharmacology* 3 (1981), 79-92. Aoke, T. et al. "Staphage Lysate and Lentinan as Immunomodulators and Immunopotentiators in Clinical and Experimental Systems." *Augmenting Agents in Cancer Therapy*, edited by Hirsh, E.M. et al. (New York: Raven Press, 1981), 101-111.

81. Tutton, P.J., and D.H. Barkla. "Cell Proliferation in Dimethylhydrazine-Induced Colonic Adenocarcinomata Following Cytotoxic Drug Treatment." *Virchows Archiv A: Pathological Anatomy and Histology* 28 (1978), 151-156.

82. Hast, R. et al. "Cimetidine as an Immune Response Modifier." *Medical Oncology and Tumor Pharmacotherapy* 6:1 (1989), 111-113.

83. Brockmeyer, N.H. et al. "Cimetidine and the Immuno-Response in Healthy Volunteers." *Journal of Investigative Dermatology* 93 (1989), 757-761.

84. Pitard, C.E. "Protocol for Combined Immunologic/Pharmacologic Therapy: Tagamet." Personal communications to Etienne Callebout, M.D. Knoxville, TN (1996).

85. Nowicky, J.W. et al. "Ukrain as Both an Anti-cancer and Immunoregulatory Agent." *Drugs Under Experimental and Clinical Research* XVIII:Suppl (1992), 51-54.

86. Lohninger, A., and F. Hamler. "Chelidonium Majus L. (Ukrain) in the Treatment of Cancer Patients." *Drugs Under Experimental and Clinical Research* XVIII:Suppl (1992), 73-77.

87. Staniszewski, A. et al. "Lymphocyte Subsets in Patients with Lung Cancer Treated with Thiophosphoric Acid Alkaloid Derivatives from Chelidonium Majus L (Ukrain)." *Drugs Under Experimental and Clinical Research* XVIII:Suppl (1992), 63-67.

88. Pengsaa, P. et al. "The Effect of Thiophosphoric Acid (Ukrain) on Cervical Cancer, Stage IB Bulky." *Drugs Under Experimental and Clinical Research* XVIII:Suppl (1992), 69-72.

89. Nowicky, J.W. "New Immuno-Stimulating Anti-Cancer Preparation: Ukrain." Proceedings of the 13th International Congress of Chemotherapy. Vienna, Austria (August 28-September 2, 1983).

90. Nowicky, J. "Cancer Treatment Using Anticancer Preparation Alkaloid Derivative Ukrain." Fourth Mediterranean Congress of Chemotherapy. Rhodos, Greece (October 1984). *Chemioterapia* 4:Suppl 2 (1985), 1169-1171. See also: Nowicky, J. et al. "Biological Activity of Ukrain In Vitro and In Vivo." Fifth Mediterranean Congress of Chemotherapy. Cairo, Egypt (January 26-November 1, 1986). *Chemioterapia* 6:Suppl 2 (1987), 683-685.

91. Hohenwarter, O. et al. "Selective Inhibition of In Vitro Cell Growth by the Anti-tumor Drug Ukrain." *Drugs Under Experimental and Clinical Research* 18:Suppl 1-4 (1992).

92. Liepins, A. "Ukrain as an Experimental Cytotoxic Agent." *Journal of Chemotherapy* 5:Suppl 1 (1992), 797-799.

93. Nowicky, J.W. et al. "Macroscopic UV-marking through Affinity." *Journal of Tumor Marker Oncology* 3:4 (1988), 463-465. Note: This journal was published by the American Academy of Tumor Marker Oncology until 1992.

94. Nowicky, J.W. et al. "Macroscopic UV-marking through Affinity." *Journal of Tumor Marker Oncology* 3:4 (1988), 463-465.

95. Danopoulos, E.D., and I.E. Danopoulou. "The Results of Urea Treatment in Liver Malignancies." *Clinical Oncology* 1 (1975), 341.

96. Danopoulos, E.D. et al. "Eleven Years of Oral Urea Treatment in Liver Malignancies." *Clinical Oncology* 7 (1981), 281-289.

97. Pelton, Ross, and Lee Overholser. *Alternatives in Cancer Therapy* (New York: Fireside/Simon & Schuster, 1994), Chapter 20, Footnote 1.

98. Pelton, Ross, and Lee Overholser. *Alternatives in Cancer Therapy* (New York: Fireside/Simon & Schuster, 1994), Chapter 20, Footnote 5. Tumor cell surfaces contain large amounts of surfactants (glycoproteins and other large molecular surface-active agents), which have hydrophobic and hydrophilic properties at non-polar and polar sites, respectively, producing a structured water matrix surrounding cancer cells that is markedly different from that surrounding normal cells.

99. Pelton, Ross, and Lee Overholser. *Alternatives in Cancer Therapy* (New York: Fireside/Simon & Schuster, 1994), Chapter 20, Footnote 2.

Chapter 7: Boosting the Immune System

1. Wiewel, F. Personal communications with Charles Starnes (1995).

2. Ward, Patricia Spain. "History of BCG Vaccine (Bacillus Calmette-Guerin)." *Townsend Letter for Doctors & Patients* (October 1996), 72-77.

3. Wiemann, B., and C.O. Starnes. "Coley's Toxins, Tumor Necrosis Factor and Cancer Research: A Historical Perspective." *Pharmacology & Therapeutics* 64:3 (1994), 536.

4. U.S. Congress Office of Technology Assessment. "Burton's Theory of Cancer Control Through Augmentation of the Immune System." *Unconventional Cancer Treatments* (September 1990), 130. See also: U.S. Congress Office of Technology Assessment. "The IAT Cancer Treatment Regimen." *Unconventional Cancer Treatments* (September 1990), 131.

5. Cassileth, B.R. et al. *Report of a Survey of Patients Receiving Immunoaugmentative Therapy* (University of Pennsylvania Cancer Center, 1987), unpublished. Cited in: U.S. Congress Office of Technology Assessment. "Burton's Theory of Cancer Control through Augmentation of the Immune System." *Unconventional Cancer Treatments* (September 1990), 130.

6. Springer, G.F. "T and Tn General Carcinoma Autoantigens." *Science* 224 (1984), 1198-1206. See also: Avichezer, D.B. et al. "Immunoreactivities of Polyclonal and Monoclonal Antibodies Specific for Human Thomsen-Friedenriech (T) and Tn Antigens with Human Carcinoma Cells." Abstract from the 25th Israel Immunological Society Meeting (1995).

7. Springer, G.F. "T/Tn Antigen: Two Decades of Experience in Early Immuno-detection and Therapy of Human Carcinoma." *Jung Foundation Proceedings* (Stuttgart, Germany: G. Thieme).

8. Springer, G.F. et al. "T/Tn Pancarcinoma Autoantigens: Fundamental Diagnostic and Prognostic Aspects." *Cancer Detection and Prevention* 19 (1995), 173-182.

9. Springer, G.F. "T/Tn Antigen: Two Decades of

Experience in Early Immuno-detection and Therapy of Human Carcinoma." *Jung Foundation Proceedings* (Stuttgart, Germany: G. Thieme). Note: Twelve of the 26 patients were over age 50 at the time of the operation.

10. Old, Lloyd J. "Immunotherapy for Cancer." *Scientific American* 275:3 (September 1996).

11. Lamm, D.L. "BCG Immunotherapy for Transitional-cell Carcinoma In Situ of the Bladder." *Oncology* 9:10 (1995), 947-952.

12. Livingston-Wheeler, Virginia. *The Conquest of Cancer: Vaccines and Diet* (New York: Franklin Watts, 1984), 55-56.

13. Walters, R. "Livingston Therapy." *Options: The Alternative Cancer Therapy Book* (Garden City Park, NY: Avery Publishing, 1993), 72-81. The mechanism for this microbe-cancer interaction is unknown, but Livingston speculated that it might relate to an effect on the genetic material of the cell.

14. Lerner, Michael. *Choices in Healing* (Cambridge, MA: MIT Press, 1994), 322.

15. Walters, R. "Livingston Therapy." *Options: The Alternative Cancer Therapy Book* (Garden City Park, NY: Avery Publishing, 1993), 72-81. Dr. Livingston also used the Bacillus Calmette-Guerin (BCG) vaccine, a mild tuberculin vaccine that stimulates white blood cells to kill cancer cells.

16. Livingston-Wheeler, V., and Edmond G. Addeo. *The Conquest of Cancer* (New York: Franklin Watts, 1984). Also based on personal communications with Neal Nathan, M.D., Livingston Foundation in San Diego, CA. These case histories are available from the Livingston Foundation.

17. Cheson, B.D. et al. "Tumor Vaccine Clinical Trials." *Oncology* 9:10 (1995), 929.

18. Lamm, D.L. "BCG Immunotherapy for Transitional-cell Carcinoma In Situ of the Bladder." *Oncology* 9:10 (1995), 947-952.

19. Scott, M.T. "Tumor-induced Specific Suppression: A Limitation to Immunotherapy." *Immunology Today* 3 (1982), 8-9. See also. Kamo, I., and H. Friedman. "Immunosuppression and the Role of Suppressive Factors in Cancer." *Advanced Cancer Research* 25 (1977), 271-321.

20. Serrano, R. et al. "Isolation of a Novel Tumor Protein That Induces Resistance to Natural Killer Cell Lysis." *Journal of Immunology* 145 (1990), 3516-3523.

21. Note: TNF seems to exert a dual, conflicting influence on the anticancer defenses. For more information regarding its negative role, see *Cell*

61 (1990), 361-370; or *Proceedings of the National Academy of Sciences* 87 (1990), 8781-8784.

22. Moss, R. "Russian Immunologist Reports Remarkable Results." *The Cancer Chronicles* (New York: Equinox Press, 1994), 4.

23. Enby, E. et al. "Hidden Killers: Causes of Cancer: A New Look." *The Revolutionary Medical Discoveries of Professor Gunther Enderlein* (Saratoga, CA: Sheehan Communications, 1990), 77.

24. Ibid.

25. Walters, R. "Enderlein Therapy: A Cancer Therapy that Promotes Gentle Self-healing." *Raum & Zeit* 3:1 (1991), 24-27.

26. Ibid.

Chapter 8:
Enhancing Metabolism

1. Wallach, D.F.H. "Cellular Aspects of Tumor Thermobiology." *Proceedings of the International Congress on Chemotherapy*, 13th 18 (1983), 273.

2. Warburg, O. "Preface to the Second Edition of the Lindau Lecture." *The Prime Cause and Prevention of Cancer* (Wurzburg, Germany: Konrad Triltsch, 1967), 2. Translation by Dean Burk, Ph.D., National Cancer Institute, Bethesda, MD.

3. Ibid., 6.

4. Oberley, L.W., and G.R. Buettner. "Role of Superoxide Dismutase in Cancer: A Review." *Cancer Research* 39:4 (1979), 1141-1149.

5. Von Ardenne, Manfred. *Oxygen Multistep Therapy, Physiological and Technical Foundations* (New York: Thieme Medical, 1990).

6. Altman, N. "Hydrogen Peroxide." *Oxygen Healing Therapies* (Rochester, VT: Healing Arts Press, 1995), 51.

7. Helfland, S.L. et al. "Oxygen Intermediates Are Required for Interferon Activation of NK Cells." *Journal of Interferon Research* 3:2 (1983), 143-51.

8. Dormandy, T.L. "In Praise of Peroxidation." *The Lancet* 2:8620 (1988), 1126-1128.

9. Yamazaki M., and S. Tsunawaki. "Anti-tumor Effect by Leukocyte-Derived Active Oxygens." (Japanese) *Tanpakushitsu Kakusan Koso-Protein, Nucleic Acid, Enzyme* 33:16 (1988), 3031-3036.

10. Altman, N. "Hydrogen Peroxide in Medicine." *Oxygen Healing Therapies* (Rochester, VT: Healing Arts Press, 1995), 42-43.

11. "Common Denominators in Cancer Non-reme-

dies and in Human Longevity." *Townsend Letter for Doctors & Patients* (January 1992), 48-50.

12. Stark, H.R. "Cause and Treatment of Malignancy." *The Koch Treatment* (Asheville, NC: Christian Medical Research League, 1950), 103.

13. Nathan, C.F. et al. "Administration of Recombinant Interferon Gamma to Cancer Patients Enhances Monocyte Secretion of Hydrogen Peroxide." *Proceedings of the National Academy of Sciences* 82:24 (1985), 8686-8690.

14. Helfland, S.L. et al. "Oxygen Intermediates Are Required for Interferon Activation of NK Cells." *Journal of Interferon Research* 3:2 (1983), 143-151.

15. Apffel C.A. "Nonimmunological Host Defenses: A Review." *Cancer Research* 36:5 (1976), 1527-1537.

16. Farr, C.H. "The Therapeutic Use of Intravenous Hydrogen Peroxide." Monograph. (Oklahoma City, OK: Genesis Medical Center, 1987).

17. Holman, R.A. "A Method of Destroying a Malignant Tumor In Vivo." *Nature* 179 (1957), 1033.

18. Wirth, W. "The Effects of Hydrogen Peroxide on Ehrlich Carcinoma in Laboratory Mice." Lecture at St. Thomas Institute. Cincinatti, Ohio (November 15, 1982). Cited in: Pelton, R. *Hydrogen Peroxide: Alternatives in Cancer Therapy* (New York: Simon & Schuster, 1994), 113.

19. Nathan, C.F., and Z.A. Cohn. "Antitumor Effects of Hydrogen Peroxide In Vivo." *Journal of Experimental Medicine* 154 (1981), 1539-1553.

20. Mealey, J. "Regional Infusion of Vinblastine and Hydrogen Peroxide in Tumor-Bearing Rats." *Cancer Research* 25 (1965), 1839-1843.

21. Kaibara, N.T. et al. "Experimental Studies on Enhancing the Therapeutic Effect of Mitomycin-C with Hydrogen Peroxide." *Japanese Journal of Experimental Medicine* 41 (1971), 323-329.

22. Oliver, T.H., and D.V. Murphy. "Influenzal Pneumonia: The Intravenous Use of Hydrogen Peroxide." *The Lancet* (February 21, 1920), 432-433.

23. Pelton., R. "Hydrogen Peroxide." *Alternatives in Cancer Therapy* (New York: Simon & Schuster, 1994), 117.

24. Donsbach, K.W. *Oxygen-Peroxides-Ozone* (Tulsa, OK: Rockland Corporation, 1993), 66.

25. Ibid.

26. Farr, C.H. *Oxidative Therapy* (Oklahoma City, OK: International Bio-Oxidative Medicine Foundation, 1993), 3.

27. Zanker, K.S. "In Vitro Synergistic Activity of 5-fluorouracil with Low-dose Ozone Against Chemoresistant Tumor Cell Line and Fresh Human Cells." *International Journal of Experimental and Clinical Chemotherapy* 36 (1990).

28. Sweet, J. et al. "Ozone Selectively Inhibits Growth of Human Cancer Cells." *Science* 209 (1980), 931-933.

29. Bocci, V. "Ozonization of Blood for the Therapy of Viral Diseases and Immunodeficiencies: A Hypothesis." *Medical Hypotheses* 39:1 (1992), 30-34.

30. Varro, J. "Ozone Applications in Cancer Cases." *Medical Applications of Ozone*, edited by LaRaus, J. (Norwalk, CT: International Ozone Association Pan American Committee, 1983), 97-98.

31. Howell, E. *Enzyme Nutrition: The Food Enzyme Concept* (Garden City Park, NY: Avery Publishing, 1985), 130.

32. Wrba, H., and O. Pecher. *Enzyme: Wirkstoff der Zukunft Mitt der Enzymtherapie das Immunsystem Starken* (Vienna: Verlag Orac, 1993).

33. Cichoke, A.J. "The Effect of Systemic Enzyme Therapy on Cancer Cells and the Immune System." *Townsend Letter for Doctors & Patients* (November 1995), 30-32.

34. Wolf, M., and K. Ransberger. *Enzyme Therapy* (Los Angeles: Regent House, 1972), 156-166, 193-194.

35. Nydegger, U.E., and J.S. Davis. "Soluble Immune Complexes in Human Disease." *Critical Reviews in Clinical Laboratory Sciences* 12 (1980), 123.

36. Boik, John. *Cancer & Natural Medicine* (Princeton, MN: Oregon Medical Press, 1995).

37. Bland, J. *Glandular-Based Food Supplements: Helping to Separate Fact from Fiction* (Tacoma, WA: Bellevue-Redmond Medical Laboratory, Department of Chemistry, University of Puget Sound, 1980), 20-21.

38. Stretch, Eileen, N.D. "DHEA & Cancer Prevention in Women: Friend or Foe?" *Townsend Letter for Doctors & Patients* (October 1996), 144-145.

39. Pashko, L.L. "Cancer Chemoprevention with Adrenocortical Steroid Dehydroepiandrosterone and Structural Analogs." *Journal of Cell Biochemistry* Suppl 17G (1993), 73-79.

40. Li, S. et al "Prevention by Dehydroepiandrosterone of the Development of Mammary Carcinoma Induced by 7, 12-dimethylbenzy(a)anthra-cene (DMBA) in the Rat." *Breast Cancer Research and Treatment* 29:2 (1994), 203-217.

41. Caroleo, M. et al. "Melatonin as

Immunomodulator in Immunodeficient Mice." *International Journal of Immunopharmacology* 23 (1992), 81-89. See also: Hadden, J.W. "T-cell Adjuvants." *International Journal of Immunopharmacol-ogy* 16:9 (1994), 703-710.

42. Neri, B. et al. "Effects of Melatonin Administration on Cytokine Production in Patients with Advanced Solid Tumors." *Oncology Reports* 2 (1995), 45-47. See also: Del Gobbo, V. et al. "Pinealectomy Inhibits IL-2 Production and NK Activity in Mice." *International Journal of Immunopharmacology* 11 (1989), 567-577.

43. Lissoni, P. et al. "Immunotherapy with Subcutaneous Low-dose Interleukin-2 Plus Melatonin vs. Chemotherapy with Cisplatin and Etoposide as First-Line Therapy for Advanced Non-Small-Cell Lung Cancer." *Tumori* 80 (1994), 464-467.

44. Lissoni, P. et al. "A Randomized Study with the Pineal Hormone Melatonin Versus Supportive Care Alone in Patients with Brain Metastases Due to Solid Neoplasms." *Cancer* 73:3 (1994), 699-701.

45. Lissoni, P. et al. "Subcutaneous Therapy with Low-dose Interleukin-2 Plus the Neurohormone Melatonin in Metastatic Gastric Cancer Patients with Low-performance Status." *Tumori* 79:6 (1993), 401-404.

46. Barni, S. et al. "A Randomized Study of Low-dose Subcutaneous Interleukin-2 Plus Melatonin Versus Supportive Care Alone in Metastatic Colorectal Cancer Patients Progressing Under 5-Fluorouracil and Folates." *Tumori* 78:6 (1992), 383-387.

47. Blask, D.E. "Melatonin Modulates Growth Factor Activity in MCF-7 Human Breast Cancer Cells." *Journal of Pineal Research* 17:1 (1994), 25-32.

48. Lissoni, P. et al. "Immunoendocrine Therapy with Low-dose Subcutaneous Interleukin-2 Plus Melatonin of Locally Advanced or Metastatic Endocrine Tumors." *Oncology* 52:2 (1995), 163-166.

49. Pierpaoli, W., and W. Regelson. "A Powerful Protector and Treatment Against Cancer." *The Melatonin Miracle* (New York: Simon & Schuster, 1995), 113-129.

50. Garaci, E. et al. "Combination Treatment Using Thymosin Alpha 1 and Interferon after Cyclophosphamide Is Able to Cure Lewis Lung Carcinoma in Mice." *Cancer Immunology and Immunotherapy* 32 (1990), 154-160.

51. Cohen, M.H. et al. "Thymosin Fraction V and Intensive Combination Chemotherapy. Prolonging the Survival of Patients with Small-Cell Lung Cancer." *Journal of the American Medical Association* 241 (1979), 1813-1815.

52. Drozdova, T.S. et al. "Immunologic Correction Using Thymus Gland Preparation (T-Activin) in the Programmed Treatment of Patients with Non-lymphoid Leukemia." *Gematologiia I Transfuziologiia* 35:1 (1990), 14-16. Cited in: Boik, J. "Thymostimulin." *Cancer and Natural Medicine* (Princeton, MN: Oregon Medical Press, 1995), 76-77.

53. Langer, S.E. et al. *Solved: The Riddle of Illness* (New Canaan, CT: Keats, 1984).

54. Quillan, P. *Beating Cancer With Nutrition* (Tulsa, OK: Nutrition Times Press, 1994), 117.

Chapter 9: Physical Support Therapies

1. The Burton Goldberg Group. *Alternative Medicine: The Definitive Guide* (Tiburon, CA: Future Medicine Publishing, 1995), 3.

2. Straus, Howard. "Coffee Corner." *Gerson Healing Newsletter* 11:5 (1996), 9-11.

3. Singer, Sidney R., and Soma Grismaijer. *Dressed to Kill: The Link Between Breast Cancer and Bras* (New York: Avery Publishing, 1995).

4. Steinman, D., and S.S. Epstein. *The Safe Shopper's Bible* (New York: Macmillan, 1994).

5. Wittlinger, Gunther, and Hildegard Wittlinger. *Textbook of Dr. Vodder's Manual Lymph Drainage Vol. 1: Basic Course* 4th Edition (Brussels: Editions Haug International, 1992), 10-36.

6. Thomas, G. *Into the Unknown: Dr. Issels and His Revolutionary Cancer Treatment* (New York: Peter H. Wyden, 1973), 94.

7. Issels, J. *More Cures for Cancer* (Bad Homburg, Germany: Helfer Publishing, 1995), 5.

8. Ibid., 11.

9. Cranton, E.M., and J.P. Frackelton. "Free Radical Pathology in Age-Associated Diseases: Treatment with EDTA Chelation, Nutrition and Antioxidants." *Journal of Holistic Medicine* 6:1 (1984), 6-36.

10. Thomas, G. *Into the Unknown: Dr. Issels and His Revolutionary Cancer Treatment* (New York: Peter H. Wyden, 1973), 96.

11. Anonymous. *Cancer: A Healing Crisis* (Los Angeles: Cancer Resource Center, 1980), 13.

12. Royal, Daniel F., D.O. "Health Hazard in Your Teeth," *Alternative Medicine Digest* 13 (1996), 40-44.

13. Castleman, M. "Aromatherapy." *Nature's Cures* (Emmaus, PA: Rodale Press, 1996), 39. Castleman notes that heliotropin is a close relative of vanilla oil.

14. Dewhirst, M., Professor of Radiation Oncology

and Director of the Duke Hyperthermia Program at the Duke University Medical Center, Durham, North Carolina. Personal communications (1996).

15. Ibid.
16. The Burton Goldberg Group. *Alternative Medicine: The Definitive Guide* (Tiburon, CA: Future Medicine Publishing, 1995), 6.
17. Ibid., 7.
18. Ibid., 8.
19. Ibid., 10.
20. Ibid., 13.
21. Ibid., 14.
22. Ibid., 15.
23. Dibell-Hope, S. "Moving Toward Health: A Study of the Use of Dance-Movement Therapy in the Psychological Adaptation to Breast Cancer." University of California School of Professional Psychology Dissertation (1989).
24. The Burton Goldberg Group. *Alternative Medicine: The Definitive Guide* (Tiburon, CA: Future Medicine Publishing, 1995), 1.
25. Ibid., 2.
26. Ibid., 4.
27. Milne, Robert D., M.D., and Blake More with Burton Goldberg. *Alternative Medicine Definitive Guide to Headaches* (Tiburon, CA: Future Medicine Publishing, 1997).
28. Tomasi, et al. "Immune Parameters in Athletes before and after Strenuous Exercise." *Journal of Clinical Immunology* 2 (1982), 173-8. See also: Soppi, et al. "Effect of Strenuous Physical Stress on Circulating Lymphocyte Number and Function Before and After Training." *Journal of Clinical and Laboratory Immunology* 8 (1982), 43-46.
29. Cannon, V., and J. Kluger. "Endogenous Pyrogen Activity in Human Plasma after Exercise." *Science* 220 (1983), 617-9. See also: Cannon, V., and C. Dinarello. "Interleukin I Activity in Human Plasma." *Federation Proceedings* 43 (1984), 462.
30. Ballard-Barbash, R. et al. "Physical Activity and Risk of Large Bowel Cancer in the Framingham Study." *Cancer Research* 50:12 (1990), 3610-3613.
31. Frisch, R.E. et al. "Lower Prevalence of Breast Cancer in Cancers of Reproductive System among Former College Athletes Compared to Non-Athletes." *British Journal of Cancer* 52 (1985), 885-891.
32. Blair, S.N. et al. "Physical Fitness and All-cause Mortality." *Journal of the American Medical Association* 262:17 (1989), 2395.
33. Oliveria, S. et al. "The Association between Cardiorespiratory Fitness and Prostate Cancer."

Medicine and Science in Sports and Exercise 28:1 (1996), 97.
34. "Chinese Display *Qigong* Energy for U.S. Doctors." *Brain Mind Bulletin* 11:6 (March 3, 1986), 1. In addition, subjects showed measurable changes in brain states during *qigong* practice. When a *qigong* master directed his *qi* at a crystal for 15 minutes, light was diffracted differently through it afterward.
35. Lee, R.H. *Scientific Investigations into Chinese Qigong* (San Clemente, CA: China Healthways Institute, 1992).
36. Yi, Y. et al. "The Effect of Self-Controlling *Qigong* Therapy on the Immune Function of Cancer Patients." Second World Conference on Academic Exchange of Medical *Qigong* (September 15, 1993), 128.
37. Hongmei, A., and B. Jingnan. "Curative Effect Analysis of 122 Tumor Patients Treated by the Intelligence *Qigong*." Second World Conference on Academic Exchange of Medical *Qigong* (September 15, 1993), 130.
38. Chang, S. *The Complete System of Self-Healing: Internal Exercises* (San Francisco: Tao Publishing, 1986).
39. Jahnke, R. *The Most Profound Medicine* (Santa Barbara, CA: Health Action Books, 1990).
40. Yao, W. et al. "The Effect of Traditional Chinese Medicine on Cancer Rehabilitation." Fourth International Symposium on *Qigong*. Shanghai, China (September 1992), 76.
41. Ibid.
42. Shouzhang, W. et al. "A Clinical Study of the Routine Treatment of Cancer Coordinated by *Qigong*." Second World Conference on Academic Exchange of Medical *Qigong* (September 15, 1993), 129.
43. Li-da, F. "The Effects of External *Qi* on Bacterial Growth Patterns." *China Qi Gong* 1 (1983), 36.

Chapter 10:
Energy Support Therapies

1. Filshie, J. et al. "Report on Acupuncture-induced Pain Relief for Cancer Patients." International Medical Acupuncture Conference. London, England (1986).
2. Wu, B. et al. "Effect of Acupuncture on Interleukin-2 and NK Cell Immunoactivity of Peripheral Blood of Malignant Tumor Patients." *Chung-Kuo Chung Hsi I Chieh Ho Tsa Chih* 14:9 (1994), 37-39.
3. Clark, James Hoyt, B.Sc., M.Sc. *Computerized Electro Dermal Screening & The Life Information System* (Orem, UT: Biosource, 1994), 34.

4. Dr. Voll reported four principles as a result of his research: 1) the body's resistance is not uniform; 2) meridians (energy pathways) show electrical fields; 3) meridians actually generate the body's energy; and 4) the skin is a semi-insulator with respect to the external environment. Dr. Voll's first instrument to measure body energy signals by point testing was called the Diatherapuncteur and was exhibited in 1955 as part of an electroacupuncture demonstration. A more sophisticated version was renamed Dermatron and released by the Pitterling Electronic Company of Munich, Germany, in the 1970s. Dr. Voll discovered that higher or lower readings than normal at a particular acupuncture point indicate a problem in the organ that corresponds to that acupoint; a higher reading generally means there is irritation or inflammation in the organ, while a lower reading usually indicates fatigue or degeneration.

5. Clark, James Hoyt, B.Sc., M.Sc. *Computerized Electro Dermal Screening & The Life Information System* (Orem, UT: Biosource, 1994), 27-33.

6. The Burton Goldberg Group. *Alternative Medicine: The Definitive Guide* (Tiburon, CA: Future Medicine Publishing, 1995), 192.

7. Ibid., 330.

8. Philpott, W.H. "Cancer Prevention and Reversal." *Journal of the Bio-Electro-Magnetics Institute* 2:3 (1990), 12-16.

9. Riviere, M. et al. "Test with Lymphosarcoma on Mice." *Comptes Rendus de'l'Academie des Sciences* (March 1, 1965).

10. Troeng, I. Commenting on the study's results. Laholm, Sweden (July 1984). See: Riviere, M. et al. "Test with Lymphosarcoma on Mice." *Comptes Rendus de'l'Academie des Sciences* (March 1, 1965).

11. The Burton Goldberg Group. *Alternative Medicine: The Definitive Guide* (Tiburon, CA: Future Medicine Publishing, 1995), 319.

12. Ibid., 2.

13. Ibid., 3.

14. Ibid., 5.

15. Ibid., 9.

16. Ibid., 10.

17. Ibid., 11.

18. Ibid., 16. See also: "Holistic Physician-Asthma." *Alternative Medicine Digest* 8 (1995), 13.

19. Symonds, W.C., and B. Bremner. "A Ray of Hope for Cancer Patients: Photodynamic Therapy May Stop Early-stage Tumors." *Business Week* (June 10, 1996), 104-106.

20. Ibid.

21. Ibid.

Index

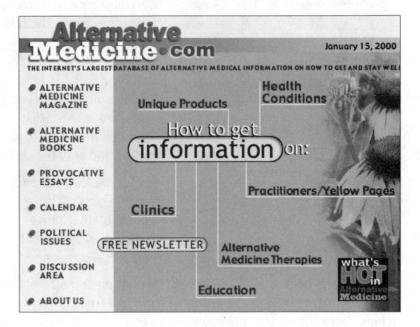

We provide the best and most important information from the world of alternative medicine, distilling complicated and technical medical jargon so that you can understand and actually use it to improve your health and the quality of your life.

■ *Search the largest database of alternative medical information on the Internet*

■ *Use our Yellow Pages to locate an alternative medical practitioner*

■ *Shop for the best supplements and health products*

www.alternativemedicine.com

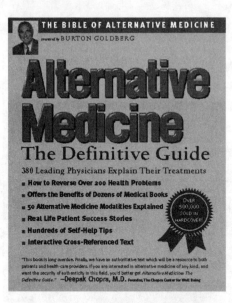

THE BIBLE OF ALTERNATIVE MEDICINE

presented by BURTON GOLDBERG

Alternative Medicine
The Definitive Guide

380 Leading Physicians Explain Their Treatments

- How to Reverse Over 200 Health Problems
- Offers the Benefits of Dozens of Medical Books
- 50 Alternative Medicine Modalities Explained
- Real Life Patient Success Stories
- Hundreds of Self-Help Tips
- Interactive Cross-Referenced Text

OVER 500,000 SOLD IN HARDCOVER!

"This book is long overdue. Finally, we have an authoritative text which will be a resource to both patients and health-care providers. If you are interested in alternative medicine of any kind, and want the security of authenticity in this field, you'd better get *Alternative Medicine: The Definitive Guide*." —Deepak Chopra, M.D. *Founder, The Chopra Center for Well Being*

Millions of people are searching for a better way to health—this is the book they're reaching for. *Alternative Medicine: The Definitive Guide* is an absolute must for anyone interested in the latest information on how to get healthy and stay that way.

At 1,100 pages, this encyclopedia puts all the schools of alternative medicine—50 different therapies—under one roof.

The *Guide* is packed with lifesaving information and alternative treatments from 380 of the world's leading alternative physicians. Our contributors give you the safest, most affordable, and most effective remedies for over 200 serious health conditions.

The *Guide* does something no other health book has ever done. It combines the best clinical information from doctors with the most practical self-help remedies all in a format that is easy-to-read, practical, and completely user-friendly.

The *Guide* gives you the knowledge you need today so you can make intelligent choices about the future of your health.

Now available in Spanish

To order, call 800-333-HEAL or visit www.alternativemedicine.com.
You can also find our books at your local health food store or bookstore.

national book network

We digest it for you—*Alternative Medicine Magazine* tracks the entire field—all the doctor's journals, research, conferences, and newsletters. Then we summarize what is essential for you to know to get better and stay healthy. We're your one-stop read for what's new and effective in alternative medicine.

TO ORDER, CALL 800-333-HEAL

THE BOOK
THAT EVERYONE WITH
CANCER NEEDS

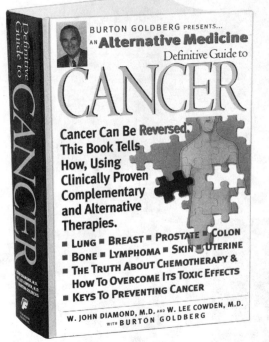

There has never been a book like this about cancer. The message is simple, direct, and lifesaving: cancer can be successfully reversed using alternative medicine. This book shows how.

The clinical proof is in the words and recommendations of 37 leading physicians who treat and restore life to thousands of cancer patients. Read 55 documented patient case histories and see how alternative approaches to cancer can make the difference between life and death.

This book includes the complete cancer protocols of 23 alternative physicians. These doctors bring to alternative cancer care decades of careful study and practice. They know that there is no magic bullet cure for cancer. They also know that many factors contribute to the development of cancer and many modalities and substances must be used to reverse it.

Hardcover ∎ISBN 1-887299-01-7 ∎ 6" x 9" ∎ 1,116 pages

TO ORDER, CALL 800-333-HEAL

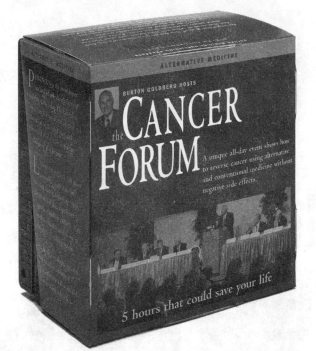

The Cancer Forum—five hours of lifesaving information from leading alternative medicine physicians who show you how to reverse cancer using alternative and conventional medicine without negative side effects.

Prevention is the most important and reliable cancer-fighting tool that exists today. The fact that cancer can be treated and reversed and that it can be detected early and prevented are the most significant messages of this forum.

Learn the latest proven, safe, nontoxic, and successful treatments for reversing cancer, including herbs, nutrition and diet, supplements, enzymes, glandular extracts, home-opathic remedies, and more, in this groundbreaking video.

TO ORDER, CALL 800-333-HEAL

BOOKS *your health* depends on

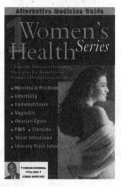
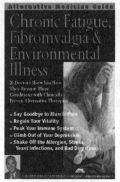
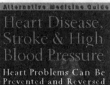
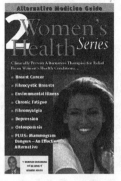
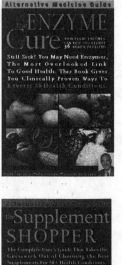

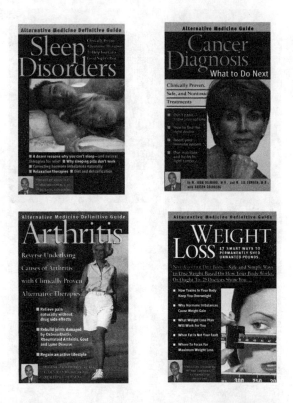

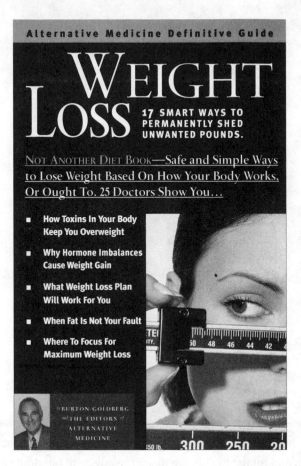

Alternative Medicine Definitive Guide

WEIGHT LOSS

17 SMART WAYS TO PERMANENTLY SHED UNWANTED POUNDS.

NOT ANOTHER DIET BOOK—Safe and Simple Ways to Lose Weight Based On How Your Body Works, Or Ought To. 25 Doctors Show You…

- How Toxins In Your Body Keep You Overweight
- Why Hormone Imbalances Cause Weight Gain
- What Weight Loss Plan Will Work For You
- When Fat Is Not Your Fault
- Where To Focus For Maximum Weight Loss

by BURTON GOLDBERG *and* THE EDITORS *of* ALTERNATIVE MEDICINE

Unlike any other weight loss book ever published, this book shows readers how to lose weight based on how their particular body biochemistry works. We show them how to determine their body type, then how to individualize their diet and exercise program to fit their type. In addition, 25 leading physicians reveal the keys to permanent weight loss—nutrition, enzymes, supplements, colon cleansing, liver detoxification, overcoming psychological obstacles, and more.

TO ORDER, CALL 800-333-HEAL